Federated Learning and Privacy-Preserving in Healthcare AI

Umesh Kumar Lilhore
School of Computing, Galgotias University, Greater Noida, India

Sarita Simaiya
School of Computing, Galgotias University, Greater Noida, India

Manoharan Poongodi
Hamad Bin Khalifa University, Qatar

Vishal Dutt
Department of Computer Science and Engineering, Chandigarh University, India

IGI Global
PUBLISHER of TIMELY KNOWLEDGE

A volume in the Advances in Healthcare Information Systems and Administration (AHISA) Book Series

Published in the United States of America by
IGI Global
Medical Information Science Reference (an imprint of IGI Global)
701 E. Chocolate Avenue
Hershey PA, USA 17033
Tel: 717-533-8845
Fax: 717-533-8661
E-mail: cust@igi-global.com
Web site: http://www.igi-global.com

Library of Congress Cataloging-in-Publication Data

Names: Lilhore, Umesh Kumar, 1982- editor. | Simaiya, Sarita, 1986- editor. | Poongodi, Manoharan, 1988- editor. | Dutt, Vishal, Dr., editor.
Title: Federated learning and privacy-preserving in healthcare AI / edited by Umesh Kumar Lilhore, Sarita Simaiya, Manoharan Poongodi, Vishal Dutt.

Description: Hershey, PA : Medical Information Science Reference, [2024] | Includes bibliographical references and index.
Identifiers: LCCN 2023056805 (print) | LCCN 2023056806 (ebook) | ISBN 9798369318744 (hardcover) | ISBN 9798369318751 (ebook)
Subjects: MESH: Machine Learning | Confidentiality--ethics | Artificial Intelligence | Medical Informatics--methods
Classification: LCC R859.7.A78 (print) | LCC R859.7.A78 (ebook) | NLM W 26.55.A7 | DDC 610.285--dc23/eng/20231220
LC record available at https://lccn.loc.gov/2023056805
LC ebook record available at https://lccn.loc.gov/2023056806

This book is published in the IGI Global book series Advances in Healthcare Information Systems and Administration (AHISA) (ISSN: 2328-1243; eISSN: 2328-126X)

British Cataloguing in Publication Data
A Cataloguing in Publication record for this book is available from the British Library.

All work contributed to this book is new, previously-unpublished material. The views expressed in this book are those of the authors, but not necessarily of the publisher.

For electronic access to this publication, please contact: eresources@igi-global.com.

Advances in Healthcare Information Systems and Administration (AHISA) Book Series

Anastasius Moumtzoglou
Hellenic Society for Quality & Safety in Healthcare and P. & A. Kyriakou Children's Hospital, Greece

ISSN:2328-1243
EISSN:2328-126X

Mission

The **Advances in Healthcare Information Systems and Administration (AHISA) Book Series** aims to provide a channel for international researchers to progress the field of study on technology and its implications on healthcare and health information systems. With the growing focus on healthcare and the importance of enhancing this industry to tend to the expanding population, the book series seeks to accelerate the awareness of technological advancements of health information systems and expand awareness and implementation.

Driven by advancing technologies and their clinical applications, the emerging field of health information systems and informatics is still searching for coherent directing frameworks to advance health care and clinical practices and research. Conducting research in these areas is both promising and challenging due to a host of factors, including rapidly evolving technologies and their application complexity. At the same time, organizational issues, including technology adoption, diffusion and acceptance as well as cost benefits and cost effectiveness of advancing health information systems and informatics applications as innovative forms of investment in healthcare are gaining attention as well. **AHISA** addresses these concepts and critical issues.

Coverage

- E-Health and M-Health
- IT Applications in Physical Therapeutic Treatments
- Clinical Decision Support Design, Development and Implementation
- Decision Support Systems
- Measurements and Impact of HISA on Public and Social Policy
- Pharmaceutical and Home Healthcare Informatics
- Role of informatics specialists
- IT Applications in Health Organizations and Practices
- Virtual health technologies
- Telemedicine

IGI Global is currently accepting manuscripts for publication within this series. To submit a proposal for a volume in this series, please contact our Acquisition Editors at Acquisitions@igi-global.com or visit: http://www.igi-global.com/publish/.

The Advances in Healthcare Information Systems and Administration (AHISA) Book Series (ISSN 2328-1243) is published by IGI Global, 701 E. Chocolate Avenue, Hershey, PA 17033-1240, USA, www.igi-global.com. This series is composed of titles available for purchase individually; each title is edited to be contextually exclusive from any other title within the series. For pricing and ordering information please visit http://www.igi-global.com/book-series/advances-healthcare-information-systems-administration/37156. Postmaster: Send all address changes to above address.

Titles in this Series

For a list of additional titles in this series, please visit: http://www.igi-global.com/book-series/advances-healthcare-information-systems-administration/37156

Emerging Technologies for Health Literacy and Medical Practice
Manuel B. Garcia (University of the Philippines Diliman, Philippines) and Rui Pedro Pereira de Almeida (University of Algarve, Portugal)
Medical Information Science Reference • copyright 2024 • 462pp • H/C (ISBN: 9798369312148) • US $325.00 (our price)

Pioneering Smart Healthcare 5.0 with IoT, Federated Learning, and Cloud Security
Ahdi Hassan (Global Institute for Research Education and Scholarship, The Netherlands) Vivek Kumar Prasad (Nirma University, India) Pronaya Bhattacharya (Amity University Kolkata, India) Pushan Kumar Dutta (Amity University Kolkata, India) and Robertas Damaševičius (Center of Real Time Computer Systems, Kaunas University of Technology, Lithuania)
Medical Information Science Reference • copyright 2024 • 352pp • H/C (ISBN: 9798369326398) • US $375.00 (our price)

Perspectives on Social and Material Fractures in Care
Colleen R. Greer (Bemidji State University, USA (Emerita)) and Debra F. Peterson (California Polytechnic State University, USA)
Medical Information Science Reference • copyright 2024 • 314pp • H/C (ISBN: 9798369300152) • US $345.00 (our price)

Ethics for Mental Health Professionals
S. Jack Olszewski (Yorkville University (retired), Canada)
Medical Information Science Reference • copyright 2024 • 257pp • H/C (ISBN: 9781668486078) • US $315.00 (our price)

Transformative Approaches to Patient Literacy and Healthcare Innovation
Manuel B. Garcia (University of the Philippines Diliman, Philippines) and Rui Pedro Pereira de Almeida (University of Algarve, Portugal)
Medical Information Science Reference • copyright 2024 • 400pp • H/C (ISBN: 9798369336618) • US $495.00 (our price)

Federated Learning and AI for Healthcare 5.0
Ahdi Hassan (Global Institute for Research Education and Scholarship, The Netherlands) Vivek Kumar Prasad (Nirma University, India) Pronaya Bhattacharya (Amity University Kolkata, India) Pushan Dutta (Amity Univer-

IGI Global
PUBLISHER of TIMELY KNOWLEDGE

701 East Chocolate Avenue, Hershey, PA 17033, USA
Tel: 717-533-8845 x100 • Fax: 717-533-8661
E-Mail: cust@igi-global.com • www.igi-global.com

Table of Contents

Detailed Table of Contents

AI might conduct screening and assessment in the event that medical expertise is lacking in a setting with limited resources. Because algorithms are involved, even the most rapid AI decisions are methodical in comparison with human decision-making. In this chapter, the authors provide a thorough literature review on data privacy for healthcare AI system development. In order to facilitate safer translational AI research, they offer a comprehensive review of the privacy issues data owners have when sharing datasets with researchers. They go over the many forms of attacks and how they might jeopardize user privacy. They also go into detail about several possible ways to fix these privacy problems.

Modern bioinformatics and artificial intelligence technologies are coming together to transform the process of developing pharmaceuticals, marking the beginning of an entirely novel phase in pharmaceutical discovery at the nexus of computational research and biological sciences. This work examines the relationship between statistics and biological processes, emphasizing the promise of significant change by combining artificial intelligence (AI) with bioinformatics methods to improve drug research. Incorporating computational methods, mathematical models, and machine learning procedures in computational biology tools improves our ability to understand biological phenomena's intricacies. The chapter examines the incorporation of few-shot and zero-shot learning approaches in drug discovery, emphasizing their significant potential in overcoming the obstacles related to scarce data and expediting the finding of novel targets for treatment. The review introduces the principle of few-shot learning and its practical implementation in drug research.

Escalating unhealthy lifestyles has led to a surge in common health diseases, notably cardiovascular ailments, a leading cause of human mortality with over 17 million annual fatalities. This study focuses on conducting data analytics within the domain of heart disease, which has become a progressively popular predictive field. The expanding availability of data in this area further emphasizes the significance of in-depth analysis for comprehensive insights and informed decision-making. Diverse strategies and methods have been explored by other researchers. Employing algorithms encompassing KNN, decision tree, and random forest, the authors prognosticate patient illnesses. The support vector machine (SVM) demonstrated superior accuracy among all algorithms. This research enhances heart disease prediction through varied algorithms, underscoring SVM's efficacy and data-driven approaches in addressing escalating health concerns.

Bioinformatics is an interdisciplinary field that develops methods and software tools for understanding biological data. Bioinformatics is an interdisciplinary field of study that combines computer science, mathematics, statistics, and engineering to analyze and comprehend biological data. Researchers faced a major issue in describing this new topic in a methodical, scientific manner and drawing attention to its potential uses and capabilities. This chapter will discuss the immense quantity of data generated in the biological area and how bioinformatics can manage, examine, and preserve them, along with a few algorithms that can be applied over bioinformatics data. In many bioinformatics studies and applications, machine learning is applied. This chapter will also provide a clear overview of the field's definition, goals, applications, related technologies, and future directions.

This research explores the integration of privacy-preserving federated learning techniques in the context of biomedical image analysis within the metaverse. The metaverse, a virtual shared space, has witnessed remarkable advancements in various fields, including healthcare. However, ensuring the confidentiality of sensitive medical data poses a significant challenge. This study proposes a novel approach to address this concern by employing federated learning, a collaborative machine learning paradigm that enables model training across decentralized devices without compromising individual data privacy. The investigation focuses on the application of these techniques to enhance biomedical image analysis within the metaverse, aiming to facilitate medical research and diagnosis. Through the implementation of secure and privacy-preserving federated learning, the authors aim to strike a balance between technological innovation and safeguarding sensitive health information in the evolving landscape of the metaverse.

The main idea behind this work is to present three-dimensional (3D) image visualization through two-dimensional (2D) images that comprise various images. 3D image visualization is one of the essential methods for excerpting data from given pieces. The main goal of this work is to figure out the outlines of the given 3D geometric primitives in each part, and then integrate these outlines or frames to reconstruct 3D geometric primitives. The proposed technique is very useful and can be applied to many kinds of images. The experimental results showed a very good determination of the reconstructing process of 2D images.

This chapter presents a comprehensive exploration of federated learning's real-world applications in healthcare contexts across four diverse regions: China, India, Spain, and the United States. The authors delve into how this innovative approach addresses the critical need for patient data privacy while advancing disease diagnosis, personalized treatment, and healthcare quality. From improving diagnostics through local data utilization in China to enhancing healthcare access in India, the chapter showcases the practical benefits and challenges of implementing federated learning. It also sheds light on collaborative drug development in Spain and navigating stringent data privacy regulations in the United States, emphasizing the global significance of Federated Learning in healthcare AI.

Current intrusion detection models based on machine learning require reliable datasets, but the public dataset updates are typically delayed after new attacks, which slows down the model's update speed. Also, to train the existing model, the data needs to be shared; hence, it lacks data integrity. To address this issue, this project implements a never-ending learning (NEL) framework for intrusion detection that utilizes multi-task and transfer learning to continuously acquire knowledge from private datasets, regardless of sharing them publicly. The NEL framework also integrates serendipitous learning, which updates the model by identifying and classifying new attack categories from the suspected traffic of attacked devices. The project also enhances various continuous learning training methods with federated learning to safeguard user privacy, ensuring that user data is not transmitted directly.

Preface

Welcome to the intersection of revolutionary advancements in healthcare and cutting-edge artificial intelligence. As editors of *Federated Learning and Privacy-Preserving in Healthcare AI*, we, Umesh Kumar Lilhore, Sarita Simaiya, Manoharan Poongodi, and Vishal Dutt, are delighted to present this meticulously curated reference book.

In the age of data-driven medicine, artificial intelligence has become indispensable for healthcare practitioners. AI facilitates accurate illness diagnosis, personalized therapy recommendations, and streamlined healthcare processes. However, this transformative technology has brought forth a critical need to handle sensitive patient data with the utmost care. Privacy, security, and trust in medical AI systems have emerged as pivotal concerns in the pursuit of technological advancements.

This edited publication explores the revolutionary concept of Federated Learning, a paradigm that stands as a beacon for patient data protection. Federated Learning, which trains models on local devices or servers while keeping data decentralized, addresses the privacy concerns associated with centralized data repositories. By ensuring that patient data never leaves its original location, Federated Learning significantly reduces the risks of breaches and misuse.

The book is a compilation of insights from leading experts in healthcare, AI, and data privacy. Through comprehensive chapters, readers will embark on a journey to gain foundational knowledge about federated learning and its application in healthcare AI, explore the algorithms, designs, and tactics employed in federated learning systems, delve into real-world applications of federated learning, specifically in radiology and genomics, and understand and address the challenges associated with implementing federated learning in healthcare.

AI in healthcare holds immense potential, but the critical concern of patient privacy often impedes its widespread adoption. Federated Learning emerges as a solution that enables doctors to harness the power of AI without compromising the integrity of patient data. This book provides unique insights and deep dives into one of the most crucial aspects of modern healthcare technology, catering to data scientists, medical professionals, policymakers, and those intrigued by the confluence of healthcare and AI.

Furthermore, the book goes beyond the immediate horizon, inviting readers to imagine privacy-preserving methods in healthcare AI beyond federated learning. As the use of AI in healthcare continues to evolve, addressing patient data security concerns is paramount, aligning with ethical principles and privacy regulations.

This book aims to provide technical insights beyond surface-level explanations, guiding readers on implementing and optimizing federated learning systems by analyzing algorithms and structures. It also intends to bridge the gap between theory and application by demonstrating real-world case studies that showcase the practical pros and cons of federated learning in healthcare. Additionally, the book seeks to foster collaboration across disciplines, encouraging varied perspectives to overcome the challenges in healthcare AI.

The book serves as a comprehensive source, consolidating foundational and advanced knowledge on federated learning and healthcare. It bridges the gap between academic research and practical applications, introducing theoretical insights alongside their healthcare applications. By celebrating successes and critically analyzing drawbacks, the book contributes to building more robust and efficient systems. It not only explains the current state but also proposes a future vision, guiding scholars and practitioners.

This book is designed for a diverse audience, including healthcare professionals, doctors, clinicians, medical researchers, AI and data science professionals, data scientists in healthcare, tech policymakers, ethicists, students, academics, industry stakeholders, healthcare IT leaders, tech entrepreneurs, and general enthusiasts

The book is structured into 18 chapters, covering a range of topics from the introduction to federated learning and privacy preservation to challenges and future directions in the field. Each chapter contributes to a comprehensive understanding of federated learning in healthcare AI, addressing technical aspects, real-world applications, ethical considerations, and collaborative strategies between healthcare and AI communities.

We invite you to embark on this enlightening journey through the realms of federated learning and privacy-preserving techniques in healthcare AI. May this book inspire curiosity, facilitate learning, and contribute to the ethical advancement of AI in healthcare.

Chapter 1: A Comparative Analysis of Federated Learning and Privacy-Preserving Techniques in Healthcare AI

In this chapter, authored by Yogesh Kumar Sharma, Deepika Amol Ajalkar, Smitha Nayak, and Jayashri Prashant Shinde, the focus lies on the meticulous examination of privacy concerns in the development of healthcare AI systems. Through an extensive literature review, the chapter addresses data privacy issues encountered by data owners when sharing datasets with researchers. Various forms of attacks compromising user privacy are explored, accompanied by an in-depth discussion on potential solutions to mitigate these privacy challenges.

Chapter 2: Advanced Learning and Bioinformatics in Innovative Drug Discovery Towards Bridging Biology

Authored by Yogesh Kumar Sharma, Sunayana Kundan Shivthare, Avinash Godharam Chaure, and Shital Vaibhav Ghotekar, this chapter explores the transformative intersection of modern bioinformatics and artificial intelligence in the realm of pharmaceutical development. The authors delve into the relationship between statistics and biological processes, emphasizing the potential of combining AI with bioinformatics methods. The chapter further discusses the incorporation of Few-shot and

Zero-shot learning approaches in drug discovery, highlighting their significance in overcoming data scarcity challenges.

Chapter 3: A Comparative Analysis of Heart Disease Prediction Using Machine Learning Approaches

Khushi, Sonia Deshmukh, and Rohit Vashisht from KIET Group of Institutions delve into the growing concern of heart diseases, providing a comprehensive data analytics perspective. The chapter evaluates diverse machine learning approaches such as KNN, Decision Tree, and Random Forest for heart disease prediction, with the Support Vector Machine emerging as the most accurate. The research aims to enhance heart disease prediction through various algorithms, emphasizing the efficacy of data-driven approaches in addressing health concerns.

Chapter 4: A Comprehensive Study of Bio-Informatics With Machine Learning

Rohit Vashisht and Gagan Thakral from KIET Group of Institutions present a comprehensive exploration of the interdisciplinary field of bioinformatics. The chapter defines the field, discusses its goals, applications, and related technologies, emphasizing the role of machine learning in bioinformatics studies and applications. The authors provide insights into handling and analyzing the vast biological data generated, offering a clear overview of the field's potential and future directions.

Chapter 5: Securing Privacy in the Metaverse Advancing Biomedical Image Analysis Through Federated Learning

Authored by Parveen Kumar Sharma, Ramesh B, Farrukh Arslan, Anshumali Parashar, and Malarvizhi N, this chapter addresses the integration of privacy-preserving federated learning techniques in biomedical image analysis within the metaverse. Focusing on the challenges of confidentiality in handling sensitive medical data, the authors propose a novel approach using federated learning. The study explores the application of these techniques to enhance biomedical image analysis, aiming to contribute to medical research and diagnosis while safeguarding individual health information.

Chapter 6: An Efficient Technique to Perform 3D Visualization on Clinical Image Datasets

Prabhjyot Haryal and Punam Rattan from Lovely Professional University present an innovative approach to three-dimensional (3D) image visualization through two-dimensional (2D) images. The chapter outlines the main idea of reconstructing 3D geometric primitives from given 2D images, demonstrating its utility across various image types. The proposed technique shows promising results in the reconstruction process, providing a valuable contribution to 3D visualization in clinical image datasets.

Chapter 7: Case Studies in Federated Learning for Healthcare

Authored by Javier Prieto, this chapter offers a global perspective on the real-world applications of federated learning in healthcare across China, India, Spain, and the United States. The author explores how federated learning addresses the critical need for patient data privacy while advancing disease diagnosis, personalized treatment, and healthcare quality. Through case studies, the chapter highlights the practical benefits and challenges of implementing federated learning in diverse healthcare contexts.

Chapter 8: Federated Learning Approach to Safeguard User Privacy

Aryan Bansal and A Karmel from Vellore Institute of Technology propose a Never-Ending Learning (NEL) framework for intrusion detection, integrating multi-task and transfer learning to continuously acquire knowledge from private datasets. The chapter enhances various continuous learning training methods with federated learning to safeguard user privacy. The NEL framework, incorporating serendipitous learning, aims to update models by identifying and classifying new attack categories from suspected traffic, ensuring continuous learning without compromising data integrity.

Chapter 9: Federated Learning for Privacy Preservation in Healthcare: A Comprehensive Introduction

Hari Kondaveeti, Chinna Simhadri, Srileakhana Mangapathi, and Valli Vatsavayi from Vellore Institute of Technology present a comprehensive introduction to federated learning and its applications in healthcare privacy preservation. Emphasizing the importance of privacy in healthcare data, the chapter explores the history, significance, and techniques of federated learning. Real-world examples illustrate the application of federated learning in healthcare scenarios, addressing technical and ethical challenges. The chapter envisions federated learning as a promising solution to balance patient data protection with AI advancements in healthcare.

Chapter 10: Federated Learning for Private AI Diagnosis of Schizophrenia

Authored by Kunal, Santosh Kumar Sahu, Mohammed Azam, Manuj Takkar, Jatin Bansal, and Dr. Jyoti Prasad Patra, this chapter focuses on federated learning's application in the private and accurate AI diagnosis of schizophrenia. Leveraging distributed datasets without compromising individual privacy, the research employs advanced AI algorithms for schizophrenia diagnosis. The results highlight the potential of federated learning as a secure and efficient approach for enhancing diagnostic capabilities in mental health, specifically in the context of schizophrenia.

Chapter 11: Real-World Applications of Explainable AI in Healthcare

Yash Mahajan, Muskan Sharma, and Inderjeet Singh from Chandigarh University explore the impact of Explainable Artificial Intelligence (XAI) in the healthcare sector. The chapter emphasizes XAI's role in elevating diagnostics, treatment modalities, and patient outcomes. By demystifying decision-making processes in AI algorithms, particularly deep learning neural networks, the chapter showcases practical applications of XAI in healthcare. It aims to equip healthcare professionals with actionable insights while addressing ethical concerns associated with opaque AI systems.

Chapter 12: Federated Learning for Private Cancer Diagnosis With Exascale Computing

Vembu N R, Niladri Maiti, Kadiervel K, Amarendranath Choudhury, and Rajasekhar Pinnamaneni contribute to the intersection of federated learning, privacy preservation, and exascale computing in cancer diagnosis. The chapter addresses the imperative need for collaborative yet privacy-conscious approaches to healthcare data analysis, focusing on human cancer diagnosis and detection. Leveraging the power of exascale computing, the proposed methodology ensures privacy by design, enabling secure model training without centralized data aggregation.

Chapter 13: Revolutionizing Healthcare Harnessing IoT-Integrated Federated Learning for Early Disease Detection and Patient Privacy Preservation

Authored by C.V. Suresh Babu, Surendar V, Dheepak N, Shiraj S, and Praveen K from Hindustan Institute of Technology and Science, this chapter explores the transformative potential of IoT-integrated federated learning in optimizing healthcare privacy and detection. The chapter focuses on early disease detection, personalized treatment planning, remote patient monitoring, and clinical trial enhancement. It demonstrates how wearable and home IoT devices, processed through federated learning models, can identify health anomalies before symptoms manifest, driving a patient-centric future in healthcare.

Chapter 14: Healthcare Services Enhancement in the Smart City Using 5G

Manjula Rao, Gururaj Rao, Priyanka H, Hemant Reddy, Ch Kumar, and Shaun Noronha contribute to the exploration of the impact of 5G in Health Care Services (HCS) within the context of a smart city. The chapter analyzes the effects and ramifications of 5G in HCS, emphasizing the technological setting, financial advantages, and a suggested model for HCS in a 5G-enabled smart city. It underscores the role of 5G in providing higher data rates, increased traffic capacity, ultra-low latency, and high connection density for enhancing healthcare services in a smart city.

Chapter 15: Healthcare 5.0 Unveiling the Future of Integrated Medicine

Shanthalakshmi Revathy J. and Mangaiyarkkarasi J. delve into the concept of Healthcare 5.0, which signifies a transformative shift from traditional to integrated healthcare. The chapter explores technology, patient empowerment, interdisciplinary collaboration, data-driven decision-making, and preventive healthcare. It discusses the role of AI in diagnostics and treatment, the use of big data for improved outcomes, and the impact of virtual reality and augmented reality on medical practices. The chapter provides insights into the future of integrated medicine in the Healthcare 5.0 era.

Chapter 16: Overview of Federated Learning and Its Advantages

Authored by Alisha Kakkar and Sudesh Kumar from Banasthali Vidyapith, this chapter explores the fundamental principles of Federated Learning (FL). It elucidates FL's foundational technologies and structures, categorizing its applications in data analytics, medical care, learning, and business. The chapter discusses research frontiers in tackling Federated Learning, contributing to a progressive understanding of FL for future enhancements.

Chapter 17: AI in Mental Health Federated Learning and Privacy

Shyelendra Pardeshi and Dinesh Jain explore the integration of artificial intelligence (AI) in mental health, focusing on the application of federated learning to ensure privacy and confidentiality. The chapter delves into the challenges of implementing AI-driven solutions in mental health contexts while prioritizing the protection of sensitive patient information. By leveraging federated learning, a decentralized machine learning approach, the research aims to enhance the accuracy and efficacy of mental health diagnostics without compromising individual privacy.

Chapter 18: Secure and Privacy-Preserving Federated Learning With Explainable Artificial Intelligence for Smart Healthcare Systems

Authored by Rita Komalasari from Yarsi University, Indonesia, this chapter addresses challenges in data privacy, security, and model interpretability in healthcare applications of Deep Learning (DL) and Federated Learning (FL). The research proposes robust frameworks for secure, privacy-preserving federated learning with explainable artificial intelligence in smart healthcare systems. The goal is to enhance the security, performance, and privacy of healthcare systems, ensuring resilience and efficiency in real-world scenarios. The comprehensive approach establishes a foundation for the future development of smart healthcare systems, fostering trust, transparency, and efficiency in healthcare decision-making processes.

As editors of *Federated Learning and Privacy-Preserving in Healthcare AI*, we are pleased to present this comprehensive reference book that explores the intersection of healthcare advancements and cutting-edge artificial intelligence. In an era dominated by data-driven medicine, the transformative potential of AI in healthcare is indisputable. However, it comes with the critical responsibility of handling sensitive patient data with the utmost care. Privacy, security, and trust in medical AI systems have become central concerns in the quest for technological progress.

This meticulously curated publication delves into the revolutionary concept of Federated Learning, a paradigm that serves as a beacon for patient data protection. By training models on local devices or servers while keeping data decentralized, Federated Learning addresses the privacy concerns associated with centralized data repositories. This book is a compilation of insights from leading experts in healthcare, AI, and data privacy, offering readers a profound journey into foundational knowledge about federated learning and its applications in healthcare AI.

We extend our gratitude to the contributors, each an expert in their field, who have provided in-depth explorations of topics ranging from the comparative analysis of privacy-preserving techniques to advanced learning in drug discovery. The chapters not only cover theoretical aspects but also present real-world applications of federated learning, addressing challenges and envisioning future directions in healthcare.

We invite you to embark on this enlightening journey through the realms of federated learning and privacy-preserving techniques in healthcare AI. May this book inspire curiosity, facilitate learning, and contribute to the ethical advancement of AI in healthcare.

Umesh Kumar Lilhore
School of Computing, Galgotias University, Greater Noida, India

Sarita Simaiya
School of Computing, Galgotias University, Greater Noida, India

Manoharan Poongodi
Hamad Bin Khalifa University, Qatar

Vishal Dutt
Department of Research and Development, AVN Innovations, India

Chapter 1
A Comparative Analysis of Federated Learning and Privacy-Preserving Techniques in Healthcare AI

Yogesh Kumar Sharma
https://orcid.org/0000-0003-1934-4535
Koneru Lakshmaiah Education Foundation, India

Deepika Amol Ajalkar
G.H. Raisoni College of Engineering and Management, Pune, India

Smitha Nayak
Muscat College, University of Stirling, Oman

Jayashri Prashant Shinde
G.H. Raisoni College of Engineering and Management, Pune, India

ABSTRACT

AI might conduct screening and assessment in the event that medical expertise is lacking in a setting with limited resources. Because algorithms are involved, even the most rapid AI decisions are methodical in comparison with human decision-making. In this chapter, the authors provide a thorough literature review on data privacy for healthcare AI system development. In order to facilitate safer translational AI research, they offer a comprehensive review of the privacy issues data owners have when sharing datasets with researchers. They go over the many forms of attacks and how they might jeopardize user privacy. They also go into detail about several possible ways to fix these privacy problems.

1. INTRODUCTION

When computers are able to mimic human intellect in some way, it's known as artificial intelligence (AI). John McCarthy first used the phrase in 1956. In simpler terms, AI is the practice of creating computer

DOI: 10.4018/979-8-3693-1874-4.ch001

systems that function in a way that is seemingly human. But for AI to reach its maximum potential, massive amounts of data and processing power are needed. Data is what has allowed AI to do everything that it has accomplished so far, while processing power has undoubtedly helped in AI's comeback (Shivthare, S. K. et al., 2023).

There has been a massive uptake of software solutions driven by AI in the last few years. The analysis of vast volumes of data in support of complicated choices is becoming the norm in many industries, and here is where AI really shines. People can't keep up with the rate of data creation, let alone process, understand, and apply it to timely, non-trivial judgments. So, AI is useful in a wide variety of contexts. This remarkable breakthrough of our times will help almost every sector (Nair et al., 2023).

When it comes to healthcare, AI is opening up new doors by improving medicine in ways no one could have predicted and by addressing some of the world's most pressing healthcare issues. As an example, the protein folding issue has impeded essential advances in biology and medicine for the last half-century, but a new algorithm driven by AI called Alpha-Fold has solved it. Similarly, advances like In Silicon Trailing enable pharmaceutical firms to replicate clinical trials for medication development on broader population models with improved control and fewer resource limitations, ultimately leading to the development of superior medicinal formulations Pradeep S. et al. (2023).

Artificial intelligence has tremendous potential in the medical field. Figure 1 shows the main healthcare specialities that have been trying to use digital solutions based on artificial intelligence. Unfortunately, ethical considerations about the possible abuse of these advancements are present. The most potent nerve agents and forty thousand potentially deadly compounds were found using artificial intelligence drug discovery in six hours [3]. Everyone agrees that AI has the potential to revolutionize healthcare in many ways, including cutting down on needless outpatient sessions that might cost the economy billions of dollars and speeding up diagnosis (Patel P. et al., 2023).

For AI systems trained using ML to achieve human-level performance on pattern-matching tasks, massive volumes of high-quality data are necessary. Data privacy is a significant problem since algorithms rely on it. This is particularly true when the data needed to train AI contains sensitive patient information. Patients, medical professionals, and software suppliers might all suffer significantly in the event of a data breach or abuse. When dealing with healthcare datasets, it is imperative that strict rules, such as the "European Union's" (EU) "General Data Protection Regulation" (GDPR), be adhered to. These requirements primarily pertain to patient information. For its artificial intelligence solution developed to detect individuals at risk of severe kidney damage, Google was lately the target of a class-action lawsuit alleging that the tech company violated UK data privacy rules (Dasaradharami Reddy, K., & Gadekallu, T. R. (2023).

The healthcare industry is highly motivated to revamp current data management processes and develop new ways to use healthcare data in order to advance artificial intelligence research while protecting patient privacy. Users' privacy is significantly compromised in the event of an assault on medical services resources and AI models that enable the adversary to get sensitive and secret information like location, health records, or identification details (Guleria et al., 2020).

The confidentiality and safety of data must be adequately handled in order for AI to realize its promise in healthcare, regardless of how well it outperforms humans. The deployment of AI-based solutions, particularly in healthcare, raises privacy concerns, according to many recent studies. As an example, if the data and technology used for telehealth are not correctly secured and patients' privacy is not adequately protected, healthcare professionals, as well as patients, would lose trust in these solutions(Swapna et al., 2023). In the era of AI-enabled ophthalmology, data security is crucial. Finding a happy medium between privacy and creativity was the writers' primary concern. With an emphasis on the potential impact of IoT on patient privacy in healthcare settings, Research brought attention to the privacy issues surrounding the IoT (Ramesh, T. R. et al., 2022). Table 1 presents the critical taxonomy of Federated Learning with AI.

The complete chapter is organized as follows. Section 2 covers the Foundations of Healthcare AI, Section 3 covers Federated learning, Section 4 covers Privacy-preserving machine learning (PPML), Section 5 covers comparative analysis, Use cases in healthcare, and ethical considerations and Section 6 covers issues and future direction. The last section covers the Conclusion and future works.

2. NEED OF PRIVACY-PRESERVING IN HEALTHCARE

Protecting the privacy of individuals' health information is known as medical or health privacy. It includes protecting the privacy of patient's medical records as well as their interactions with their healthcare providers. Both concepts may also relate to patients' right to physical seclusion from other patients and healthcare professionals while they are receiving treatment, as well as to patients' right to modesty in such environments. An issue of modern concern is the level of disclosure to parties such as employers, insurance providers, and others. There has to be a balance between the additional privacy issues brought forth by PCMS and EHR and the initiatives to reduce medical mistakes and service duplication (Butt M. et al., 2023).

Protecting against adversarial attacks that aim to deduce sensitive information from the target and cause data leaks unintentionally is what privacy means in the context of big data and machine learning. As its impacts become more widespread, big data has changed the digital world. More and more businesses are depending on big data analytics to carry out their daily operations. Our ability to control the storage, updating, and sharing of our data is essential to our privacy in the modern digital age (Swapna M. et al., 2020).

The advent of robust data mining techniques accessible via the Internet has made privacy a critical issue in modern society. Because of the big data boom and the beginning of AI, data privacy and personal information management are more critical than ever before; vital parts of privacy protection and AI increase the dangers to individual privacy. One of the most effective ways to evaluate big data sets in a reasonable amount of time is with the use of advanced AI techniques like DL, which are inherently incredible at doing so(Lilhore U. K. et al., 2023).

Concern regarding Deep Learning Security There is a risk that traditional machine learning methods may break regulations protecting user privacy and data secrecy since they require centralizing all data, usually in a cloud data centre. These days, user privacy rules in many regions make it mandatory for

Table 1. The critical taxonomy of federated learning with AI

Federated Learning With AI										
Data Partition		Different Learning						Privacy Level	Communication Architecture	
Horizontal	Vertical	Supervised			Semi-Supervised		Unsupervised	Raw Data Protection	Centralized	Decentralized
		Linear	SVM	Decision Tree	Federated Match	Logistic Regression	Federated GAN Network			

computer corporations to handle user data with the utmost care (Li H. et al., 2023). An innovative method for protecting privacy while training a Deep Neural Network Model using data from many clients is federated learning. This issue is addressed by federated machine learning, which integrates distributed machine learning with encryption and security, as well as economic and game-theoretic ideas for designing incentive mechanisms. So, federated learning has the potential to become the backbone of the future generation of machine learning, which will address both the technical and social requirements for the ethical creation and use of AI (CU, O. K. et al., 2023).

2 FEDERATED LEARNING METHODS

Centralized models are trained on decentralized data using Federated Learning. With minimal latency and privacy preservation, they are hyper-personalized for the user. The purpose of this article is to serve as a basic introduction to Federated Learning (Torkzadehmahani et al., 2022). Figure 1 presents the architecture of Federated Learning.

3.1 Why Is Federated Learning Necessary?

Big Data is the result of the proliferation of interconnected gadgets such as smartphones, wearables, and driverless cars. More and more data has to be stored and processed locally, moving computation away from the cloud and toward the edge because of the rapidly rising processing capacity of these devices and privacy concerns (Sai S. et al., 2023). Big Data cannot be fully used without Artificial Intelligence.

Figure 1. Architecture of federated learning

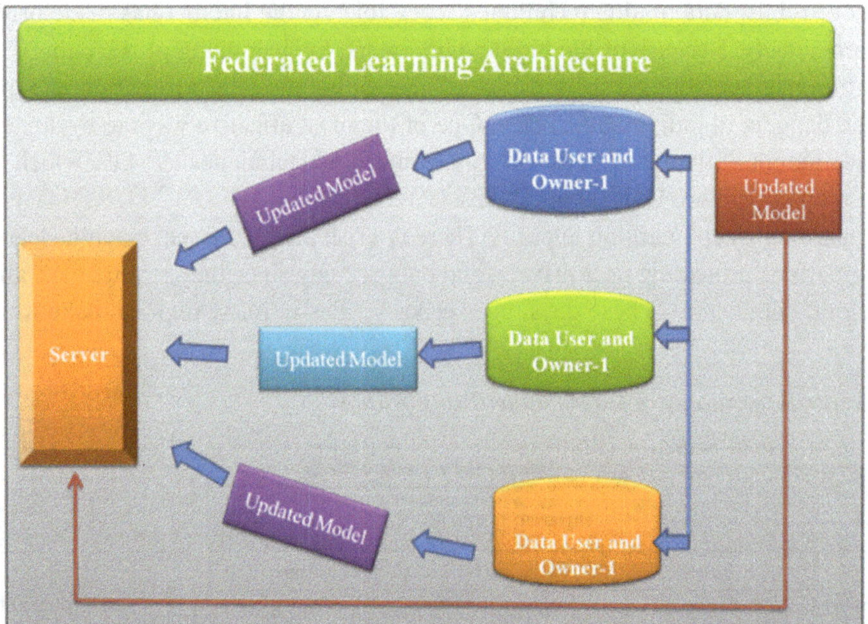

When it comes to picture recognition on the widely used ImageNet dataset, for instance, deep neural network designs have beaten humans (Tian, Y. et al., 2023).

For learning reasons, classic AI models often need users to exchange individual information with a master network. The security of users' data is a significant issue with these methods. When it comes to handling privacy and security concerns while generating decisions based on large amounts of data spread out across many training nodes, FL shines. In order to make predictions, machine learning models are trained utilizing data that has been obtained from various sources. Still, it's not feasible to send raw data to a central place due to concerns about bandwidth, security, and storage facilities (Jalali, N. A., & Chen, H. 2023).

To guarantee optimum learning, practical usage of obtained raw data, and transmission to a centralized site, FL serves as a distributed learning model. According to the authors (Kumar, N., Verma, H., & Sharma, Y. K., 2023), FL is also crucial to the development of smart cities. For efficient administration of priority assets, policymakers in urban smart cities may use FL to transfer sensitive information acquired from IoT sensors. Users may access data without obtaining personal information about other clients using the FL framework. At some point, the server updates its global model and sends it out to all clients (Iqbal et al., 2023). After that, customers learn about interference on their own devices by downloading the latest global model and distributing it across the cloud (Nayak, S., & Sharma, Y. K. (2023).

3.2 Federated Machine Learning (FML) Steps

In addition to facilitating learning at the edge, federated learning allows for the distribution of data from millions of devices to train models. Also, from the centre, you may improve the outcomes that were produced in the peripheral (Rahman, A. et al., 2023). FML is based on the following steps.

- Pick a model that hasn't been trained or one that has been pre-trained on the central server.
- After that, the first model, which might be devices or local servers, should be sent to the customers.
- The training process is ongoing on-site for each customer, utilizing their local data. Crucially, this training data may include private information such as images, emails, health measurements, or conversation logs. Gathering such data in cloud-based settings could be difficult, if not impossible (Awan K. A. et al., 2023).
- Encrypted communication channels are used to send the locally trained models back to the central server with any updates. It should be noted that the server does not get any actual data but rather the model's learned parameters, such as neural network weights. In order to improve the correctness of the shared model, all of the clients' changes are averaged and combined. (Stephanie, V. et al., 2022).
- Ultimately, this model is sent back to every server and device (Pradeep S. et al., 2023).

One neat thing about federated learning is that iterative training is used. In other words, participants may continuously exchange information while the server and clients communicate the updated parameters back and forth several times Rauniyar, A. et al. (2023).

3 APPLICATION OF FEDERATED LEARNING

Federated learning approaches are essential when it comes to privacy-sensitive apps that use dispersed training data at the edge. Autonomous cars that can adjust to pedestrian behaviour, mobile phone activity, sentiment, and semantic location are all examples of federated learning applications. Wearable gadgets may also be used to forecast health events, such as the risk of heart attacks (Rieyan S. A. et al., 2024). Prominent federated learning applications come in several forms:

- **Smartphones:** The use of statistical models to understand user behaviour over a broad pool of mobile phones enables applications like next-word prediction, facial identification, and voice recognition. Users may choose not to consent to data sharing in order to safeguard their privacy or reduce their phone's data use or battery life. Using federated learning, predictive features on smartphones may be enabled without compromising user privacy or reducing the quality of the user experience (Kumar, N., Verma, H., & Sharma, Y. K. (2023).
- **Organizations:** Entire institutions or organizations may likewise be seen as "devices" in the context of federated learning. One kind of institution that stores a great deal of patient data suitable for predictive healthcare applications is the hospital. The healthcare industry is susceptible to patient information and may be compelled to keep some records locally due to ethical, legal, or administrative considerations. Federated learning is a solution for such applications because it allows for private learning across different devices/organizations and reduces pressure on the network (Ullah I. et al., 2023).
- **Internet of Things:** Sensors allow modern IoT networks like smart homes, autonomous cars, and wearable devices to gather and respond to incoming data in real time. For instance, in order for an autonomous car fleet to function securely, it may be necessary to have an up-to-date model of construction, pedestrian, or traffic patterns. Nevertheless, it can be challenging to construct aggregate models in such situations owing to privacy issues and the restricted connection of every device. In order to train models that can effectively adapt to changes in these systems while respecting user privacy, federated learning approaches are used Singh S. et al. (2022).

4 APPLICATIONS OF PPML IN THE HEALTHCARE INDUSTRY

One distributed collaborative AI approach that has great potential in intelligent healthcare is federated learning. This paradigm enables many clients, like hospitals, to work together on AI training without requiring them to share local data (Wang R. et al., 2022). Consequently, we have compiled an in-depth study of FL's capabilities in cutting-edge healthcare. To start, we provide an overview of the most recent FL developments, the rationale for their use in innovative healthcare, and the necessary conditions for their implementation (Wang T. et al., 2023). Figure 2 presents the role of PPML in Healthcare.

Data analytics is all the rage right now, especially in the healthcare industry. The importance of healthcare data for data analysis has grown in recent years (Nayak, S., & Sharma, Y. K. (2023). This includes information on patients, healthcare professionals, prescription supplies, insurance companies, and other relevant businesses. Nevertheless, information about the healthcare industry is scattered. They don't share a standard format, and the data is sensitive since it pertains to the healthcare sector Eltaras T. et al. (2023). Information related to the insurance industry is particularly delicate and cannot be shared

Figure 2. Role of PPML in healthcare

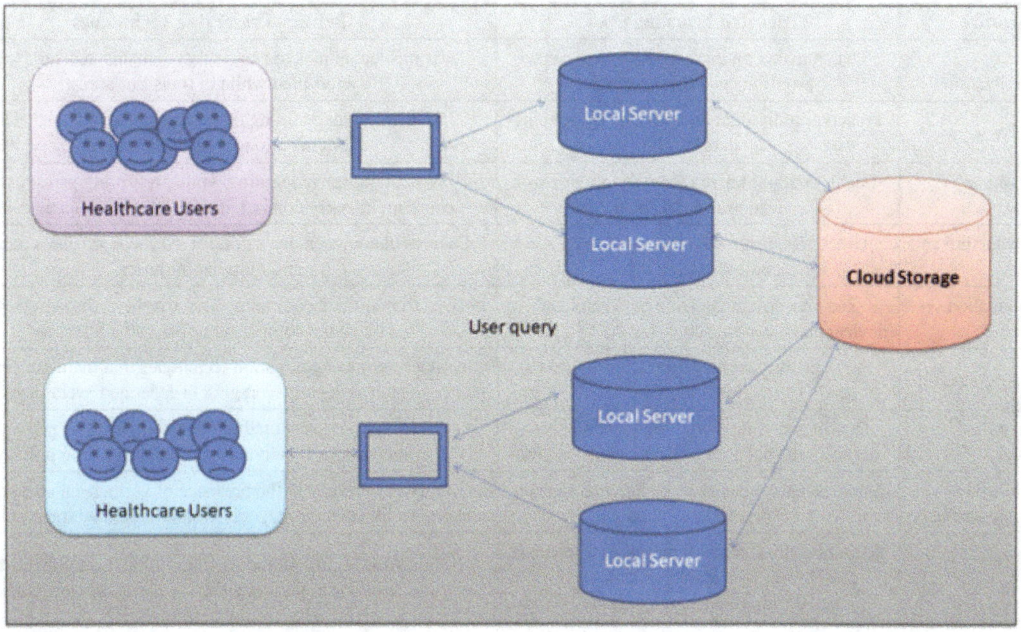

across other sectors. There is a considerable hole in data analysis due to the inability to process using conventional learning and training approaches in the absence of data transmission (Singh et al., 2023). Table 2 presents a comparative analysis of PPML applications in healthcare.

5. OPEN ISSUES

Federated Learning is an ongoing procedure in which a model undergoes continual updates. That's why new difficulties emerged as a result of these advancements. Because the problems are out in the open, the researchers should be able to find practical solutions quickly. Given that the whole process takes place online, issues of confidentiality and security are perennial worries in the healthcare industry. In comparison to other types of data, health-related data is more vulnerable. Here, several technologies are being integrated into healthcare systems, including SDN, Blockchain (Wang R. et al., 2022).

Big datasets are required, however, since it is a sophisticated ML technique. For these kinds of issues, you need a suitable dataset. One drawback of this area is the difficulty of managing enormous datasets for medical situations. The user end, where the global model would be updated somewhat via distributed training, also lacks datasets. In addition to this, the health data does not provide sufficient performance due to the fact that the information domain is different and the data points include outliers. The training of machine learning models and processing of health data is a time-consuming and costly process. To this day, it is essential to discover efficient techniques.

Nevertheless, scientists are attempting to use new approaches and technology in order to improve the functionality of these systems in the pharmaceutical industry. Staff members continue to prioritize healthcare system security. In order to create intelligent healthcare systems, it is necessary to

Table 2. A comparative analysis of PPML applications in healthcare

Feature	Federated Learning (FL)	Privacy-Preserving Techniques
Data Decentralization	Data remains on local devices or servers, avoiding centralized storage	Various techniques to ensure data remains decentralized or encrypted while in transit or at rest
Data Privacy	Preserves individual data privacy by keeping data local	Focuses on maintaining data privacy through encryption, anonymization, or differential privacy
Collaborative Learning	Enables collaborative model training across decentralized devices	Allows collaborative learning while preserving privacy through secure multi-party computation or homomorphic encryption
Data Ownership and Control	Users or institutions retain ownership and control of their data	Ensures data owners have control over who accesses their data and for what purposes
Communication Overhead	Requires communication between local devices and a central server for model updates	Strives to minimize communication overhead through techniques like edge computing or federated learning
Model Aggregation	Aggregates local model updates to build a global model	Utilizes various aggregation techniques that maintain privacy, such as secure averaging or federated averaging
Computational Resources	Distributed computation on local devices, reducing the need for centralized processing	Focuses on distributed or edge computing to perform computations locally without compromising privacy
Adaptability to Heterogeneous Data	Handles heterogeneity by training models on diverse local data	Ensures privacy in the presence of various data through techniques like data homogenization or federated transfer learning
Security	Requires robust security measures to prevent model inversion attacks or data leakage during model aggregation	Emphasizes secure protocols, encryption, and authentication mechanisms to protect against various privacy attacks
Regulatory Compliance	Compliance may vary based on local regulations and data governance policies.	Aims to comply with data protection regulations by implementing privacy-preserving methods and obtaining user consent
Scalability	Potentially scalable with a large number of local devices participating	Scalability is a crucial consideration, and techniques aim to handle large-scale implementations while preserving privacy
Example Use Cases	Personalized healthcare, clinical research collaboration	Secure health data sharing, collaborative disease prediction, and patient monitoring

handle patients' personal and sensitive data. They are being made more accessible and affordable via the usage of the Internet of Medical Things. Thus, security might be provided by means of SDN, Blockchain, and NFV.

Since Federated Learning necessitates a substantial quantity of data, we may utilize data augmentation in this AI age to mimic the current datasets in order to produce more data. Discovering the sweet spot for training duration and peak performance requires more data analysis. When applied to the healthcare industry, the present state of machine learning models' generalizability falls short of expectations. Here is an opportunity to develop and test a CNN improvement. It is recommended to use statistical approaches for the cost analysis of the models before putting them into practice (T. et al., 2023).

Analyzing healthcare system data pertaining to medical diseases or the medical industry is a crucial concern. But doctors' records are very private, and if anything were to be altered, the whole system would suffer a catastrophic loss. By combining federated learning with the blockchain mechanism, a safe and effective model for the intelligent healthcare system may be created. This model will make use of advanced learning and training algorithms without exposing sensitive data to the network. The protected Blockchain stores the starting parameters, the number of rounds, and the keys to the public one for every client for the secure aggregation. Clients or local models receive parameters, while an alternative block is created when the verification operation is finished. As a result, the safety of patient records is guaranteed by means of Federated Learning and the Blockchain, and a practical model is guaranteed.

6. FUTURE DIRECTION OF FLM

6.1 Impact of FL on Data Science

The present system's growing reliance on approaches based on the IoT results in massive data collection across all sectors. Right now, this is what data scientists are up against. With less memory in the sensors linked to the IoT-based mechanism, data security becomes one of the most critical concerns. The data they produce every millisecond is enormous, however. This makes the crucial but challenging task of storing or transmitting this data quickly. The advantage of using FL in this case is that the data storage method is not used and is instead spread across many clients. Additionally, the confidentiality of individual data is guaranteed since the data is trained locally on each client (Wang R. et al., 2022).

6.2 Integrating AI and Blockchain for Security

When it comes to all kinds of applications, artificial intelligence is the most potent agent. In several cases, AI mediates between theoretical concepts and practical implementations. In contrast, blockchain technology may provide a distributed ledger for potentially susceptible parts [241]. Additionally, BC provides a temporary catalogue that may be used to execute security and confidentiality criteria effectively. In order to carry out their operations in the application settings, AI applications need a secure platform. Working together, BC and AI provide superior performance for the target system. During conversations, AI agents in the BC environment are only ever connected. Together, they provide an exceptionally safe setting that will be able to serve its customers far into the future.

6.3 Automated Robot Control With FL-AI

Robots are utilized in many industries in today's technology world to do risky jobs that people used to do. Once again, agents powered by AI can perform diverse data transactions with ease and efficiency. In addition, the current cloud storage technology makes it possible to store data and information effectively with extensive memory storage on the cloud. Thanks to rapid data retrieval from many sources, continuous learning and training are now within reach. The significance of autonomous agents has increased in the modern era of Industry 4.0. Quite a few hotels, among other places, use robots, as do schools, the military, and hospitals. It is critical to provide safe data collection for training, nevertheless, as training an agent requires gathering massive volumes of data from many sources. To provide data privacy while retaining the efficiency of the autonomous system, FL is a good fit since it prohibits the primary demanding job, data transmission, in this case.

6.4 Using Big Data Analytics With FL

Data volume, velocity, and diversity are the three pillars upon which Big Data rests. A diverse dataset, including data from a variety of sources, is the primary goal of broad data analysis, which entails collecting data from a variety of sources. This is now much simpler because of advancements in wireless networking resources like 5G and 6G, the Internet of Things (IoT), and Industry 4.0. These innovations all work better in a real-time setting and with data collecting. Big data comes from many places, including heterogeneous ones, and the industrial sector is no exception. This method is challenging because sensitive user information is at risk of being compromised at any point along the data flow from source to destination. FL is an emerging field of artificial intelligence that uses locally trained ML models that are fed data from the local system. Using the source data guarantees continuous training and meets the criterion for meaningful data. This eliminates the need to transfer sensitive user data across several locations, thus ensuring data privacy.

6.5 FL Using Blockchain for Applications in Industry 5.0

The integration of smart devices and the population at large is the fundamental objective of the future IR 5.0. By connecting disparate devices via the Internet of Things, data may be acquired from even the most inaccessible places and then used to set up communication with no effort on the part of the owner. Nevertheless, the data that has been collected is in its raw form and may not be in a computer-friendly format that allows it to comprehend its nature. The AI powering the ML algorithm comes into play at this point. We use AI algorithms to do the heavy lifting, and then we use edge computing to analyze the results of our investigation quickly. However, preventing an intruder's assault on sensitive data is a difficulty. Potentially vulnerable to intrusion at the data hub's nodes due to data exchange between devices. Using FL and blockchain technology, a solution might be found where both parties' data is gathered, taught, and processed locally before being sent to the server. After that, for safe transmission, the initial parameters went across the Blockchain's blocks.

6.6 Using FL-Blockchain to Get Access to Patient Records

Analyzing healthcare system data pertaining to medical diseases or the medical industry is a crucial concern. But doctors' records are very private, and if anything were to be altered, the whole system would suffer a catastrophic loss. By combining federated learning with the blockchain mechanism, a safe and effective model for the intelligent healthcare system may be created. This model will make use of advanced learning and training algorithms without exposing sensitive data to the network. The protected Blockchain stores the starting parameters, the number of rounds, and the keys—the public one for every client—for the secure aggregation. Clients or local models receive parameters, while an alternative block is created when the verification operation is finished. With the help of Federated Learning and the Blockchain, the confidentiality of medical data is guaranteed, and an efficient model may be achieved.

6.7 FL in Smart Industrial IoT With Healthcare

Many sectors are making use of IoT devices as their popularity grows; they include healthcare, education, data science, analytics, and more. In the age of intelligent IIoT, data from a variety of sources can be readily collected and transmitted to a central server for analysis in the healthcare system. This includes MRI images, disease test samples, information about hospitalized patients, and even data from hospital employees or management. However, with the development of these tools, data collection has emerged as the primary motivation for cybercriminals. Consequently, an attacker may easily acquire control of the system by intercepting these data as they are being sent from the source to the destination. Since FL ensures data security on the local computer while processing activities are executed at each client, it might be a good fit for this situation. After that, the results are securely sent back to the central server for further analysis.

6.8 AI-FL in Smart Healthcare Using Large Data

Data collection, processing, and the creation of results are all areas where uniformity is highly sought after. The healthcare business stands to benefit a great deal from a platform that can autonomously collect data from many sources, execute a job, resolve critical issues, or make a judgment. AI plays a crucial role in healthcare by helping computer systems comprehend human thought processes and by developing and implementing efficient AI-based algorithms to simplify complex tests for medical personnel.

Using electronic health records to forecast mortality and length of hospital stay, with the help of the FL model's secure data collection and the development of an intelligent AI model, we can aggregate data using FL and smart wearables with AI benefits to create a safe and philosophical system.

7. CONCLUSION

The research community and FL are very interested in integrating AI into the required networks, thanks to the recent advancements in healthcare. This study sifts through mountains of data in four new areas: Federated learning, Healthcare, and Machine Learning. Our discussion also delves into the latest innovations in clever healthcare applications using FL and AI. Much work has gone into integrating FL-AI, FL-Healthcare, and AI-Healthcare. Additionally, we handle other matters related to security, privacy, dependability, scalability, and secrecy by using the concepts that we have already described. While we have examined and classified FL and AI-XAI methods for healthcare systems into distinct categories, it is essential to note that healthcare encompasses more than just these two approaches. Lots of issues and difficulties that still need fixing. Next, the presentation of taxonomies, unresolved problems, advantages of integration, state-of-the-art debate, and security advances, the subsequent Research evaluates these topics. Furthermore, we have provided some recommendations for further studies in this area.

REFERENCES

Ali, M., Naeem, F., Tariq, M., & Kaddoum, G. (2022). Federated learning for privacy preservation in smart healthcare systems: A comprehensive survey. *IEEE Journal of Biomedical and Health Informatics*, *27*(2), 778–789. doi:10.1109/JBHI.2022.3181823 PMID:35696470

Awan, K. A., Din, I. U., Almogren, A., & Rodrigues, J. J. (2023). Privacy-Preserving Big Data Security for IoT With Federated Learning and Cryptography. *IEEE Access : Practical Innovations, Open Solutions*, *11*, 120918–120934. doi:10.1109/ACCESS.2023.3328310

Butt, M., Tariq, N., Ashraf, M., Alsagri, H. S., Moqurrab, S. A., Alhakbani, H. A. A., & Alduraywish, Y. A. (2023). A Fog-Based Privacy-Preserving Federated Learning System for Smart Healthcare Applications. *Electronics (Basel)*, *12*(19), 4074. doi:10.3390/electronics12194074

CU, O. K., Gajendran, S., Bhavadharini, R. M., Suguna, M., & Krithiga, R. (2023). EHR privacy preservation using federated learning with DQRE-Scnet for healthcare application domains. *Knowledge-Based Systems*, *275*, 110638. doi:10.1016/j.knosys.2023.110638

Dahiya, N., Sharma, Y. K., Rani, U., Hussain, S., Nabilal, K. V., Mohan, A., & Nuristani, N. (2023). Hyper-parameter tuned deep learning approach for effective human monkeypox disease detection. *Scientific Reports*, *13*(1), 15930. doi:10.1038/s41598-023-43236-1 PMID:37741892

Dasaradharami Reddy, K., & Gadekallu, T. R. (2023). A Comprehensive Survey on Federated Learning Techniques for Healthcare Informatics. *Computational Intelligence and Neuroscience*, *2023*, 2023. doi:10.1155/2023/8393990 PMID:36909974

Eltaras, T., Sabry, F., Labda, W., Alzoubi, K., & Malluhi, Q. (2023). Efficient Verifiable Protocol for Privacy-Preserving Aggregation in Federated Learning. *IEEE Transactions on Information Forensics and Security*, *18*, 2977–2990. doi:10.1109/TIFS.2023.3273914

Guleria, K., Sharma, A., Lilhore, U. K., & Prasad, D. (2020). Breast cancer prediction and classification using supervised learning techniques. *Journal of Computational and Theoretical Nanoscience*, *17*(6), 2519–2522. doi:10.1166/jctn.2020.8924

Iqbal, S., Qureshi, A. N., Alhussein, M., Aurangzeb, K., Javeed, K., & Ali Naqvi, R. (2023). Privacy-preserving collaborative AI for distributed deep learning with cross-sectional data. *Multimedia Tools and Applications*, 1–23.

Jalali, N. A., & Chen, H. (2023). Federated Learning Security and Privacy-Preserving Algorithm and Experiments Research Under Internet of Things Critical Infrastructure. *Tsinghua Science and Technology*, *29*(2), 400–414. doi:10.26599/TST.2023.9010007

Khalid, N., Qayyum, A., Bilal, M., Al-Fuqaha, A., & Qadir, J. (2023). Privacy-preserving artificial intelligence in healthcare: Techniques and applications. *Computers in Biology and Medicine*, *158*, 106848. doi:10.1016/j.compbiomed.2023.106848 PMID:37044052

Kumar, N., Verma, H., & Sharma, Y. K. (2023). Adversarial Attacks on Graph Neural Network: Techniques and Countermeasures. In Concepts and Techniques of Graph Neural Networks (pp. 58-73). IGI Global.

Kumar, N., Verma, H., & Sharma, Y. K. (2023). Graph Convolutional Neural Networks for Link Prediction in Social Networks. In Concepts and Techniques of Graph Neural Networks (pp. 86-107). IGI Global. doi:10.4018/978-1-6684-6903-3.ch007

LEAF: A Federated Learning-Aware Privacy Preserving Framework for Healthcare Ecosystem. (2023) *IEEE Transactions on Network and Service Management*.

Li, H., Li, C., Wang, J., Yang, A., Ma, Z., Zhang, Z., & Hua, D. (2023). Review on security of federated learning and its application in healthcare. *Future Generation Computer Systems*, *144*, 271–290. doi:10.1016/j.future.2023.02.021

Lilhore, U. K., Manoharan, P., Sandhu, J. K., Simaiya, S., Dalal, S., Baqasah, A. M., Alsafyani, M., Alroobaea, R., Keshta, I., & Raahemifar, K. (2023). Hybrid model for precise hepatitis-C classification using improved random forest and SVM method. *Scientific Reports*, *13*(1), 12473. doi:10.1038/s41598-023-36605-3 PMID:37528148

Lilhore, U. K., Poongodi, M., Kaur, A., Simaiya, S., Algarni, A. D., Elmannai, H., Vijayakumar, V., Tunze, G. B., & Hamdi, M. (2022). Hybrid model for detection of cervical cancer using causal analysis and machine learning techniques. *Computational and Mathematical Methods in Medicine*, *2022*, 2022. doi:10.1155/2022/4688327 PMID:35572826

Moulahi, T., Jabbar, R., Alabdulatif, A., Abbas, S., El Khediri, S., Zidi, S., & Rizwan, M. (2023). Privacy-preserving federated learning cyber-threat detection for intelligent transport systems with blockchain-based security. *Expert Systems: International Journal of Knowledge Engineering and Neural Networks*, *40*(5), e13103. doi:10.1111/exsy.13103

Nair, A. K., Sahoo, J., & Raj, E. D. (2023). Privacy preserving Federated Learning framework for IoMT based big data analysis using edge computing. *Computer Standards & Interfaces*, *86*, 103720. doi:10.1016/j.csi.2023.103720

Nayak, S., & Sharma, Y. K. (2023). A modified Bayesian boosting algorithm with weight-guided optimal feature selection for sentiment analysis. *Decision Analytics Journal*, *8*, 100289. doi:10.1016/j.dajour.2023.100289

Onyema, E. M., Lilhore, U. K., Saurabh, P., Dalal, S., Nwaeze, A. S., Chijindu, A. T., Ndufeiya-Kumasi, L. C., & Simaiya, S. (2023). Evaluation of IoT-Enabled hybrid Model for genome sequence analysis of patients in healthcare 4.0. *Measurement. Sensors*, *26*, 100679. doi:10.1016/j.measen.2023.100679

Pradeep, S., Sharma, Y. K., Lilhore, U. K., Simaiya, S., Kumar, A., Ahuja, S., Margala, M., Chakrabarti, P., & Chakrabarti, T. (2023). Developing an SDN security model (EnsureS) based on lightweight service path validation with batch hashing and tag verification. *Scientific Reports*, *13*(1), 17381. doi:10.1038/s41598-023-44701-7 PMID:37833379

Pradeep, S., Sharma, Y. K., Lilhore, U. K., Simaiya, S., Kumar, A., Ahuja, S., Margala, M., Chakrabarti, P., & Chakrabarti, T. (2023). Developing an SDN security model (EnsureS) based on lightweight service path validation with batch hashing and tag verification. *Scientific Reports*, *13*(1), 17381. doi:10.1038/s41598-023-44701-7 PMID:37833379

Rahman, A., Hossain, M. S., Muhammad, G., Kundu, D., Debnath, T., Rahman, M., Khan, M. S. I., Tiwari, P., & Band, S. S. (2023). Federated learning-based AI approaches in smart healthcare: Concepts, taxonomies, challenges and open issues. *Cluster Computing*, *26*(4), 2271–2311. doi:10.1007/s10586-022-03658-4 PMID:35996680

Ramesh, T. R., Lilhore, U. K., Poongodi, M., Simaiya, S., Kaur, A., & Hamdi, M. (2022). Predictive analysis of heart diseases with machine learning approaches. *Malaysian Journal of Computer Science*, **•••**, 132–148.

Rauniyar, A., Hagos, D. H., Jha, D., Håkegård, J. E., Bagci, U., Rawat, D. B., & Vlassov, V. (2023). Federated learning for medical applications: A taxonomy, current trends, challenges, and future research directions. *IEEE Internet of Things Journal*.

Rieyan, S. A., News, M. R. K., Rahman, A. M., Khan, S. A., Zaarif, S. T. J., Alam, M. G. R., Hassan, M. M., Ianni, M., & Fortino, G. (2024). An advanced data fabric architecture leveraging homomorphic encryption and federated learning. *Information Fusion*, *102*, 102004. doi:10.1016/j.inffus.2023.102004

Sai, S., Hassija, V., Chamola, V., & Guizani, M. (2023). Federated Learning and NFT-Based Privacy-Preserving Medical Data Sharing Scheme for Intelligent Diagnosis in Smart Healthcare. *IEEE Internet of Things Journal.*

Shivthare, S. K., Sharma, Y. K., & Patil, R. D. (2023). Multi-modal Biometric in Computer Vision. *Multi-modal Biometric and Machine Learning Technologies: Applications for Computer Vision*, 1-29.

Singh, K., Kumar, A., Sharma, Y. K., & Rai, A. K. (2023). AIoT-based e-commerce. *AIoT Technologies and Applications for Smart Environments*, 215.

Singh, S., Rathore, S., Alfarraj, O., Tolba, A., & Yoon, B. (2022). A framework for privacy-preservation of IoT healthcare data using Federated Learning and blockchain technology. *Future Generation Computer Systems*, *129*, 380–388. doi:10.1016/j.future.2021.11.028

Stephanie, V., Khalil, I., Atiquzzaman, M., & Yi, X. (2022). Trustworthy privacy-preserving hierarchical ensemble and federated learning in healthcare 4.0 with Blockchain. *IEEE Transactions on Industrial Informatics.*

Swapna, M., Sharma, Y. K., & Prasad, B. M. G. (2020). A survey on face recognition using convolutional neural network. In *Data Engineering and Communication Technology: Proceedings of 3rd ICDECT-2K19* (pp. 649–661). Springer Singapore. doi:10.1007/978-981-15-1097-7_54

Swapna, M., Sharma, Y. K., & Prasadh, B. M. G. (2020). CNN Architectures: Alex Net, Le Net, VGG, Google Net. *Res Net. Int. J. Recent Technol. Eng*, *8*(6), 953–960. doi:10.35940/ijrte.F9532.038620

Tian, Y., Wang, S., Xiong, J., Bi, R., Zhou, Z., & Bhuiyan, M. Z. A. (2023). Robust and privacy-preserving decentralized deep federated learning training: Focusing on digital healthcare applications. *IEEE/ACM Transactions on Computational Biology and Bioinformatics.* PMID:37028039

Torkzadehmahani, R., Nasirigerdeh, R., Blumenthal, D. B., Kacprowski, T., List, M., Matschinske, J., Spaeth, J., Wenke, N. K., & Baumbach, J. (2022). Privacy-preserving artificial intelligence techniques in biomedicine. *Methods of Information in Medicine*, *61*(S 01), e12–e27. doi:10.1055/s-0041-1740630 PMID:35062032

Ullah, I., Deng, X., Pei, X., Jiang, P., & Mushtaq, H. (2023). A verifiable and privacy-preserving blockchain-based federated learning approach. *Peer-to-Peer Networking and Applications*, *16*(5), 2256–2270. doi:10.1007/s12083-023-01531-8

Wang, R., Lai, J., Zhang, Z., Li, X., Vijayakumar, P., & Karuppiah, M. (2022). Privacy-preserving federated learning for Internet of medical things under edge computing. *IEEE Journal of Biomedical and Health Informatics*, *27*(2), 854–865. doi:10.1109/JBHI.2022.3157725 PMID:35259124

Wang, T., Guo, Y., & Choo, K. K. R. (2023). *Enabling Privacy-Preserving Prediction for Length of Stay in ICU-A Multimodal Federated-Learning-based Approach.* Academic Press.

Wang, W., Li, X., Qiu, X., Zhang, X., Brusic, V., & Zhao, J. (2023). A privacy preserving framework for federated learning in smart healthcare systems. *Information Processing & Management*, *60*(1), 103167. doi:10.1016/j.ipm.2022.103167

Chapter 2
Advanced Learning and Bioinformatics in Innovative Drug Discovery Towards Bridging Biology

Yogesh Kumar Sharma
https://orcid.org/0000-0003-1934-4535
Koneru Lakshmaiah Education Foundation, India

Sunayana Kundan Shivthare
MAEER'S MIT Arts Commerce and Science College, India

Avinash Godharam Chaure
MAEER'S MIT Arts Commerce and Science College, India

Shital Vaibhav Ghotekar
MAEER'S MIT Arts Commerce and Science College, India

ABSTRACT

Modern bioinformatics and artificial intelligence technologies are coming together to transform the process of developing pharmaceuticals, marking the beginning of an entirely novel phase in pharmaceutical discovery at the nexus of computational research and biological sciences. This work examines the relationship between statistics and biological processes, emphasizing the promise of significant change by combining artificial intelligence (AI) with bioinformatics methods to improve drug research. Incorporating computational methods, mathematical models, and machine learning procedures in computational biology tools improves our ability to understand biological phenomena's intricacies. The chapter examines the incorporation of few-shot and zero-shot learning approaches in drug discovery, emphasizing their significant potential in overcoming the obstacles related to scarce data and expediting the finding of novel targets for treatment. The review introduces the principle of few-shot learning and its practical implementation in drug research.

DOI: 10.4018/979-8-3693-1874-4.ch002

1. INTRODUCTION

Making standard pharmaceuticals requires a substantial investment of time and resources. Emerging computational technologies such as artificial intelligence (AI), computational biology, and computer-aided drug design (CAD) have the potential to cut down on the time and resources required for drug development in the future. The drug discovery and pipeline procedures have been greatly enhanced in the last several years by the widespread application of computational techniques. This led to the approval of a plethora of novel therapies for sale.

Common steps in creating new medications include conducting experiments to determine their bioactivity, illness specificity, appropriate target identification, and doing preclinical testing. Despite substantial investments of time and money, clinical trials have only achieved a 15% success rate. Half of all failed drug discoveries are due to medications with poor pharmacokinetic features, which include absorption, distribution, metabolism, excretion, and toxicity. Advances in computer approaches have greatly accelerated and improved the efficiency of drug discovery. Some of the ways computational biology has helped in drug development include better understanding of the molecular processes by which ligands bind to targets, better localization of binding and active sites, and improved binding poses of the ligand-target complexes. We anticipate that the majority of these methods will effectively pinpoint the binding and active sites of the target protein.

To design novel protein interactions, it is possible to direct optimization and modification of the initial lead chemical according to specific residues of these binding sites. To investigate the harmful activity, it isn't usually sufficient to engage the active site. Additional factors that might contribute to pathogenesis include mutations that are not located at the active site, structural changes, resistance to therapy, and abnormalities in expression levels.

Computational biology's bio-macromolecular simulation exposes the target protein's molecular mechanism and may inspire novel drug development strategies.Pharmaceutical companies employ molecular dynamics (MD) simulations to accurately display the location and velocity of each atom in a system using Newtonian physics. This method may reveal target protein structural changes, binding, and unbinding to assist experiments. MD simulations can develop target-ligand interaction kinetics, thermodynamics, and free energy profiles. We can use this data to boost lead molecule binding affinity. MD simulations enhance docking data accuracy and binding affinity. Virtual screening (VS) may explore ligand-target atomic-electronic interactions using QM methods like DFT and initio computing. Computing complexity renders these quantitative methods inappropriate for VS in many business settings.

Computer-aided drug design reduces costs, development time, and failure rates. It identifies, synthesizes, and tests biologically comparable active chemicals and therapy possibilities. The CADD frequently finds new drugs to test in small molecule libraries. These findings come from VS, molecular docking, pharmacophore modeling, and QSAR. When it comes to exploring huge chemical databases for novel hit compounds with the desired features, VS has shown to be the most successful strategy so far. Two methods exist for categorizing VS: structure-based VS (SBVS) and ligand-based VS (LBVS). With VS, less time is spent testing compounds in the wet lab, which speeds up drug development. Furthermore, VS is critical for optimizing candidate drugs, speeding up drug design and development, and repositioning and repurposing medications.

Improved drug identification success rates may be possible with the use of AI learning and detecting pharmacological massive data in drug development. Artificial intelligence (AI) may be able to learn and find new rules for data interpretation using big datasets in biology. The usage of AI has allowed top pharmaceutical firms to increase the effectiveness of its medicinal prospects while also decreasing the amount of testing and synthesis that is not essential. Both the structure-based VS and the ligand-based VS have shown improvements in similarity searching efficiency and mining screening data dependability after including deep learning and machine learning into the VS process. Additionally, new compounds may be produced using these techniques.

The purpose of this chapter is to provide an overview of several computational methodologies used in the drug development process. Molecular docking, QM, DL, VS, pharmacophore modeling, ML, and constructed coarse-grained models are all part of this set of methods. It also delves at methods to speed up drug development by expanding the chemical universe of possible lead compounds using VS and other computational tools.

2. RELATED WORK

The purpose of this section is to examine and compare the findings of prior research that employed machine learning as well as deep learning in order to discover novel medications.

2.1 Drug-Correlation Synergy Forecast

The last several decades have seen the development of a variety of different tactics that have been presented with the intention of boosting the synergistic effects of pharmaceutical combinations (Bran, A. M., & Schwaller, P. 2023). The exact label that is assigned to the existing methods, which may be potentially context-aware or multi-way connection approaches, is determined by the data type.

Pharmaceutical, gene, and drug and cell type data are used in multi-way interaction techniques to predict drug pairing synergy (Sharma, Y. K., & Rokade, M. D. 2019). Context-aware techniques predicted drug-drug, medication-gene, gene-gene, and cellular environment relationships using chemical and gene data from pharmaceuticals and cell types. High performance is often accomplished by employing many properties on typical tissues. Due to data and biological characteristic shortages, uncommon tissue cell lines cannot use most techniques. Li, H. et al. (2023) add unique tissues with substantial data and biological properties to a typical tissue prediction model using transfer learning. Abnormal tissues without data and biological components are excluded (Balyan A. K. et al., 2022).

2.2 Zero-Shot and Few-Shot Structured Statistics

Zhang et al. (2023) imply that standard supervised learning methods may struggle to obtain enough labeled data for classification. This statement was made because the problem is difficult to solve. "Few-shot learning" is a new topic of study that aims to solve this issue by training computers with a few instances rather than a lot of labeled data. To remedy the issue, this was done. This method taught computers to learn. To solve the situation, this action was taken. This step was essential to solve the problem. Onyema, E. M. et al. (2023) define "meta-learning" as a few-shot learning method. This is supported by the researchers' findings. The model may rapidly learn to tackle new problems with less training data since it is trained on a specific set of tasks. It learns to solve issues faster. Because of this, the model can resolve difficulties faster. Thus, the model may be utilized more effectively. The model will become more efficient after training, improving its performance. Swapna M. and her colleagues' 2020 research found that data augmentation involves creating new instances to update existing data. This technique creates new instances. Using this technique may indicate an extra data collecting method.

Rokade et al. (2021) suggest that language simulations, or LLMs, may be a useful but underutilized method. LLMs are utilized multiple times. The above approach is used to employ existing information in a corpus of words as a prediction feature. TabLLM is a good framework example since it meets all of these needs. TabLLM, a model that meets these criteria, is a good example. This is the next step after turning mathematical data to English. We employed TabLLM in Jadhav D. and others' 2020 study to determine whether LLMs are beneficial in physiologically based few-shot training sessions. We conducted this investigation to see whether LLMs are applicable.

2.2 Language Model for Bimolecular Molecules Pattern Identification

Language modeling in bimolecular molecules unit patterning examination is an innovative method to genomics that makes use of natural language processing (NLP) tools to extract complicated data from medical records (Deng Y. et al., 2022). This approach was developed by Deng Y. and colleagues. Deng Y. and his colleagues were the researchers that came up with this approach. According to Chen Y. et al. (2023), these mathematical models are able to adequately portray the complicated relationships that occur between DNA, RNA, and protein patterns. This is made possible by the use of transformer structures. Using sequence-to-sequence modeling, language models are able to grasp the environmental and operational importance of certain motifs in great detail, as stated by Sanchez-Fernandez et al. (2022). This is because sequence-to-sequence modeling allows for the construction of language models.

The analysis of input patterns, as well as the production of appropriate predictions and designs, provide the means by which this objective is realized. In order to further enhance the multimodal evaluation of bimolecular facts, it is feasible to combine language models with other statistical methodologies and expert graphs. This is a possibility. This, in turn, makes a contribution to the identification of health indicators and encourages research in the field of operational genomics (Qiu J. et al., 2023). (Jadhav and colleagues, 2019) There is a continuing need for improvements to be made to new procedures in medical research, as well as for an increasing use of these methodologies in practical settings. This is because there are ongoing problems with the effectiveness of data, the avoidance of bias, and the interpretability of the data. The research that was conducted by Xu H. and his colleagues in the year 2023 revealed that natural language processing and bimolecular analysis have the ability to work together in order to hasten the progression of genomics and bioinformatics.

The use of computational models of language towards biomolecular pattern recognition received increasing attention, and a particular method has been proposed for the development of Few-shot and Zero-shot learning-based language modelling using bimolecular facts (Lilhore, U. K. et al., 2022). These algorithms acquire the linguistic patterns of bimolecular, particularly DNA RNA, including protein patterns, in a manner analogous to how GPT-2 accepts patterns in human discourse. Table 1 presents a comparative analysis of existing research.

3. ADVANCED LEARNING IN DRUG DISCOVERY

The field of drug discovery experienced a significant change with the incorporation of sophisticated training methods (Dou B. et al., 2023). The term "molecular anatomy" (MA) refers to a technique de-

Table 1. Comparison of existing research

References	Method Used	Key Findings	Dataset	Key Outcomes	Limitations
Varshney, N., et. al., 2023	Transfer Learning (TL) with Graph Neural Network (GNN)	Cutting-edge performance in predicting interactions and identifying new pairings	An extensive dataset of drug-target interactions, along with supplementary molecular properties.	Precision in forecasting relationships, Expedited drug development	The dependence on existing datasets and the limited comprehension of deep learning algorithms.
Veríssimo, G. C., et. al., 2022	Algorithm for clustering based on network analysis.	Potential targets for therapy for cancer subgroups with distinct biological features	The TCGA dataset consists of multiple types of omics data, including transcriptomics, genomic, and epigenomic statistics.	Recognizing cancer diversity, better classification of patients	Dependence on TCGA statistics, Clustering method variable sensitivity
Chundawat, et., al., 2023	Used CNN-based deep learning	Obtained a precision rate of 85% in forecasting novel drug-target combinations.	Databases containing information on drug-target interactions that are accessible to the public.	Enhancing drug discovery by prioritizing possible interactions.	The deep learning algorithms have a restricted ability to be interpreted, and there is a possibility of data biases.
Qiu, Y., & Wei, G. W. (2023)	Utilized a comprehensive analysis method that merged genetics with epigenomics primarily.	Discovered new types of cancer with unique biological features.	The TCGA dataset includes multiple types of omics data, such as transcriptomic, genomic, and epigenomic statistics.	Enhanced categorization of patients for tailored treatment methods.	The clustering method's sensitivity to essential variables and reliance on TCGA statistics.
Zeng, X., et al., 2022	Explored ethical dilemmas surrounding the utilization of biomedical research.	Diverse bioethics and medical statistics	Highlighted the significance of obtaining informed permission and practising responsible utilization of data.	Principles for conducting research with ethical standards and promoting community consciousness.	The difficulties in establishing universally relevant ethical principles and the changing nature of morality issues.

signed to control molecules in a manner that is roughly in conformity with the principles of classical mechanics. This approach is an alternative to the quantum mechanical computations that are known as quantum mechanics, which are known to be computationally intensive. Over the past several decades, the MM approach has been crucial for improving leads, understanding ligand-protein structures and interactions, and other pertinent topics.

The MA potential energy function, which represents the sum of several energy components, or "force fields," is responsible for its effective accomplishment of this job. Several sampling methods employ potential energy functions, including Monte Carlo (MCL) and MCL. Developing novel medications typically involves MDD simulations. There are several sampling algorithms; however MDD is one of the most used. The interpretation of the traditional Newton's equation of motion is accomplished by the use of a number of different integration techniques, such as Verlet's Algorithm, Leap-frog Algorithm, and Beeman's Algorithm. Because of this, it is able to explore the trajectories, motions, and interactions that take place inside a specific molecular system.

It is possible to employ MDD to get properties that are dependent on the passage of time. Both the environment in which the biomacromolecule is located and the biomacromolecule itself, which may be an enzyme or a protein, are components of the system. Experiments are carried out in order to arrive at a conclusion about the original protein structure of this enzyme or protein system. Following that, it is feasible that we will go on to use various approaches in order to explain the structure. As soon as the model is complete, it will be feasible to begin the simulations. It is possible to get experimental proof of the three-dimensional structure of a protein by using X-ray crystallography.

This is a technique that has been discovered. When it comes to membrane proteins, obtaining high-quality protein structures via the use of X-rays is an exceptionally difficult task. The reason for this is because the production of crystals is essential, and the resolution of the structure is determined by the quality of the crystals. In order to circumvent this problem, cryo-electron microscopy is able to do so without the need for crystal formation. Cryo-electron microscopy makes it feasible to resolve membrane protein structures that are very delicate and difficult to manipulate. This is made possible by the use of high-speed electron microscopy. The cryo-EM treatment, on the other hand, will not solve all of your problems. When it comes to the identification of the high-resolution structure as seen using cryo-electron microscopy, there is still a large level of dependence put on the quality of the material.

It is important to either model or predict the structure of the experiment in order to conduct the experiment when there is no experimental structure on hand. Examples of techniques that are well regarded for the aim of creating the first protein structure are homology modeling and "Deep-Mind's Alpha-Fold" (DMAF). Both of these approaches belong to the category of methods. It is possible for the molecular dynamics simulation to capture the dynamic characteristics of the system by analyzing the interactions that occur between the atoms and molecules that make up the system during a period of time that has been set. In the majority of cases, atoms move along the paths that are established by Newton's laws of motion for them to follow.

3.1 Few-Shot Learning Methods

Few-shot learning Methods (FSLM) may help train algorithms with less labeled data (Seidl P. et al., 2022). To assist drug developers understand Few-Shot Learning, this section explains its ideas, methodologies, and applications. Few-Shot Learning method utilizes data shortage management in pharmaceutical research. Its effectiveness and versatility may help new treatments. Figure 1 presents a Few-Shot Problem Overview.

3.1.1 Few-Shot Drug Discovery Procedure

The process of developing innovative approaches to drug discovery which utilize the use of advanced methods of machine learning includes the use of Few-Shot Learning techniques as a component of the procedure. It was determined that the Few-shot Algorithm was used in order to ascertain the presence of unique drugs; Algorithm 2 displays the testing operations, and Algorithm 1 demonstrates the training (Meier, J., Rao et al., 2021).

3.2 Zero-Shot Learning

In advanced learning, Zero-Shot Learning (ZSL) appears as a trailblazing technique that transforms how models manage situations in which some classes' worth of data are absent throughout training. This part explores the fundamental principles, practices, and real-world uses of Zero-Shot Learning, highlighting its importance in drug research (Hayat N. et al., 2021). Figure 2 Presents the working of Zero-Shot Learning.

Figure 1. Few-shot problem overview

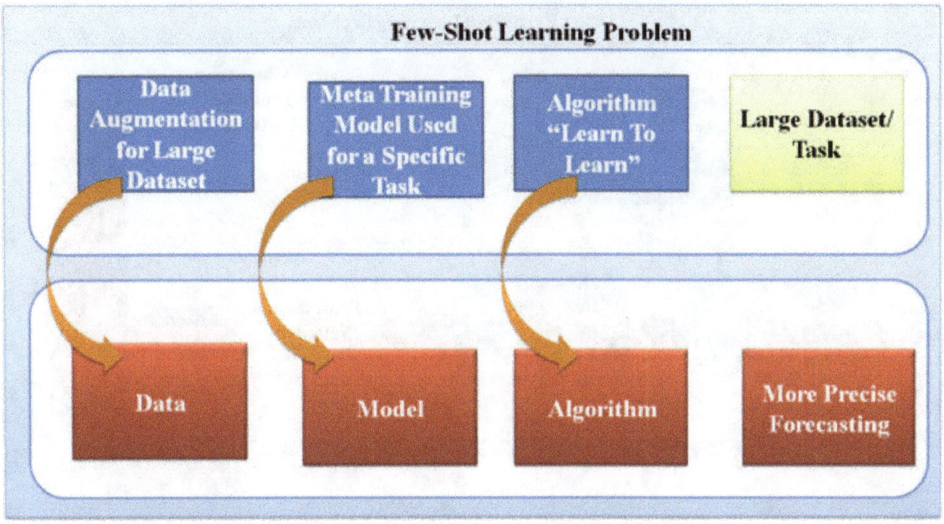

Table 2. Meta-training algorithm for few-shot learning for training

Algorithm 1: Meta-Training Algorithm for Few-Shot Learning for Training
Input: Data samples with a specific problem Outcome: The final outcome is a categorization model that has been trained on a wide range of data and can quickly adjust to new categories using just a few beginning examples.
Step 1: Partition the datasets in meta-training operations, Step 2: Each task consists of a reference set (a small number of instances per category). Step 3: Define a search set. Step 4: Using the search set and labels, train the model on the drug dataset, emphasizing adaptation to novel classes with few instances.

Table 3. Meta-testing algorithm for few-shot learning for testing

Algorithm 2: Meta-Testing Algorithm for Few-Shot Learning for Testing
Input: A new assignment consisting of a supporting set containing many instances per group and a search set. Output: Forecasts for new cases using the adjusted model.
Step 1: Refine the meta-trained network by training it further using the reference set of the new assignment. Step 2: Assess the optimized model's performance on the set of queries to make predictions for new instances.

3.2.1 Fundamental Ideas and Approaches

Zero-shot learning is derived through the human intellectual capacity to extrapolate to categories not addressed throughout the training phase. This subsection explores the fundamental ideas and techniques that form the basis of Zero-Shot Learning. It explains how Zero-Shot Training enables the prediction of consequences in drug discovery contexts involving wholly new and unexpected classes (Prabhakar C. et al., 2021).

Figure 2. The working of zero-shot learning

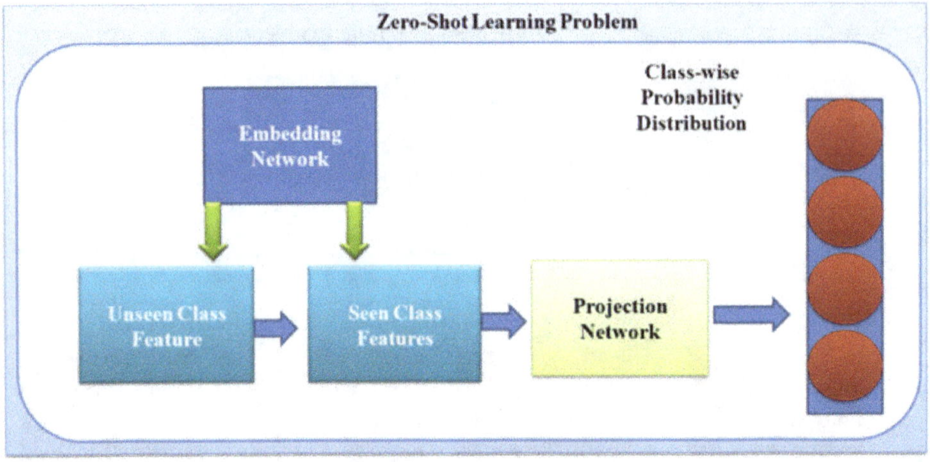

3.2.2 Components Which Are of Utmost Significance

In order for the Zero-Shot Algorithm to perform its intended functions, it is necessary to have a number of core components.

- **Semantic Embeddings:** Within the framework of Zero-Shot Learning, semantic embeddings are an important component. The reason for this is because they provide categorization models with assistance in grasping the links that exist between different categories.
- **Knowledge Transmission:** In terms of the dissemination of information: It is important to take into consideration the idea of learning transfer, which is when the computer uses the knowledge it has learned from previous classes in order to make predictions about what the classes that will come after it will be like.

3.2.2 Application

Based on the findings of Workman et al. (2023), this is considered to be the most significant application of the Zero-Shot Method (ZSM).

- **Novel Drug Response Forecasting:** Utilizing zero-shot learning, we are able to make predictions about the ways in which new pharmaceuticals are going to communicate with the body. This provides us with valuable information into the potential efficacy of these medications as a treatment. This may be highly useful in a number of areas, including the prediction of how new drugs will function.
- **Unveiling Novel Drug-Target Relationships:** The purpose of this demonstration is to showcase the significance of Zero-Shot Learning in determining drug-target interactions that have not been identified before, hence expanding the bounds of drug discovery. The discovery of new drug-target connections will be facilitated by approach.

3.2.3 Issues and Considerations That Need to Be Considered

However, despite this, there are a number of obstacles that need to be overcome before the potential of zero-shot learning can be used in an efficient manner (Sanchez-Fernandez et al., 2022).

- **Semantic gap:** The topic of bridging the "semantic gap," which refers to the divide that exists between classes that are familiar and those that are not, is at the center of the conversation that is taking place around the transfer of data. On because of this, models have a significant obstacle when it comes to effectively bridging this difference.
- **Data quality:** In order for Zero-Shot Learning to function properly, it is very essential to maintain the data in a condition of an exceptionally high quality. Furthermore, it has a direct influence on the accuracy with which the algorithm can estimate outcomes for categories especially in circumstances when the particulars are unknown. When it comes to assessing this, one of the most important factors to consider is the degree of accuracy of the tagged data for the classes that were actually seen.

3.2.4 Zero-Shot Learning Method for Drug Discovery

Sharma, Y. K., et al., 2019, discussed a Novel drug discovery approach, which incorporate the use of ZSLM, make use of machine learning techniques that are regarded as being at the level of the most advanced methods now available. On the other hand, the Zero-shot Algorithm is shown in Algorithm 4 during the testing phase, and it is demonstrated in Algorithm 3 during the training phase, both of which are for the goal of drug discovery.

4. INTEGRATING BIOINFORMATICS

Due to the use of sophisticated bioinformatics learning methods like Few-Shot Learning and Zero-Shot Learning, drug discovery challenges caused by a lack of annotated data have been overcome. This sec-

Table 4. Semantic embeddings algorithm for zero-shot learning for training

Algorithm 3: Semantic Embeddings Algorithm for Zero-Shot Learning for Training
Input: Data samples with a specific problem Outcome: Method with trained labelled.
Step 1: Set a high-dimensional region. Step 2: Incorporate semantic knowledge and generate semantic embedded data for each category.

Table 5. Knowledge transfer algorithm for zero-shot learning for testing

Algorithm 4: Knowledge Transfer Algorithm for Zero-Shot Learning for Testing
Input: labeled examples from recognized classes and fresh examples from unidentified courses. Output: The final product will be a method which can make predictions for cases in classes that weren't part of the training set.
Step 1: Develop a drug discovery model to learn from known categories and use semantic embedded data to predict new instances. Step 2: Assess the optimized model's performance on the drug dataset

tion examines how advanced learning and bioinformatics relate. M. Swapna et al., 2020 We show how these two academic domains complement each other to speed up the discovery of new treatment targets and improve our understanding of complicated biological processes.

3.1 Applying Few-Shot Learning in Bioinformatics

Markus B. et al 2023 suggested a Few-Shot Training has been found to solve problems with huge biological database systems and plenty of labeled data in bioinformatics.

3.1.1 Fundamentals of the Relationship

FSLM's capacity to learn from few instances is useful in bioinformatics. Integration recommendations include Xu, H., and colleagues (2023).

Data augmentation techniques: It improve the quality of limited labeled data by introducing synthetic occurrences, using the adaptive nature of few-shot learning. The adaptable nature of few-shot learning is used to achieve this. The few-shot learning method often employs both of these techniques simultaneously. The goal of these optimizations is to maximize the residual use of these methods in bioinformatics as much as is practically possible.

- **Cross-domain learning: Utilizing** few-shot learning algorithms that have been trained in several domains and applied to bioinformatics data is known as cross-domain learning. This is what the term "cross-domain learning" refers to. By using this approach, one may get valuable insights and predictions, which subsequently streamlines the talent transfer process.

3.1.2 Applications in Bioinformatics

According to the findings of a study that was conducted in 2022 by Deng Y. and colleagues, the combination of bioinformatics and FSLM makes it possible to provide new prospects for the extraction of significant data from biological products statistics.

- **Forecasting of Protein Functions:** The method of forecasting protein functions with a small number of occurrences employing FSLM, which permits a more in-depth grasp of the operating properties of cells may be referred to as Protein Function Forecasting.
- **Operational Labelling of Genomic Sequences:** The assigning of functional qualities to genomic sequences is accomplished via the process of functional genetic sequence categorization, which is a method that makes use of approaches from the Few-Shot Learning methodology.

3.2 Implementing in Bioinformatics Revealed Discoveries

Bioinformatics FSLM illuminates complicated biological processes and overcomes labeled data limits to help solve problems. This expands problem-solving and understanding chances. According to Dalkıran A. and colleagues (2023), FSLM is often employed in bioinformatics to provide significant results.

3.2.1 Uninterrupted System Integration Approaches

Li et al.'s 2023 study ZSLM must be combined with biological goods and understanding of technology using ways that bridge the gap among public and private knowledge. This is crucial for success.

- **Constructing semantic embeddings**: By developing semantic embeddings that truly portray the intricacies of biological interactions, it is likely that we may be able to aid people in migrating their knowledge from one category to another in the real world. This would be a significant step forward in the field of knowledge transfer.
- **Improved Transfer of Knowledge for New Bimolecular Connections:** Using ZSLM to create predictions about new biomolecular linkages, our goal is to discover previously undiscovered biological connections and to make it simpler for individuals to interact with one another and share their knowledge in this area. As part of an attempt to improve the sharing of data in the search for novel biomolecular interactions related with the following: In the process of expecting new biomolecular links, we have the ability to discover unique biological correlations via the use of zero-shot learning. If we do this, we may be able to locate patterns that we were previously unaware of. It is possible that the flow of information in this industry might be simplified by adopting technique.

3.2.2 Bioinformatics Applications

The integration of Zero-Shot Learning with genomics workflows expands the range of comprehension of biological frameworks (Bran, A. M., & Schwaller, P. 2023)

- **Predicting Novel Pathways:** Utilising zero-shot learning, we aim to anticipate unique biological processes, which should offer essential insights into possible pharmacological targets underlying disease causes.
- **Functional Labelling of Proteins:** Utilising Zero-Shot Learning to assign operational characteristics to proteins based on standard features, enhancing our understanding of protein activities.

5. FUTURE DIRECTIONS AND CONCLUSION

The article provides an in-depth analysis of the potential of Few-shot along with Zero-shot learning, when utilized alongside bioinformatics, to revolutionize the field of medicinal product discovery. The comprehensive analysis offered acts as a guide for the researchers and professionals aiming to leverage the combined benefits of advanced learning along with bioinformatics to expedite the creation of innovative treatments. The incorporation of sophisticated learning techniques, specifically Few-Shot Learning along with Zero-Shot Learning, into the field of bioinformatics signifies a revolutionary strategy in the area of developing drugs. These techniques, known for their capacity to function with a restricted amount of labelled data and extrapolate to new instances, provide an unparalleled understanding of genomics, the field of proteomics, and biological ecosystems.

The combination of computational techniques and biology helps overcome the problem of limited data and speeds up the discovery of new therapeutic targets. Responsible AI practices rely on ethical factors, accessibility, and collaborative interaction across computational and biological disciplines. Future research must focus on creating hybrid frameworks, ensemble methods, and tactics to enhance data quality, close the semantic gap, and promote cross-disciplinary learning. The fusion of digital data and biological sciences offers excellent potential in determining the future of pharmaceutical research, introducing a period of groundbreaking and influential therapeutic progress. The fusion of Few-Shot Learning and Zero-Shot Learning through bioinformatics is positioned to influence the trajectory of drug research profoundly. Projected trajectories encompass:

- **Ensemble Approaches:** Investigating the incorporation of ensemble approaches that merge the advantages of sophisticated learning techniques, bioinformatics, and conventional methodologies.
- **Implementing cross-disciplinary training:** It aims to provide scholars with the necessary expertise to navigate computational and life sciences convergence.

REFERENCES

Allaway, E., & McKeown, K. (2020). Zero-shot stance detection: A dataset and model using generalized topic representations. *arXiv preprint arXiv:2010.03640.* doi:10.18653/v1/2020.emnlp-main.717

Balyan, A. K., Ahuja, S., Sharma, S. K., & Lilhore, U. K. (2022, February). Machine learning-based intrusion detection system for healthcare data. In 2022 IEEE VLSI Device Circuit and System (VLSI DCS) (pp. 290-294). IEEE. doi:10.1109/VLSIDCS53788.2022.9811465

Bran, A. M., & Schwaller, P. (2023). Transformers and Large Language Models for Chemistry and Drug Discovery. *arXiv preprint arXiv:2310.06083.*

Chen, Y., Wang, Z., Wang, L., Wang, J., Li, P., Cao, D., Zeng, X., Ye, X., & Sakurai, T. (2023). Deep generative model for drug design from protein target sequence. *Journal of Cheminformatics*, *15*(1), 38. doi:10.1186/s13321-023-00702-2 PMID:36978179

Chundawat, V. S., Tarun, A. K., Mandal, M., & Kankanhalli, M. (2023). Zero-shot machine unlearning. *IEEE Transactions on Information Forensics and Security*, *18*, 2345–2354. doi:10.1109/TIFS.2023.3265506

Dahiya, N., Sharma, Y. K., Rani, U., Hussain, S., Nabilal, K. V., Mohan, A., & Nuristani, N. (2023). Hyper-parameter tuned deep learning approach for effective human monkeypox disease detection. *Scientific Reports*, *13*(1), 15930. doi:10.1038/s41598-023-43236-1 PMID:37741892

Dalkıran, A., Atakan, A., Rifaioğlu, A. S., Martin, M. J., Atalay, R. Ç., Acar, A. C., Doğan, T., & Atalay, V. (2023). Transfer learning for drug–target interaction prediction. *Bioinformatics (Oxford, England)*, *39*(Supplement_1), i103–i110. doi:10.1093/bioinformatics/btad234 PMID:37387156

Deng, R., Cui, C., Liu, Q., Yao, T., Remedios, L. W., Bao, S., . . . Huo, Y. (2023). Segment anything model (sam) for digital pathology: Assess zero-shot segmentation on whole slide imaging. *arXiv preprint arXiv:2304.04155.*

Deng, Y., Qiu, Y., Xu, X., Liu, S., Zhang, Z., Zhu, S., & Zhang, W. (2022). META-DDIE: Predicting drug–drug interaction events with few-shot learning. *Briefings in Bioinformatics*, *23*(1), bbab514. doi:10.1093/bib/bbab514 PMID:34893793

Dou, B., Zhu, Z., Merkurjev, E., Ke, L., Chen, L., Jiang, J., Zhu, Y., Liu, J., Zhang, B., & Wei, G. W. (2023). Machine learning methods for small data challenges in molecular science. *Chemical Reviews*, *123*(13), 8736–8780. doi:10.1021/acs.chemrev.3c00189 PMID:37384816

Dou, B., Zhu, Z., Merkurjev, E., Ke, L., Chen, L., Jiang, J., Zhu, Y., Liu, J., Zhang, B., & Wei, G. W. (2023). Machine learning methods for small data challenges in molecular science. *Chemical Reviews*, *123*(13), 8736–8780. doi:10.1021/acs.chemrev.3c00189 PMID:37384816

Hayat, N., Lashen, H., & Shamout, F. E. (2021, October). Multi-label generalized zero shot learning for the classification of disease in chest radiographs. In *Machine learning for healthcare conference* (pp. 461–477). PMLR.

Jadhav, D., Sharma, Y. K., & Arora, D. P. (2020, April). Profound Learning Approach for Shot Boundary Location. *2nd International Conference on Communication & Information Processing (ICCIP)*. 10.2139/ssrn.3645409

Jadhav, M., Kumar Sharma, Y., & Bhandari, G. M. (2019, December). Currency identification and forged banknote detection using deep learning. In *2019 International Conference on Innovative Trends and Advances in Engineering and Technology (ICITAET)* (pp. 178-183). IEEE. 10.1109/ICITAET47105.2019.9170225

Kojima, T., Gu, S. S., Reid, M., Matsuo, Y., & Iwasawa, Y. (2022). Large language models are zero-shot reasoners. *Advances in Neural Information Processing Systems*, *35*, 22199–22213.

Košprdić, M., Prodanović, N., Ljajić, A., Bašaragin, B., & Milošević, N. (2023). Zero-and Few-Shot Machine Learning for Named Entity Recognition in Biomedical Texts. In *4th Belgrade Bioinformatics Conference* (*Vol. 4*, pp. 38-38). Belgrade: Institute of molecular genetics and genetic engineering.

Kumar, N., Verma, H., & Sharma, Y. K. (2023a). Adversarial Attacks on Graph Neural Network: Techniques and Countermeasures. In Concepts and Techniques of Graph Neural Networks (pp. 58-73). IGI Global.

Kumar, N., Verma, H., & Sharma, Y. K. (2023b). Graph Convolutional Neural Networks for Link Prediction in Social Networks. In Concepts and Techniques of Graph Neural Networks (pp. 86-107). IGI Global. doi:10.4018/978-1-6684-6903-3.ch007

Li, H., Zou, L., Kowah, J. A. H., He, D., Liu, Z., Ding, X., Wen, H., Wang, L., Yuan, M., & Liu, X. (2023). A compact review of progress and prospects of deep learning in drug discovery. *Journal of Molecular Modeling*, *29*(4), 117. doi:10.1007/s00894-023-05492-w PMID:36976427

Li, Y., Yang, J., Zhang, Z., Wen, J., & Kumar, P. (2022). Healthcare data quality assessment for cybersecurity intelligence. *IEEE Transactions on Industrial Informatics*, *19*(1), 841–848. doi:10.1109/TII.2022.3190405

Lilhore, U. K., Manoharan, P., Sandhu, J. K., Simaiya, S., Dalal, S., Baqasah, A. M., Alsafyani, M., Alroobaea, R., Keshta, I., & Raahemifar, K. (2023). Hybrid model for precise hepatitis-C classification using improved random forest and SVM method. *Scientific Reports*, *13*(1), 12473. doi:10.1038/s41598-023-36605-3 PMID:37528148

Lilhore, U. K., Simaiya, S., Pandey, H., Gautam, V., Garg, A., & Ghosh, P. (2022). Breast cancer detection in the IoT cloud-based healthcare environment using fuzzy cluster segmentation and SVM classifier. *Ambient Communications and Computer Systems Proceedings of RACCCS, 2021*, 165–179.

Mahadevkar, S. V., Khemani, B., Patil, S., Kotecha, K., Vora, D., Abraham, A., & Gabralla, L. A. (2022). A review on machine learning styles in computer vision-techniques and future directions. *IEEE Access : Practical Innovations, Open Solutions*, *10*, 107293–107329. doi:10.1109/ACCESS.2022.3209825

Markus, B., Andreas, K., Arkadij, K., Stefan, L., Gustav, O., Elina, S., & Radka, S. (2023). Accelerating Biocatalysis Discovery with Machine Learning: A Paradigm Shift in Enzyme Engineering, Discovery, and Design. *ACS Catalysis*, *13*(21), 14454–14469. doi:10.1021/acscatal.3c03417 PMID:37942268

Meier, J., Rao, R., Verkuil, R., Liu, J., Sercu, T., & Rives, A. (2021). Language models enable zero-shot prediction of the effects of mutations on protein function. *Advances in Neural Information Processing Systems*, *34*, 29287–29303. doi:10.1101/2021.07.09.450648

Mendonça, S. S., de Sousa Vitória, A. R., de Lima, T. W., Galvão Filho, A. R., & Andrade, C. H. (2023). Exploring new horizons: Empowering computer-assisted drug design with few-shot learning. *Artificial Intelligence in the Life Sciences*, *4*, 100086. doi:10.1016/j.ailsci.2023.100086

Muhasina, K. M., Ghosh, P., Swaroop, A. K., Selvaraj, J., Prajapati, B. G., Duraiswamy, B., & Palaniswamy, D. S. (2023). 7 Machine Data Mining Learning and. *Artificial Intelligence in Bioinformatics and Chemoinformatics*, 117.

Nayak, S., & Sharma, Y. K. (2023). A modified Bayesian boosting algorithm with weight-guided optimal feature selection for sentiment analysis. *Decision Analytics Journal*, *8*, 100289. doi:10.1016/j.dajour.2023.100289

Onyema, E. M., Lilhore, U. K., Saurabh, P., Dalal, S., Nwaeze, A. S., Chijindu, A. T., Ndufeiya-Kumasi, L. C., & Simaiya, S. (2023). Evaluation of IoT-Enabled hybrid model for genome sequence analysis of patients in healthcare 4.0. *Measurement. Sensors*, *26*, 100679. doi:10.1016/j.measen.2023.100679

Pandey, M., Fernandez, M., Gentile, F., Isayev, O., Tropsha, A., Stern, A. C., & Cherkasov, A. (2022). The transformational role of GPU computing and deep learning in drug discovery. *Nature Machine Intelligence*, *4*(3), 211–221. doi:10.1038/s42256-022-00463-x

Prabhakar, C., Sekuboyina, A., Paetzold, J. C., Li, H., Amiranashvili, T., & Kleesiek, J. (2021). *Improving Generalized Zero-Shot Learning for Multi-LabelChest X-ray Classification Using Knowledge Graphs*. Academic Press.

Pradeep, S., & Sharma, Y. K. (2019, February). A pragmatic evaluation of stress and performance testing technologies for web based applications. In *2019 Amity International Conference on Artificial Intelligence (AICAI)* (pp. 399-403). IEEE. 10.1109/AICAI.2019.8701327

Pradeep, S., Sharma, Y. K., Lilhore, U. K., Simaiya, S., Kumar, A., Ahuja, S., Margala, M., Chakrabarti, P., & Chakrabarti, T. (2023). Developing an SDN security model (EnsureS) based on lightweight service path validation with batch hashing and tag verification. *Scientific Reports*, *13*(1), 17381. doi:10.1038/s41598-023-44701-7 PMID:37833379

Qiu, J., Li, L., Sun, J., Peng, J., Shi, P., Zhang, R., Dong, Y., Lam, K., Lo, F. P.-W., Xiao, B., Yuan, W., Wang, N., Xu, D., & Lo, B. (2023). Large ai models in health informatics: Applications, challenges, and the future. *IEEE Journal of Biomedical and Health Informatics*, *27*(12), 6074–6087. doi:10.1109/JBHI.2023.3316750 PMID:37738186

Qiu, Y., & Wei, G. W. (2023). Artificial intelligence-aided protein engineering: From topological data analysis to deep protein language models. *Briefings in Bioinformatics*, *24*(5), bbad289. doi:10.1093/bib/bbad289 PMID:37580175

Rokade, M. D., & Sharma, Y. K. (2021, March). MLIDS: A machine learning approach for intrusion detection for real-time network dataset. In *2021 International conference on emerging smart computing and informatics (ESCI)* (pp. 533-536). IEEE. 10.1109/ESCI50559.2021.9396829

Sachi, S., Singh, A. K., Jain, A., Devi, S., Sharma, Y. K., & Athithan, S. (2023, July). Hate Speech Detection Using the GPT-2 and Natural Language Processing. In *2023 Intelligent Methods, Systems, and Applications (IMSA)* (pp. 276-280). IEEE.

Sanchez-Fernandez, A., Rumetshofer, E., Hochreiter, S., & Klambauer, G. (2022, April). Contrastive learning of image-and structure-based representations in drug discovery. ICLR2022 Machine Learning for Drug Discovery.

Seidl, P., Renz, P., Dyubankova, N., Neves, P., Verhoeven, J., Wegner, J. K., Segler, M., Hochreiter, S., & Klambauer, G. (2022). Improving few-and zero-shot reaction template prediction using modern hopfield networks. *Journal of Chemical Information and Modeling*, *62*(9), 2111–2120. doi:10.1021/acs.jcim.1c01065 PMID:35034452

Sharma, Y. K., Athithan, S., Sachi, S., Singh, A. K., Jain, A., & Devi, S. (2023, July). Copy and Move Forged Image Detection by Deep Learning. In *2023 World Conference on Communication & Computing (WCONF)* (pp. 1-6). IEEE. 10.1109/WCONF58270.2023.10235115

Sharma, Y. K., & Khatal Sunil, S. (2019). Health Care Patient Monitoring using IoT and Machine Learning. *IOSR Journal of Engineering (IOSR JEN) National Conference on "Recent Innovations in Engineering and Technology" MOMENTUM-19*.

Sharma, Y. K., & Rokade, M. D. (2019). Deep and machine learning approaches for anomaly-based intrusion detection of imbalanced network traffic. *IOSR Journal of Engineering*, 63-67.

Singh, K., Kumar, A., Sharma, Y. K., & Rai, A. K. (2023). AIoT-based e-commerce. *AIoT Technologies and Applications for Smart Environments*, 215.

Swapna, M., Sharma, Y. K., & Prasad, B. M. G. (2020). A survey on face recognition using convolutional neural network. In *Data Engineering and Communication Technology: Proceedings of 3rd ICDECT-2K19* (pp. 649–661). Springer Singapore. doi:10.1007/978-981-15-1097-7_54

Varshney, N., & Mishra, A. K. (2023). Deep Learning in Phosphoproteomics: Methods and Application in Cancer Drug Discovery. *Proteomes*, *11*(2), 16. doi:10.3390/proteomes11020016 PMID:37218921

Veríssimo, G. C., Serafim, M. S. M., Kronenberger, T., Ferreira, R. S., Honorio, K. M., & Maltarollo, V. G. (2022). Designing drugs when there is low data availability: One-shot learning and other approaches to face the issues of a long-term concern. *Expert Opinion on Drug Discovery*, *17*(9), 929–947. doi:10.1080/17460441.2022.2114451 PMID:35983695

Workman, T. E., Goulet, J. L., Brandt, C. A., Warren, A. R., Eleazer, J., Skanderson, M., Lindemann, L., Blosnich, J. R., O'Leary, J., & Zeng-Treitler, Q. (2023). Identifying suicide documentation in clinical notes through zero-shot learning. *Health Science Reports*, *6*(9), e1526. doi:10.1002/hsr2.1526 PMID:37706016

Xu, H., Wang, Y., Li, Y., & Hong, P. (2023). Asymmetric Contrastive Multimodal Learning for Advancing Chemical Understanding. *arXiv preprint arXiv:2311.06456.*

Zeng, X., Wang, F., Luo, Y., Kang, S. G., Tang, J., Lightstone, F. C., Fang, E. F., Cornell, W., Nussinov, R., & Cheng, F. (2022). Deep generative molecular design reshapes drug discovery. *Cell Reports Medicine*, *3*(12), 100794. doi:10.1016/j.xcrm.2022.100794 PMID:36306797

Zhang, J., Liu, S., Chen, M., Chu, H., Wang, M., Wang, Z., Yu, J., Ni, N., Yu, F., Chen, D., Yang, Y. I., Xue, B., Yang, L., Liu, Y., & Gao, Y. Q. (2023). Unsupervisedly Prompting AlphaFold2 for Accurate Few-Shot Protein Structure Prediction. *Journal of Chemical Theory and Computation*, *19*(22), 8460–8471. doi:10.1021/acs.jctc.3c00528 PMID:37947474

Chapter 3
A Comparative Analysis of Heart Disease Prediction Using Machine Learning Approaches

Khushi
KIET Group of Institutions, Ghaziabad, India

Sonia Deshmukh
KIET Group of Institutions, Ghaziabad, India

Rohit Vashisht
KIET Group of Institutions, Ghaziabad, India

ABSTRACT

Escalating unhealthy lifestyles has led to a surge in common health diseases, notably cardiovascular ailments, a leading cause of human mortality with over 17 million annual fatalities. This study focuses on conducting data analytics within the domain of heart disease, which has become a progressively popular predictive field. The expanding availability of data in this area further emphasizes the significance of in-depth analysis for comprehensive insights and informed decision-making. Diverse strategies and methods have been explored by other researchers. Employing algorithms encompassing KNN, decision tree, and random forest, the authors prognosticate patient illnesses. The support vector machine (SVM) demonstrated superior accuracy among all algorithms. This research enhances heart disease prediction through varied algorithms, underscoring SVM's efficacy and data-driven approaches in addressing escalating health concerns.

A. INTRODUCTION

Cardiovascular disease, commonly known as heart disease, encompasses pathologies affecting both heart and blood vessels. It manifests through a range of aetiologies, including infectious agents, genetic predisposition, and life style factors; however, congenital cases also exist. Predominantly, coronary artery

DOI: 10.4018/979-8-3693-1874-4.ch003

disease, often culminating in myocardial infarction, represents a prototypical manifestation. Additionally, cardiac anomalies might compromise valvular integrity, while impaired cardiac pumping can lead to heart failure. Atherosclerotic plaque deposition within arterial walls is instrumental. Modifiable risk factors such as smoking, suboptimal dietary habits, and physical inactivity significantly elevate susceptibility.

Diabetes, hypertension, and dyslipidemia further compound the likelihood of incidence. Globally, cardiovascular diseases (CVD) accounted for a notable 30 percent of mortality in 2015, translating to approximately 58 million deaths. Remarkably, this proportion aligns with the collective impact of malnutrition, infectious diseases, and maternal conditions. Worth noting is the substantial subset almost 46 percent of individuals succumb to CVD before reaching 70 years, a phase of maximal productivity (Salhi et al.,2021). Between 2015 and 2021, a notable increase of 17 percent in fatalities was observed, and these were primarily attributed to non-communicable diseases. Approximately half of these cases specifically encompassed cardiovascular disease, highlighting a concerning trend in the health landscape. In contrast, mortality stemming from infectious diseases, nutritional deficiencies, and maternal and prenatal conditions collectively exhibited a decline of 3 percent. This underscores the pressing need for precise prognostic analysis of cardiac diseases, as even minor inaccuracies can have profound repercussions on human life. Consequently, the development of accurate methodologies and strategies for both the prevention and treatment of heart disease assumes paramount importance, given its substantial impact on public health.

To unveil discernible patterns and glean actionable insights for healthcare decision-making, data mining proves to be a highly effective approach. This method involves scrutinizing extensive repositories of patient-centric data, enabling the extraction of valuable information. By adeptly applying data mining techniques, researchers can identify crucial risk determinants and forecast outcomes. This is achieved through meticulous analysis of electronic health records, allowing for the development of personalized therapeutic regimens. This study leverages a diverse compilation of individual health profiles within the dataset, fostering a domain-specific exploration enriched by comprehensive data mining methodologies

In recent years, significant traction has been garnered by big data tools, finding extensive utility among diverse healthcare practitioners for the anticipatory analysis of multifarious ailments. Machine learning is dedicated to the formulation of data processing techniques and models that enable computers to autonomously glean insights from data with explicit programming. To elucidate, machine learning empowers computers to identify correlations and patterns within datasets, subsequently harnessing these patterns for prediction and decision-making. Through iterative exposure to data, machine learning algorithms, adept at experiential learning, progressively enhance their precision and operational efficacy.

Machine learning algorithms categorically fall into three distinct types: supervised learning, unsupervised learning, and reinforcement learning. The computer is given labelled examples of data and learns to anticipate new labels based on those examples in supervised learning. Unsupervised learning occurs when a computer is given unlabelled data and is taught to recognize patterns or groups in the data. In reinforcement learning, a computer learns to form judgments based on input from its surroundings. Machine learning exhibits widespread utility across diverse sectors including healthcare, finance, transportation, and beyond. The influx of patients has led to a substantial increase in data availability for analytical purposes. This growth has, in turn, fuelled a pursuit for elevated accuracy and precision in healthcare. Simultaneously, there has been a proliferation of algorithms tailored to meet this imperative, reflecting the escalating demand for accuracy and precision in healthcare analytics.

Jupyter Notebook has been widely used by data scientists for performing various machine learning algorithms as it combines code, graphics-, narrative text, mathematical formulas, and other rich media.

This platform facilitates the enhancement of comprehensibility, reproducibility, and sharability of research endeavours. It enables the simultaneous execution of code, result assessment, and integration of elucidations, formulas, and visual representations, all within a unified interface, thus fostering a holistic approach to research documentation and communication.

The Python programming language stands prominently as a premier choice for Machine Learning due to its inherent qualities. Its lucidity and uniformity lead to concise and legible code, facilitating the presentation process. Further bolstering its appeal, an extensive array of libraries and modules furnish a robust ecosystem, expediting software development timelines effectively.

This paper is oriented towards algorithmic comparison and subsequent identification of optimal prediction methodologies. The overarching aim is the development of a model that employs patient data to yield precise prognostications regarding cardiac disease likelihood. A performance evaluation will be carried out, focusing on both accuracy and precision. This assessment will be juxtaposed with alternative machine learning techniques that are commonly employed in medical research. The study's outcomes hold substantive implications for enhancing the precision of cardiac disease prediction, ultimately culminating in improved patient outcomes. Structured into three distinctive segments, this paper unfolds progressively. The initial section delineates pertinent antecedent research on the topic. The ensuing segment outlines our proposed approach, encapsulating multifaceted project stages. The final segment encompasses the pivotal conclusions extracted from this study.

B. RELATED WORK

Numerous research endeavours have to proficiently forecasted heart disease, predominantly within the purview of machine learning and data mining methodologies. A plethora of analysts have explored diverse algorithms, each striving for elevated accuracy levels.

The research paper "Effective Heart Disease Prediction Using Hybrid Machine Learning Techniques" (S. Mohan et al.,2019) discusses a study that used a combination of machine learning techniques to anticipate heart problems. The authors proposed a novel method that incorporates a random forest hybrid with a linear model. The research utilized a dataset comprising clinical records from heart disease patients, encompassing 11 attributes. The study assessed the hybrid model's performance in relation to individual models of each technique. The outcomes indicated that the hybrid model exhibited superior accuracy and sensitivity, thus establishing its potential as a promising avenue for heart disease forecasting hear disease.

In the research "Prediction of Heart Disease Using Machine Learning" (A. Gavhane et al., 2018) conducted by A. Gavhane et al., a multilayer perceptron algorithm is harnessed for heart disease prediction. This study employs a subset of the primary 13 attributes from the larger pool of 76 attributes, encompassing parameters such as age, gender, and blood pressure. The multilayer perceptron structure includes an entrance layer, an exit layer, and one or more intermediary concealed layers. The system's resultant output signifies the presence or absence of cardiac disease, providing a binary response. The proposed methodology holds the capability to prognosticate the cardiac condition leading to Coronary Artery Disease (CAD).

"Efficient Data Mining Techniques for Heart Disease Prediction and Comparative Analysis of Classification Algorithms" (Rahman and Salehin, 2021) by Rahman Khan et al. highlights the utilization of data mining methods in forecasting cardiovascular disease. The authors used numerous algorithms, such as Naive Bayes, Decision Tree, Random Forest, and multi-layer perceptron, to build their predictive models. Performance assessment encompassed metrics such as accuracy, sensitivity, specificity, and AUC. The findings revealed that the Random Forest algorithm attained the highest accuracy at 97.7 percent and exhibited the top AUC score, thus emerging as the optimal method for heart disease prediction. This study underscores the pivotal role of data mining strategies in the timely prognosis and identification of heart disease.

"Heart Disease Prediction Using Data Mining" (Fandavis, R et al., 2021) by Fandavis,R et al. explores heart disease prediction based on 14 distinct attributes. The literature reveals a plethora of categorization algorithms employed for this purpose, yielding commendable accuracy levels. This article delves into the deployment of two classification algorithms, Naive Bayes and decision tree, utilizing Cleveland and Statlog datasets. Notably, the Naive Bayes algorithm exhibits enhanced accuracy. Each classification methodology presents distinct advantages and limitations, motivating a hybrid approach to capitalize on strengths and enhance accuracy and scalability. Such hybrid models hold promise for extensive datasets, showcasing the capacity to be effectively applied and evaluated.

"Improving the Heart Disease Diagnosis by an Evolutionary Algorithm of PSO and Feed Forward Neural Network" (Feshki et al.,2016) by Feshki et al. introduce the application of Particle Swarm Optimization (PSO), wherein individual features are treated as particles and optimized to attain both local and global optimization. Subsequently, a Feed Forward Back Propagation (FFBP) neural network is employed for propagation, culminating in a substantially elevated prediction accuracy of 91.94 percent.

The research titled "Using Machine Learning for Heart Disease Prediction" (D. Salhi et al., 2021) by D. Salhi et al. constitutes a pivotal component of the broader inquiry into cardiac disease identification and prognosis. Leveraging machine learning algorithms, the paper attains a noteworthy accuracy of 93 percent via Neural Network experimentation. The assessment encompasses the three foremost algorithms—Neural Network, SVM, and KNN—implemented on an authentic dataset of Algerian individuals. Notably, the study's robust point lies in the algorithm's resilience analysis across varying dataset magnitudes, ultimately concluding neural networks as the superior performers. Additionally, the study delves into feature selection, employing the correlation matrix to unravel inter-attribute relationships, further bolstering the paper's analytical depth.

In "Classification Tree for Risk Assessment in Patients Suffering From Congestive Heart Failure via Long-Term Heart Rate Variability" (Melillo et al., 2013) by Paolo Melillo et al. investigate risk appraisal in individuals afflicted with congestive cardiac failure through the employment of an artificial classifier. The study employs a metric called Long-term, which proficiently differentiates individuals at lower risk from those at higher risk by monitoring the irregular rhythms of the heart. Separating patients into high- and low-risk categories is an area where the Classification and Regression Tree (CART) method excels. Additionally, the paper underscores the significance of heart rate fluctuation as a pivotal determinant of congestive cardiac failure risk.

In the paper titled "Assessment of the Risk Factors of Coronary" (A. Karaolis et al., 2021) A. Karaolis et al., evaluating the likelihood of heart risk, with the objective of mitigating Coronary Artery Disease (CAD) incidents, is bifurcated into pre-occasion and post-occasion phases. The research distinguishes between nonmodifiable and modifiable occurrences before and after instances of coronary Artery disease (CAD). The analysis of these three events utilizes the C4.5 decision tree methodology.

The paper titled "A Comparative Study on Heart Disease Prediction Using Classification Techniques" (Rovina et al., 2016) authored by Rovina et al. highlights the superiority of Support Vector Machine (SVM) over Logistic and Naive Bayes approaches, particularly for extensive datasets. The study delves into a comprehensive review of key algorithms utilized in data mining for cardiac disease prediction. The deployment of SVM holds the potential for early diagnosis of heart disease, thereby benefiting individual patients. By integrating this technology, both patients and medical practitioners can augment existing cardiac problem detection methods. The medical domain stands to significantly gain from the heightened accuracy in heart disease identification provided by this system.

The research titled "Association Rule Discovery With the Train and Test Approach for Heart Disease Prediction" (C. Ordonez, 2006) by C. Ordonez explores the utilization of association rule discovery for forecasting heart disease. The author recommends employing a train-and-validate methodology for extracting association rules from patient datasets. This approach facilitates the subsequent prognosis of the likelihood of heart disease. The study encompasses the application of this method on actual patient data and juxtaposes the results against decision tree induction and neural networks. The outcomes underscore the superior accuracy and simplicity of the association rule discovery strategy, positioning it as a preferable alternative. Collectively, the study substantiates the efficacy of the train and validates technique for prediction, further emphasizing the potential of association rule discovery as a formidable approach.

C. PROPOSED WORK

The various steps or the Knowledge Discovery Diagram of this study for the analysis are given in Figure 1.

a) Dataset Collection

Diverse data formats can be employed for datasets, yet the choice for this study was CSV format due to its inherent simplicity in retrieval and management.

The dataset underpinning this investigation originates from Kaggle as shown in Figure 2, bearing the name "Heart failure prediction dataset." This dataset encompasses 11 distinct attributes, each encapsulat-

Figure 1. Knowledge discovery diagram of this study

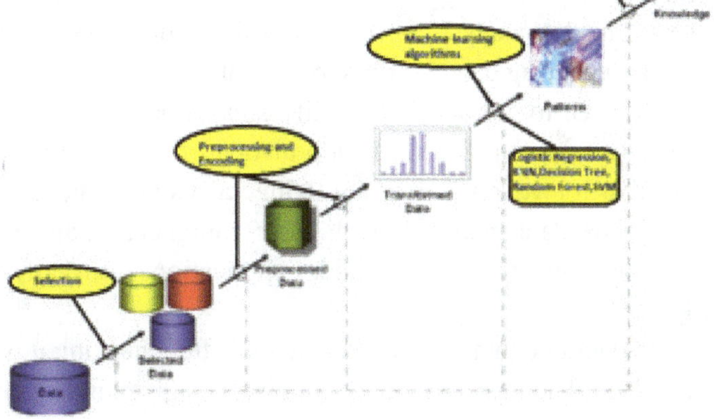

ing diverse medical records from a cohort of 918 individuals. Additionally, a crucial final target column discerns the existence or non-existence of heart disease in the respective individuals.

These attributes encompass the patient's age in years, their gender (with 'F' representing female and 'M' representing male), the type of chest discomfort they experience (categorized as 'ATA' for Atypical Angina, 'TA' for Typical Angina, 'ASY' for Asymptomatic, and 'NAP' for Non-Anginal Pain), fasting blood sugar levels (coded as '1' if fasting blood sugar is greater than 120 mg/dl, '0' otherwise), their resting blood pressure in mm Hg, serum cholesterol levels in mm/dl, the highest heart rate achieved during testing (ranging from 60 to 202), resting electrocardiogram results (classified as 'Normal' for normal, 'ST' for ST-T wave abnormality, and 'LVH' for probable or definite left ventricular hypertrophy),the presence of angina induced by physical activity ('Yes' or 'No'), a numerical value indicative of ST depression (Oldpeak), and the slope of the peak workout ST segment ('Up', 'Flat', or 'Down'). The primary target variable, Heart Disease, serves as the output class, taking on values of '1' denoting the existence of heart disease and '0' denoting a healthy heart. These attributes collectively contribute to a comprehensive evaluation and diagnosis of individuals' heart health.

The dataset employed in this study was meticulously developed through the amalgamation of pre-existing datasets that had not been previously combined. This composite dataset unites five distinct heart-related datasets, all converging on 11 shared characteristics. This comprehensive amalgamation establishes the dataset as the most extensive and all-encompassing resource available for heart disease research purposes.

The compilation incorporates data from the following five datasets: The Cleveland Dataset includes a total of 303 data points, providing a substantial amount of data for analysis. Meanwhile, the Hungarian Dataset offers 294 data points, adding to the diversity of the dataset. The Switzerland Dataset, with 123 data entries, presents a more focused set of data. The Long Beach VA Dataset contributes additional 200 data points, and finally, the Stalog (Heart) Data Set enriches the dataset with 270 data entries. When combined, these disparate parts constitute a sizable dataset for study and investigation in the area of cardiac disease prediction and diagnosis.

This aggregation yields a cumulative sum of 1190 observations, albeit with 272 instances of duplication. As a result, the ultimate dataset comprises 918 distinct observations, thus culminating in an invaluable resource for comprehensive research endeavours related to heart disease.

b) Data Pre-Processing

Data must undergo thorough pre-processing before algorithms can be effectively implemented. Pre-processing, a pivotal stage within data analysis, encompasses the critical tasks of data cleansing, conversion, and integration, thereby rendering data apt for subsequent analysis.

Data preparation is undertaken to elevate data quality and tailor it to specific analytical pursuits. In the context of data pre-processing, the foremost step involves the utilization of the Label Encoder. The transformation is crucial as it involves converting string values into a numeric (float) format. This conversion facilitates more robust data analysis, enabling a comprehensive and effective exploration of the dataset The resultant dataset, post the Label Encoder application, is visually represented in Figure 3 for reference and clarity.

We also need to see if the dataset contains any null values. After checking it is seen that this dataset does not contain any null values. The heat map of the following is given in Figure 4 & Figure 5.

Figure 2. The collected dataset

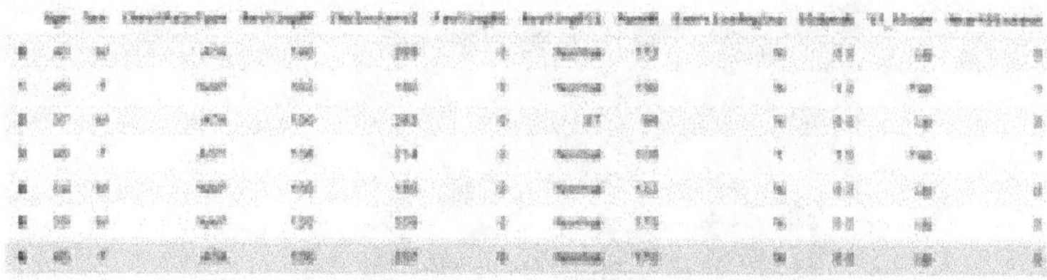

Figure 3. The dataset after applying label encoder

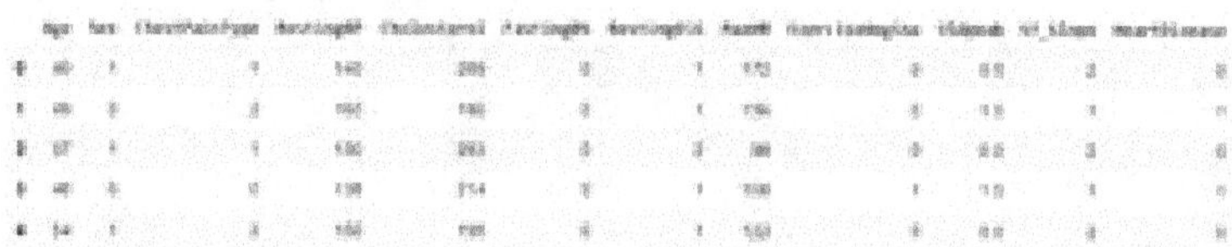

c) Methodology

After pre-processing is completed, we first divide our data into two parts - train and test data in a ratio of 80 percent and 20 percent respectively. Our second step is to apply various algorithms in order to train our heart disease prediction model. For that, we have applied different algorithms Decision Tree, Logistic regression, KNN, Random forest algorithms and SVM (Support Vector Machine). For every algorithm, we have calculated the accuracy measure, precision metric, and recall metric and performed the comparison and evaluation to check which algorithm is giving the best result.

1. **Logistic Regression:** This algorithm holds a significant position within the domain of Machine Learning, specifically categorized under Supervised Learning. Operating within this framework,

Figure 4. Sum of null values

```
Age               0
Sex               0
ChestPainType     0
RestingBP         0
Cholesterol       0
FastingBS         0
RestingECG        0
MaxHR             0
ExerciseAngina    0
Oldpeak           0
ST_Slope          0
HeartDisease      0
dtype: int64
```

Figure 5. Heat-map of null values

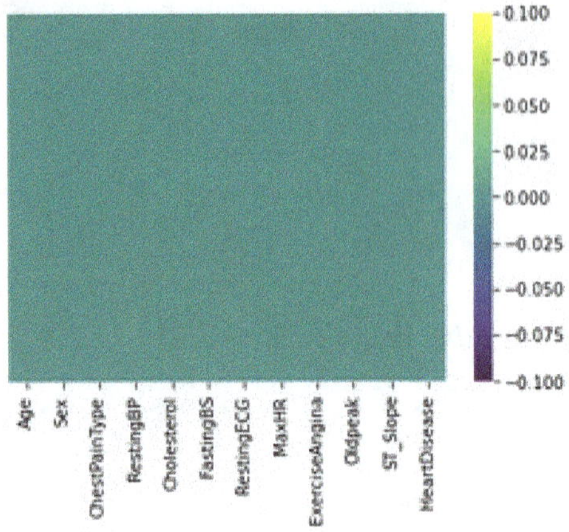

the system takes on the task of predicting the outcome of a category-dependent variable. This prediction is based on a set of independent features, and the process is essential for understanding the relationships within the dataset. Consequently, the outcomes deduced through logistic regression inherently assume a categorical or discrete nature. These outcomes may take the form of binary classifications such as Yes or No, 0 or 1, true or false, and analogous instances. Notably, in contrast to yielding precise binary values like 0 and 1, logistic regression furnishes probability readings that span the range between 0 and 1 (Zhang et al.,2020).

2. **KNN (K Nearest Neighbour):** This algorithm constitutes a pertinent approach within the realm of Machine Learning, operating distinctly under the purview of Supervised Learning. The core tenet of the KNN methodology rests upon the presumption of similarity between novel data and pre-existing instances. This methodology undertakes the classification of the new instance by aligning it with the class that bears the closest resemblance to the established categories. The KNN algorithm relies on the essential practice of retaining all accessible data. This retained data then guides the classification of new data points, determining their category based on their proximity to the preceding data points in the dataset. This mechanism culminates in the swift and effective allocation of novel data into appropriate categories (Rahmat et al., 2021).
3. **Decision tree:** While Decision Tree aligns within the domain of Supervised Learning, its prevalent utilization predominantly pertains to classification challenges, while also extending its applicability to regression scenarios. The architecture of a Decision Tree encompasses internal nodes with dataset parameters, whereas branches embody decision conditions. Ultimately, each terminal leaf node furnishes the discerned outcome. This tree based classifier's inherent structure encapsulates a succinct visualization of decision-making processes (Shouman et al., 2011).
4. **Random Forest:** The pivotal objective is to elevate the prediction accuracy of the dataset. This goal has led to the adoption of the Random Forest classification approach, a robust ensemble method known for its effectiveness in enhancing predictive performance. This methodology strategically assembles numerous decision trees, each operating on distinct fragments of the dataset. Through the aggregation of outcomes across this ensemble, Random Forest leverages the principle of averaging to enhance the predictive efficacy.

Fundamentally, the crux of the Random Forest approach resides in consolidating the projections garnered from multiple decision trees. This mechanism culminates in a final result, which is determined through a majority vote consensus. This approach contrasts with relying on the verdict of a solitary decision tree, showcasing the collaborative strength of the Random Forest classification method. The ensemble's collaborative decision-making capacity stands as a hallmark of the Random Forest methodology. (Madhumita and Smita, 2020).

5. **SVM (Support Vector Machine):** Facilitating the categorization of forthcoming data points is a primary advantage bestowed by the Support Vector Machine (SVM) . Achieved through the discernment of an optimal line that demarcates n-dimensional space, the SVM algorithm effectively undertakes classification tasks. This delineating frontier, commonly termed a hyperplane, emerges as the epitome of the optimal solution. The process of pinpointing the most apt hyperplane entails the meticulous selection of extreme vectors and points, instrumental in delineating this pivotal boundary. These instances, recognized as support vectors, are pivotal in orchestrating the hyperplane's configuration. The terminology "Support Vector Machine" encapsulates this distinctive methodology, hinging on the strategic deployment of support vectors to attain maximal classification precision (Madhu and Ramesh, 2021).

D. EXPERIMENTAL RESULTS AND DISCUSSION

Table 1 shows various comparative parameters for five different algorithms. The table clearly demonstrates that the Support Vector Machine renders the highest accuracy possible in addition to a high precision and recall score.

Figure 6 to 7 provides the confusion matrices for various algorithms used in the study. It displays the results of calculation for True Positive, False Positive, and False Negative, True Negative values.

The plot of actual vs. predicted values by Random Forest Classifier is given in Figure 8 by taking the density of the variables as a y-axis. The red lines give the actual value while the blue line gives the predicted value.

Similarly, another density-based graph between actual and predicted values is given for SVM in Figure 12. It plots with blue lines as actual values and green lines as predicted values.

A comparison analysis of the accuracy and precision of all the five algorithms applied in this study is given in Figure 13. From the plot, it is clear that SVM shows the best accuracy as well as precision of all the five algorithms. From the above analysis and results, it can be depicted that SVM is the best

Table 1. Performance comparison of various ML algorithms

Algorithms	Precision	Accuracy	Recall
Knn	71.844	75	77.894
LogisticRegression	83.928	83.695	88.679
Decision tree	82.524	84.782	89.473
Random Forest	84.761	87.5	92.708
SVM	90.163	89.13	93.220

Figure 6. Confusion matrices for logistic regression

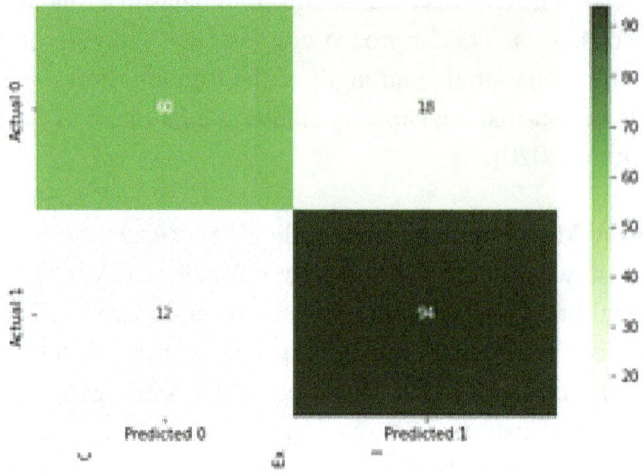

Figure 7. Confusion matrices for k-nearest neighbour

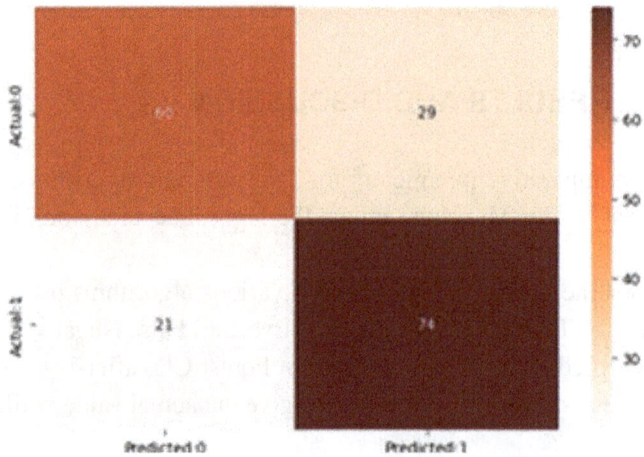

Figure 8. Confusion matrices for decision tree

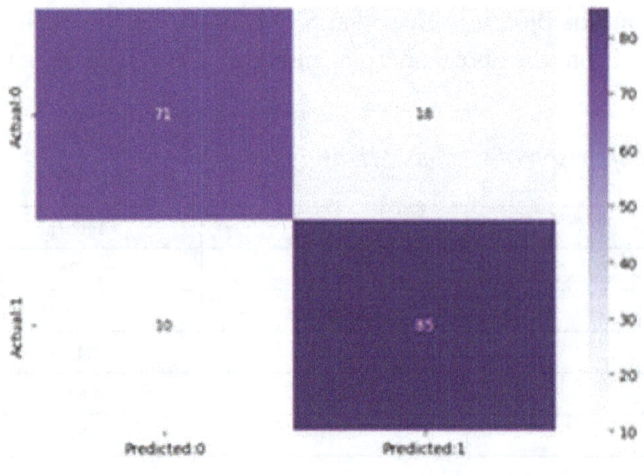

Figure 9. Confusion matrices for random forest

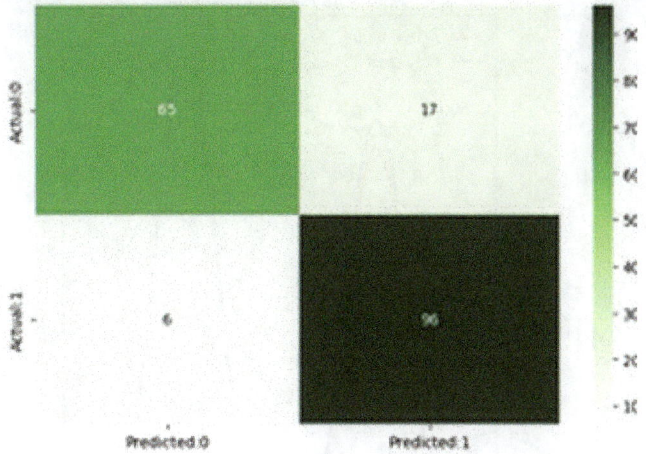

Figure 10. Confusion matrices for support vector machine

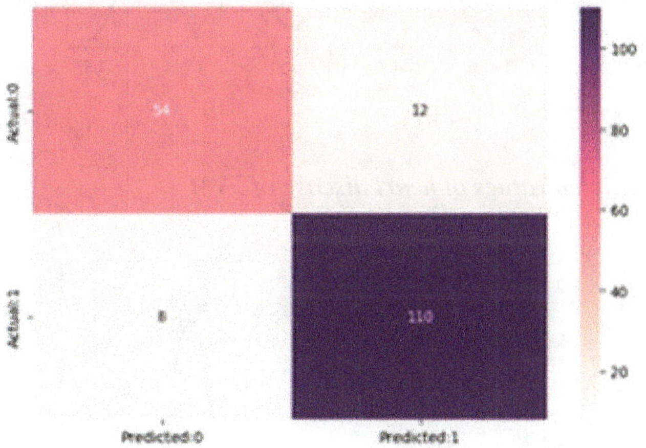

algorithm to be employed for cardiovascular disease prediction. Overall its accuracy can range between 89-91 percent.

E. CONCLUSION

This research endeavour serves to showcase the precision and accuracy underpinning heart disease prediction through an array of machine-learning methodologies. The escalating volume of data within the medical sphere underscores the pivotal need for systematic data organization. Thorough analysis becomes imperative to derive meaningful insights and ensure the effective utilization of this wealth of information for healthcare advancements. A pronounced challenge therein lies in the formulation of adept and computationally efficient algorithms, an imperative underscored by the burgeoning medical data landscape. Of notable significance within our study, the Support Vector Machine (SVM) emerges

Figure 11. Actual vs. predicted values of heart disease of random forest

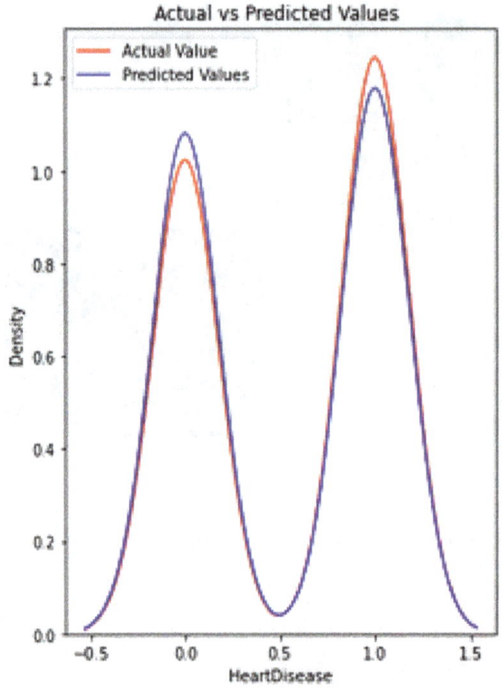

Figure 12. Actual vs. predicted values of heart disease of SVM

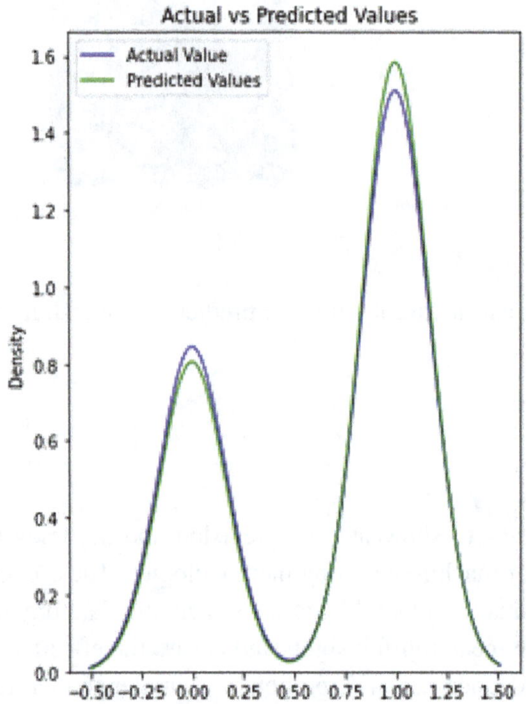

Figure 13. Comparison analysis of accuracy and prediction of various algorithms

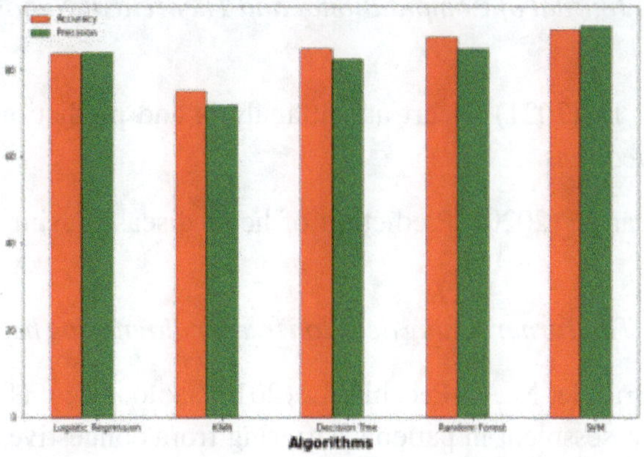

as a standout performer, manifesting optimal predictive prowess with an impressive accuracy rating of 89.13 percent. The experimental results demonstrate that by applying the predictive models to the records of arriving new patients, we may construct a brief but precise prognosis list for cardiac patients.

REFERENCES

Dbritto, R., Srinivasaraghavan, A., & Joseph, V. (2023). Hybrid model for precise hepatitis-C classification using improved random forest and SVM method. *Scientific Reports*, *13*(1), 12473. doi:10.1038/s41598-023-36605-3 PMID:37528148

Fadnavis, R., Dhore, K., Gupta, D., Waghmare, J., & Kosankar, D. (2021). Heart disease prediction using data mining. *Journal of Physics: Conference Series*, *1913*(1), 012099. doi:10.1088/1742-6596/1913/1/012099

Feshki, S., & Omid, M. (2016). *Improving the heart disease diagnosis by evolutionary algorithm of pso and feed forward neural network*. Paper presented at the artificial intelligence and robotics (IRANOPEN). 10.1109/RIOS.2016.7529489

Gavhane, A., Kokkula, G., Pandya, I., & Devadkar, K. (2018). Prediction of heart disease using machine learning. *Second International Conference on Electronics, Communication and Aerospace Technology (ICECA)*, Coimbatore, India. 10.1109/ICECA.2018.8474922

Lilhore, U. K., Poongodi, M., Kaur, A., Simaiya, S., Algarni, A. D., Elmannai, H., Vijayakumar, V., Tunze, G. B., & Hamdi, M. (2022). Hybrid model for detection of cervical cancer using causal analysis and machine learning techniques. *Computational and Mathematical Methods in Medicine*, *2022*, 2022. doi:10.1155/2022/4688327 PMID:35572826

Lilhore, U. K., Simaiya, S., Pandey, H., Gautam, V., Garg, A., & Ghosh, P. (2022). Breast cancer detection in the IoT cloud-based healthcare environment using fuzzy cluster segmentation and SVM classifier. *Ambient Communications and Computer Systems Proceedings of RACCCS*, *2021*, 165–179.

Lilhore, U. K., Simaiya, S., Prasad, D., & Guleria, K. (2020). A hybrid tumor detection and classification based on machine learning. *Journal of Computational and Theoretical Nanoscience*, *17*(6), 2539–2544. doi:10.1166/jctn.2020.8927

Madhu, H. K., & Ramesh, D. (2021). Heart attack analysis and prediction using svm. *International Journal of Computer Applications*.

Madhumita Pal & Smita Parija. (2020). Prediction of heart diseases using random forest. *Journal of Physics: Conference Series*.

Mai, S. (2011). *Rob Stocker, Tim Turner: Using decision tree for diagnosing heart disease patients*. CRPIT.

Melillo, P., De Luca, N., Bracale, M., & Pecchia, L. (2013). aolo, Luca, N., Bracale, M., Pecchia, L.: Classification tree for risk assessment in patients suffering from congestive heart failure via long-term heart rate variability. *IEEE Journal of Biomedical and Health Informatics*, *17*(3), 727–733. doi:10.1109/JBHI.2013.2244902

Minas, A. (2010). Assessment of the risk factors of coronary heart events based on data mining with decision trees. *IEEE Transactions on Information Technology in Biomedicine*.

Mohan, S., Thirumalai, C., & Srivastava, G. (2019). Effective heart disease prediction using hybrid machine learning techniques. *IEEE Access : Practical Innovations, Open Solutions*, *7*, 81542–81554. doi:10.1109/ACCESS.2019.2923707

Onyema, E. M., Lilhore, U. K., Saurabh, P., Dalal, S., Nwaeze, A. S., Chijindu, A. T., Ndufeiya-Kumasi, L. C., & Simaiya, S. (2023). Evaluation of IoT-Enabled hybrid model for genome sequence analysis of patients in healthcare 4.0. *Measurement. Sensors*, *26*, 100679. doi:10.1016/j.measen.2023.100679

Ordonez, C. (2006). Association rule discovery with the train and test approach for heart disease prediction. *IEEE Transactions on Information Technology in Biomedicine*, *10*(2), 334–343. doi:10.1109/TITB.2006.864475 PMID:16617622

Rahmat, D., Putra, H. A. A., & Setiawan, A. W. (2021). Heart disease prediction using k-nearest neighbor. *International Conference on Electrical Engineering and Informatics (ICEEI)*. 10.1109/ICEEI52609.2021.9611110

Ramesh, T. R., Lilhore, U. K., Poongodi, M., Simaiya, S., Kaur, A., & Hamdi, M. (2022). Predictive analysis of heart diseases with machine learning approaches. *Malaysian Journal of Computer Science*, 132–148.

Rathore, M. S., Poongodi, M., Saurabh, P., Lilhore, U. K., Bourouis, S., Alhakami, W., Osamor, J., & Hamdi, M. (2022). A novel trust-based security and privacy model for internet of vehicles using encryption and steganography. *Computers & Electrical Engineering*, *102*, 108205. doi:10.1016/j.compeleceng.2022.108205

Sharma, S. K., Lilhore, U. K., Simaiya, S., & Trivedi, N. K. (2021). An improved random forest algorithm for predicting the COVID-19 pandemic patient health. *Annals of the Romanian Society for Cell Biology*, 67–75.

Simaiya, S., Lilhore, U. K., Prasad, D., & Verma, D. K. (2021). MRI brain tumor detection & image segmentation by hybrid hierarchical K-means clustering with FCM based machine learning model. *Annals of the Romanian Society for Cell Biology*, 88–94.

Zhang, Y., Diao, L., & Ma, L. (2020). Logistic regression models in predicting heart disease. *Journal of Physics: Conference Series*.

Chapter 4
A Comprehensive Study of Bio-Informatics With Machine Learning

Rohit Vashisht
KIET Group of Institutions, Ghaziabad, India

Gagan Thakral
KIET Group of Institutions, Ghaziabad, India

ABSTRACT

Bioinformatics is an interdisciplinary field that develops methods and software tools for understanding biological data. Bioinformatics is an interdisciplinary field of study that combines computer science, mathematics, statistics, and engineering to analyze and comprehend biological data. Researchers faced a major issue in describing this new topic in a methodical, scientific manner and drawing attention to its potential uses and capabilities. This chapter will discuss the immense quantity of data generated in the biological area and how bioinformatics can manage, examine, and preserve them, along with a few algorithms that can be applied over bioinformatics data. In many bioinformatics studies and applications, machine learning is applied. This chapter will also provide a clear overview of the field's definition, goals, applications, related technologies, and future directions.

A. INTRODUCTION

Bioinformatics is an interdisciplinary field that develops methods and software tools for understanding biological data. Bioinformatics is an interdisciplinary field of study that combines computer science, statistics, mathematics, and engineering to analyze and understand biological data. Bioinformatics has used statistical and mathematical techniques to examine biological research in silico (Jawdat D., 2006). Computer assessments of biological data are used to derive knowledge about bioinformatics. These may also include patient information, experimental results from various sources, and scholarly literature in addition to the information included in the genetic code. A component of bioinformatics research is the

DOI: 10.4018/979-8-3693-1874-4.ch004

development of techniques for data archiving, retrieval, and analysis. Using methods and ideas from informatics, statistics, mathematics, mathematics, chemistry, biology, physics, and linguistics, bioinformatics is rapidly expanding field of biology. It has several practical applications in a variety of medical and biological disciplines (Kilhara D. et al., 2007).

In bioinformatics, information technology is used to organize, store, and analyze the massive amounts of biological data. For instance, the sequence and structure of information carriers like proteins and nucleic acids, among others, are available as the recorded data. Structures have a three-dimensional form of various sequences, while sequences can be represented in a single dimension. The various disciplines that were involved in founding bioinformatics are shown in Figure 1. It denotes that the field of bioinformatics combines biology, mathematics, statistics, information technology, and computer science to process vast amounts of biological data (Zheng Zhao et al., 2021). The four main processes of bioinformatics—collecting, processing, analyzing, and disseminating of biological data—are illustrated in Figure 2. This chapter will discuss the development of bioinformatics, its needs, its objectives, and a variety of applications of bioinformatics along with their obstacles. Finally, some of the well-known databases and tools for bioinformatics are also reviewed, along with potential future directions.

B. EMERGENCE OF BIOINFORMATICS

Paulien Hogeweg first used the term "bioinformatics" in 1978. Bio stands for biology or biological data, while informatics is the processing of data. The birth of bioinformatics is generally credited to Mendel's

Figure 1. Integrating components of bio-informatics

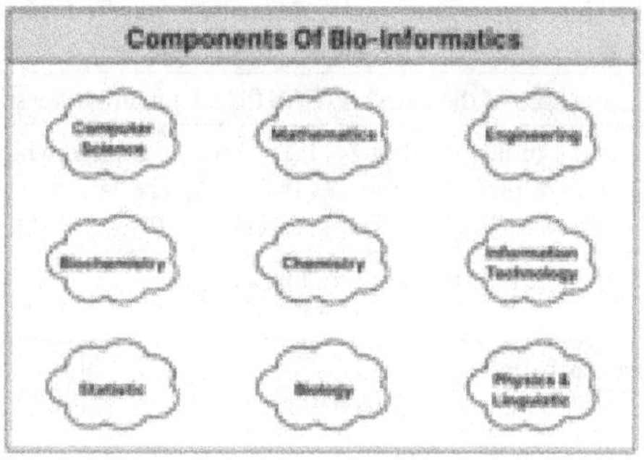

Figure 2. Process of bio-informatics

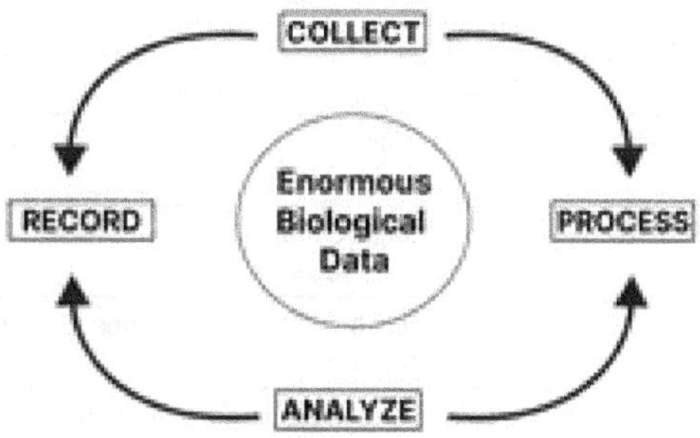

discovery of genetic inheritance in 1865. The development of bioinformatics is systematically shown in Table 1 with clarity (Gauthier et al., 2018).

Table 1. History of bioinformatics

Year	Major Findings
1951	The alpha-helix and beta-sheet structures have been proposed by Pauling and Corey.
1953	For DNA-based X-ray data, Watson and Crick developed a double helix model.
1955	S. Hanger examines the amino acid sequence of the first protein known as bovine insulin.
1958	Jack Kilby of Texas Instruments created the first integrated circuit.
1965	Margaret Dayhoff produced the atlas of protein sequences.
1968	ARPA offered packet networking switching protocols.
1970	The Neddleman-Wunsch for sequence comparison is provided in detail.
1972	Paul Berg and his team produced the first recombinant DNA molecule.
1975	Farrell announced the use of 2-D electrophoresis, which combines the separation of proteins on an SDS polyacrylamide gel with isoelectric point separation.
1976	Bell Labs is where the Unix-to-Unix Copy Protocol (UUCP) is being developed. The experimental information on the southern biot method for particular DNA sequences was published by E.M. Southern.
1980	The first complete gene sequence for an organism (FX174), which comprises of 5386 base pairs and nine proteins, has been released.
1982	While GenBank published three made-public Phagae lambda genome sequences, the Wisconsin Biological Centre created a set of molecular biological instruments.
1983	Creation of DNA clone libraries for individual chromosomes is started by the LANL (Los Alamos National Laboratory) and LLNL (Lawrence Livermore National Laboratory).
1986	The scientific field of gene mapping, gene sequencing, and gene analysis was first referred to as genomics. Thomas Roderick was the author of the term.
1988	Pearson and Lupman are the creators of the FASTA (FAST-ALL) method for sequence algorithms. (Padole, 2005)
1990	A new algorithm called Basic Local Alignment Search Tool (BLAST) is created which refers to a group of software tools that produce alignments between nucleotide or protein sequences from a "query" and sequences from databases known as "subject" sequences. (Stephen, 2005)
1992	A published low resolution genetic linkage map of the entire human genome. The DOE and NIH released guidelines for sharing resources and data.
1996	Saccharomyces cerevisiae's genome has been sequenced. The presence of the third major branch of life on Earth is confirmed by the prossite database, according to Bairoch.
1997	The E. coli genome has been made public. The Genetic Computer Group is acquired by Oxford Molecular Group.
1999	The first human chromosome was fully sequenced on December 1st, 1999. A comprehensive DNA sequencing of 22 human chromosomes was presented.
2000	Pseudomonas aeruginosa's genome was made public. This year also saw the presentation of other biological species' genome sequencing.
2001	The human genome is published. The third human chromosome to be fully sequenced to the high standard required by the Human Genome Project is chromosome 20.
2002	A multinational group that combines structural bioinformatics and gene-formatics published the complete genomic sequence of the common house mouse.
2003	The Human Genome Project finished sequencing the human chromosome 14 in April 2003, making it the fourth chromosome to do so.
2004	The Rat Genome Sequencing Project Consortium has finished the entire genome sequence of the brown Norway laboratory rat, Rattus norvegicus.
2005	This year saw the completion of the sequencing of the rice genome.

The emergence of bioinformatics was prompted by the requirement to create large databases, such as EMBL, Japan's DNA Database and GenBank to store and compare the DNA sequence data obtained from the sequencing of the human being genome and other genomes. In today's era, bioinformatics now includes studying protein structures, genes and proteins' functions, patient data, pre-clinical and clinical studies, and many species' metabolic pathways (Gauthier et al., 2019).

C. NEED AND IMPORTANCE OF BIOINFORMATICS

Bioinformatics is used to analyze and comprehend biological data, design computer programs for swift access to, management of, and application of biological data, and produce equations and statistical methods for assessing relationships in sizable datasets. The next-generation sequencing systems generate enormous amounts of data. Data is gathered regarding sequencing performance as well as DNA sequencing results in order to aid in the identification of mistakes or repetitive sequencing. Issues with data management and storage result from this (Shahnaz et al., 2016). To process the massive amounts of data, specialized software and quick computing systems are also needed. The interpretation of data produced by next-generation sequencing, as well as the development and expansion of precision medicine, depend on specialized, trained bioinformaticists.

Bioinformatics will become more and more important as we gather more and more biodata. Understanding and drawing conclusions from biological data would be very challenging without bioinformatics and the capacity to use computer science skills to huge data (Qi., 2013). Figure 3 outlines the approach to solve a bioinformatics problem in detail.

To deal with a problem in bioinformatics, one must first have a fundamental understanding of biology, and more especially, the biological area they are working with. The problem statement required for the experimentation should be chosen in the second phase. The full operation of a bioinformatics tool should

Figure 3. Road-path to solve a problem in bioinformatics

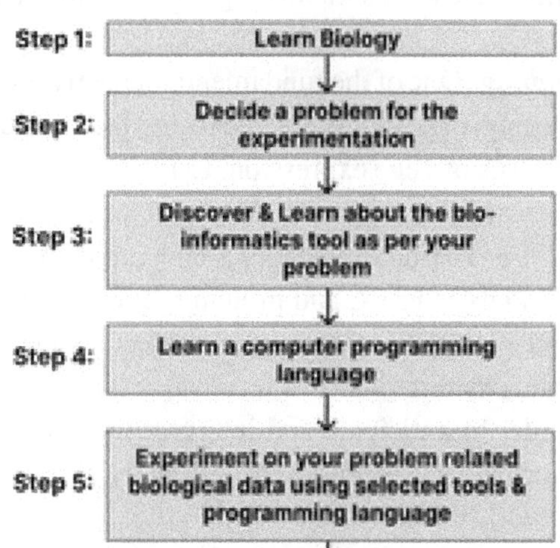

then be understood in relation to the problem statement. In later sections, the authors explain various well-known bioinformatics databases and tools. As, it is very well known, one of the key integrating elements of bioinformatics is computer science. Therefore, it is advisable to learn a programming language that is compatible with the bioinformatics tool that was learnt in the third phase. The experiments were carried out utilizing a chosen bioinformatics tool and computer programming language on biological data linked to the subject at hand in the next phase. The experimental results are finally analyzed and recorded for use in the future.

Sustainable agriculture also benefits from the use of bioinformatics. It has fundamentally changed the way we research and comprehend living systems, and its applications have broad ramifications for sustainability and food security. With the help of bioinformatics, researchers can analyze enormous volumes of biological data, find novel crop kinds, and come up with creative strategies to raise crop yields. Bioinformatics will continue to be essential for enhancing our understanding of biological processes in agriculture as data sets rise (Rajamanickam & Elanchezhian, 2012)..

Hence, bioinformatics has become an important area of contemporary biology and is predicted to continue to do so. Its applications have profound effects on human health and wellbeing and have revolutionized how humans study and comprehend living systems. Researchers can analyze enormous volumes of biological data using bioinformatics, find new pharmacological targets, and create individualized treatments. Bioinformatics will continue to be essential for enhancing our understanding of biological systems as data sets increase.

D. MAJOR OBJECTIVES OF BIOINFORMATICS

Bioinformatics' primary objectives are to organize bio-data to make it easily searchable and accessible, create software to assist with bio-data analysis and biologically-based analysis and interpretation of bio-data (Goldin L., 2006). The main objectives of bioinformatics are to use computational techniques and tools to understand biological systems, to support data-driven investigations, and to speed up improvements in a variety of areas, such as genetics, proteomics, genomics, and discovering new drugs. The following have been identified clearly as the main goals of bioinformatics.

a) *Data Management & Handling:* One of the fundamental objectives of bioinformatics is the creation of efficient methods for storing, organizing, and retrieving biological data, such as DNA sequences, protein structures, and patterns of gene expression. Large volumes of biological data are managed and curated using bioinformatics tools and databases.
b) *Study of Sequence & Structure:* To find similarities, trends, and functional components, bioinformatics compares and examines DNA, RNA, and protein sequences. Techniques used to comprehend the structure, function, and evolutions of biological molecules include sequence alignment, motif discovery, and phylogenetic examination.
c) *Structural Analysis:* In order to anticipate and interpret the 3-D structures of biomolecules like RNA and proteins, bioinformatics is essential. Additionally, it results in better drug discovery and development (Ardekani et al., 2007).
d) *Functional Interpretation:* Genes and proteins are given functional labels using bioinformatics tools and algorithms. Bioinformatics aids in predicting gene activities, finding protein domains, and comprehending molecular interactions by fusing experimental data with computer predictions.

e) *Comparative Study of Genomics:* To find parallels, differences, and evolutionary connections between different species' genomes, bioinformatics makes this comparison possible. Understanding the genetic causes of diseases, locating intact elements, and researching genome rearrangements are all made easier by the study of comparative genomics (Domokos A., 2008).
f) *Systems Biology:* By combining and evaluating massive biological data sets from fields like genomics, transcriptomics, and proteomics to comprehend biological systems as a whole, bioinformatics makes a contribution to the study of systems biology. It entails building biological networks, simulating biological systems, and modeling biological processes.
g) *Drug Design & Production:* By enabling the study of biological data to pinpoint possible therapeutic targets, forecast drug interactions, and enhance drug candidates, bioinformatics plays a crucial role in the search for drugs. It speeds up and lowers the cost of the procedure for developing drugs by assisting with virtual screening, lead selection, and validation of targets.
h) *Customized Medici nation:* In order to customize medical therapies based on a person's genetic make-up, bioinformatics permits the study of individual genomic and clinical data. It aids in the discovery of genetic risk factors for diseases, the prediction of drug reactions, and the establishment of individualized treatment plans (Chavan PR, 2008).

E. APPLICATIONS OF BIOINFORMATICS

The following are the primary applications of bioinformatics:

a) Understanding the role of genes
b) Cell organization and function
c) Analysis of drug targets
d) Examining the traits of various diseases
e) Integration and development of various tools for the management of biological databases.

The evaluation and examination of numerous categories of data consist of sequences of amino acids and nucleotides, as well as the domains of proteins and structures of proteins. The creation of new algorithms and statistics that can be used to analyze relationships between individuals in huge datasets (Bayat A., 2002). Techniques for locating genes inside sequences, foretelling proteins' structures and functions, and for classifying protein sequences into groups of related sequences are a few examples.

Next-generation sequencing technology makes it simple to identify and quantify mutations in a heterogeneous sample, enabling the administration of precision medicine—the "right drug at the right dose to the right patient at the right time"—at a reasonable cost (Kasabov N., 2004).

One method to lessen the quantity of carbon dioxide produced into the atmosphere is to study the genomes of bacteria that use CO2 as their sole source of carbon, which is regarded to be a contributing factor to global climate change. Mutations can be easily fixed thanks to the identification of genes by sequence examination and splice site prediction. It is extensively employed in cancer-causing mutations. The use of bioinformatics to monitor gene expressions over time or to compare the gene expressions of two samples taken from the same population is also beneficial. Figure 4 includes a list of further applications for bioinformatics (Ardekani et al., 2007).

Figure 4. Applications of bio-informatics

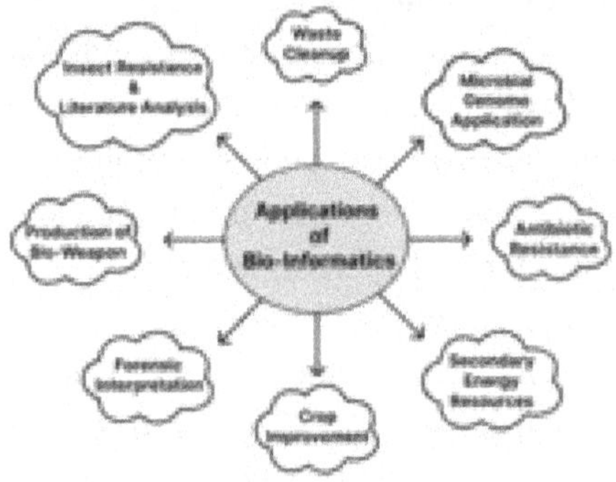

F. BIOINFORMATICS DATABASES AND TOOLS

The development of computational tools for data management and analysis was required due to the increase in biological data, and this resulted in the emergence of the new field of bioinformatics. Bioinformatics is a rapidly developing field of biology with an emphasis on the development and application of computational tools for the analysis and interpretation of biological data. Bioinformatics software, tools, and databases are used to handle, store, analyze, and interpret biological data.

Biological databases are collections of biological data like notes, pathways, genetic and protein sequences, and disease information. These databases are used to store and arrange data in a way that makes it simple to access the data. The three major categories into which biological databases can be divided as follows.

a) *Primary Databases:* These databases are assemblages of unprocessed biological data, such as unaltered structure or sequencing data. These databases serve as repositories of original data and are unaltered.
b) *Secondary Databases:* Information that has been handled or reviewed using computational or manual methods can be found in secondary databases. Based on the actual data from main sources, the information in these databases is stored.
c) *Specialized Databases:* Databases with a specialized study focus are referred to as specialized databases. These databases were made with an emphasis on a certain sort of data or organism.

Some well-known databases are outlined in depth in Table 2.

The creation and upkeep of biological databases as well as the development of software tools for studying sequencing, structure, and function are all included in bioinformatics. Bioinformatics tools are user-friendly software programs that allow researchers to explore biological data. Based on their capability, use, and difficulty, bioinformatics tools can be divided into a number of categories (Roumpeka DD et al., 2017). Tools that are widely utilized include:

a) *Sequence Analysis Tools:* These tools are used to analyze protein or nucleotide sequences. They are also utilized to find homologous sequences and understand the relationships in animal evolu-

Table 2. Bio-informatics databases

Database Name	Database Type	Description
EMBL	Primary	The European Bioinformatics Institute (EBI) is in charge of managing the nucleotide sequence database known as EMBL (European Molecular Biology Laboratory). Data on DNA and RNA, gene expression, proteins, organization, procedures, and literature are all included in this vast database of basic nucleotide sequences. (Guenter Stoesser et al., 1998)
GenBank	Primary	The National Centre for Biotechnology Information (NCBI) created GenBank, a large and well-annotated database of nucleic acid sequence data. It includes information on almost every kind of life. (Dennis A. et al., 2007)
PIR	Secondary	A database of protein informatics called Protein Information Resource is available to the general public. The Protein Sequence Database (PSD), the Non-redundant Reference (NREF), and the Integrated Protein Classification (iProClass) databases are the other three databases that PIR maintains. (Winona C. et al., 1999)
PDB	Secondary	A biological database called Protein Data Bank holds structural information on biological macromolecules. Large biological molecules including proteins, DNA, and RNA have three-dimensional structural data stored in PDB that has been obtained by experimental techniques like X-ray crystallography and NMR spectrometry. (Abola EE et al. 1996)
OMIM	Specialized	Online Mendelian Inheritance in Man (OMIM) is a freely accessible database of human genomes and genetic disorders that includes comprehensive summaries of more than 16,000 genes and all recognized Mendelian genetic disorders. (Ada Hamosh et al., 2005)
FlyBase	Specialized	A database of genetic and molecular information about Drosophila is called FlyBase. In Sybase, FlyBase is stored as a relational database. Genes, alleles (and phenotypes), aberrations, links to sequencing data, clones, stock lists, Drosophila workers, and bibliographic references are all included in the scope of FlyBase. (FlyBase, 1996)

tion. They include tools for sequence matching, motif discovery in sequence databases, phylogeny, pattern recognition, genome assembly, and comparison.

b) *Structure Analysis Tools:* These tools are used to examine the structure of proteins and nucleic acids. Structural analysis tools include tools for contrasting, classifying, and predicting the structures of nucleic acids and proteins.
c) *Function Analysis Tools:* These instruments are essential for identifying the primary disease-related pathways as well as for comprehending the functions and relationships among diverse genes and proteins. They include methods for predicting protein-protein interactions, tracking gene expression, simulating metabolic pathways, and predicting protein sub-cellular localization.

These tools can be used in a wide range of situations. Sequence analysis and phylogenetic analysis are two techniques that can be used to understand the evolutionary connections and similarities between sequences. New genes and proteins are annotated and identified, and their functions are predicted using tools for structure and functional analysis. Protein sequence analysis methods can also be used to estimate the 3-D structure of proteins. It also makes use of functional analytic tools to identify and comprehend different metabolic pathways. They are also instruments for locating prospective therapeutic targets and creating novel medications (Ramachandran et al., 2022).

G. BIOINFORMATICS AND MACHINE LEARNING

The massive amount of data conversion offered by recently acquired technology into knowledge is currently one of computational biology's most difficult tasks. Machine learning has developed into a crucial tool for implementing this shift (Pedro Larrañaga et al., 2006).

There are several uses for machine learning in a variety of sectors, from healthcare to natural language processing. The technological advancement has not ignored fields relating to biology or bioinformatics. In the past, before machine learning, these fields struggled to draw meaningful conclusions from massive biological datasets. But as of right now, ML techniques like deep learning can discover the features of complicated datasets and display them in a clear way. Six biological fields— systems biology, genomics, proteomics, evolution, microarrays and text mining—have all seen the use of machine learning (Inza, I. et al., 2010)

- ***Genomics:*** The demand for machine learning algorithms that can automatically find protein-coding genes inside a given DNA sequence is rising. Gene identification is the term used to describe this problem in computational biology. It has also been applied to the problem of multiple sequence alignment, which includes aligning various DNA or amino acid sequences in order to find similarities that would indicate a common evolutionary history.
- ***Proteomics*:** Proteomics issues including protein side-chain prediction, protein loop modeling, and protein contact map prediction have all been tackled using ML. A protein sequence's amino acids are categorized using ML into one of three structural classes (helix, sheet, or coil).
- ***Micro-Arrays:*** Using the data gathered to determine which genes are expressed is one of the primary issues in this subject. This issue is further complicated by the fact that the microarray collects data on an enormous number of genes, creating an abundance of irrelevant data that is unrelated to the objective of identifying expressed genes. The methods that are most frequently used are radial basis function networks, random forests, deep learning, decision trees and Bayesian classification (Aljarah, I. et al., 2018).
- ***Text Mining:*** The extraction of additional information from biomedical literature is usually necessary since protein annotations in protein databases do not always reflect the entirety of knowledge about each protein. Applications of ML include the automatic annotation of the function of genes and proteins, the determination of a protein's sub-cellular localization, DNA-expression array analysis, large-scale protein interaction analysis, and molecular interaction analysis. Given enough reference material, text mining can also be used to identify and display different DNA regions (Khattree, R., & Naik, D., 2007).
- ***System Biology:*** ML applications in systems biology include the difficulty of predicting enzyme activity, high throughput microarray data processing, analysis of genome-wide association studies to better understand disease signs, and protein function prediction.

The Support Vector Machine (SVM), Naive Bayes, and decision tree classifier are now the most widely used ML classification techniques for supervised learning and partition-based clustering and hierarchical clustering for unsupervised learning (Naresh E. et al., 2020).

H. CONCLUSION AND FUTURE DIRECTIONS

An interdisciplinary field called bioinformatics brings together expertise from various scientific fields, including math, information science, and biology, to address complex problems linked to cellular life and its complex molecular processes. This chapter provides a quick introduction to the field of bioinformatics, outlining its history, inception, and key accomplishments. It also contains a list of various bioinformatics databases and tools that are frequently used to store, display, and interpret molecular data. Although numerous research groups are producing a vast amount of genomic data from model and non-model systems, advancements in the current algorithms and bioinformatics tools are still needed, which will greatly enhance the analysis process and the accuracy of structure and function prediction. The potential future directions in the same field are as follows:

- The development of further discovery techniques based on machine learning.
- Increased use of Genome-Wide Association Studies (GWAS) to comprehend diseases and develop patient therapeutics in a better manner.
- Greater use of high-resolution sequencing techniques

The problems this will create with data management in terms of storage, transport, and processing have already been highlighted in the chapter. Data integration will also be a major hurdle. Consider omics data, where it is possible to produce a variety of data formats from the same samples in a single study. There isn't yet a standardized method for integrated analysis of those data formats in bioinformatics, though.

REFERENCES

Abola, E. E., Manning, N. O., Prilusky, J., Stampf, D. R., & Sussman, J. L. (1996, May-June). The Protein Data Bank: Current Status and Future Challenges. *Journal of Research of the National Institute of Standards and Technology*, *101*(3), 231–241. doi:10.6028/jres.101.025 PMID:27805161

Aljarah, I., Ala'M, A. Z., Faris, H., Hassonah, M. A., Mirjalili, S., & Saadeh, H. (2018). Simultaneous feature selection and support vector machine optimization using the grasshopper optimization algorithm. *Cognitive Computation*, *10*(3), 478–495. doi:10.1007/s12559-017-9542-9

Ardekani, A. M., Aslani, F., & Lakpour, N. (2007). Application ofgenomics and proteomics technologies to early diagnosis ofreproductive organ cancers. *Journal of Reproduction & Infertility*, *8*(3), 259–278.

Chavan, P. R. (2008). Application of Bioinformatics in the Field ofCancer Research. *11th Workshop on Medical Informatics &CME on Biomedical Communication*, 20-22.

Chelliah, R., Banan-MwineDaliri, E., Khan, I., Wei, S., Elahi, F., Yeon, S.-J., Selvakumar, V., Ofosu, F. K., Rubab, M., Ju, H. H., Rallabandi, H. R., Madar, I. H., Sultan, G., & Oh, D. H. (2022, March). A review on the application of bioinformatics tools in food microbiome studies. *Briefings in Bioinformatics*, *23*(2), bbac007. Advance online publication. doi:10.1093/bib/bbac007 PMID:35189636

Domokos, A. (2008). Bioinformatics and Computational Biology. *Bulletin of University of Agricultural Sciences and Veterinary Medicine Cluj-Napoca, 6527*, 571 – 574.

FlyBase. (1996, January 1). The *Drosophila* Database. *Nucleic Acids Research*, *24*(1), 53–56. doi:10.1093/nar/24.1.53 PMID:8594600

Gauthier, J., & Antony, T. (2019, November). A brief history of bioinformatics. *Briefings in Bioinformatics*, *20*(6), 1981–1996. doi:10.1093/bib/bby063 PMID:30084940

Gauthier, J., Vincent, A., Charette, S., & Derome, N. (2018). A Brief History of Bioinformatics. *Briefings in Bioinformatics*, *2018*, 1–16. doi:10.1093/bib/bby063 PMID:30084940

Goldin, L. (2006). Bioinformatics Integration for Cancer Research-Goal Question analysis. *Information Technology: Research and Education. ITRE'06. International Conference on*, 248-252. 10.1109/ITRE.2006.381575

Hamosh, Scott, Amberger, Bocchini, & McKusick. (2005). Online Mendelian Inheritance in Man (OMIM), a knowledgebase of human genes and genetic disorders. *Nucleic Acids Research*, *33*(1), D514–D517. doi:10.1093/nar/gki033

Inza, I., Calvo, B., Armañanzas, R., Bengoetxea, E., Larrañaga, P., & Lozano, J. A. (2010). Machine learning: an indispensable tool in bioinformatics. In *Bioinformatics methods in clinical research* (pp. 25–48). Humana Press. doi:10.1007/978-1-60327-194-3_2

Jawdat, D. (2006). The Era of Bioinformatics. Information and Communication Technologies, 1, 1860-1865. doi:10.1109/ICTTA.2006.1684672

Kasabov, N. (2004). Bioinformatics: a knowledge engineering approach. *Intelligent Systems, 2004 Proceedings. 2004 2nd International IEEE Conference*, 19-24.

Khattree, R., & Naik, D. (2007). Machine Learning Techniques for Bioinformatics. In Computational Methods in Biomedical Research (pp. 57-88). Chapman and Hall/CRC.

Kihara, D., Yang, Y. D., & Hawkins, T. (2007). Bioinformatics resources for cancer research with an emphasis on gene function and structure prediction tools. *Cancer Informatics*, *2*, 25–35. PMID:19458756

Larrañaga, P., Calvo, B., Santana, R., Bielza, C., Galdiano, J., Inza, I., Lozano, J. A., Armañanzas, R., Santafé, G., Pérez, A., & Robles, V. (2006, March). Machine learning in bioinformatics. *Briefings in Bioinformatics*, *7*(1), 86–112. doi:10.1093/bib/bbk007 PMID:16761367

Lilhore, U. K., Manoharan, P., Sandhu, J. K., Simaiya, S., Dalal, S., Baqasah, A. M., Alsafyani, M., Alroobaea, R., Keshta, I., & Raahemifar, K. (2023). Hybrid model for precise hepatitis-C classification using improved random forest and SVM method. *Scientific Reports*, *13*(1), 12473. doi:10.1038/s41598-023-36605-3 PMID:37528148

Lilhore, U. K., Poongodi, M., Kaur, A., Simaiya, S., Algarni, A. D., Elmannai, H., Vijayakumar, V., Tunze, G. B., & Hamdi, M. (2022). Hybrid model for detection of cervical cancer using causal analysis and machine learning techniques. *Computational and Mathematical Methods in Medicine*, *2022*, 2022. doi:10.1155/2022/4688327 PMID:35572826

Lilhore, U. K., Simaiya, S., Pandey, H., Gautam, V., Garg, A., & Ghosh, P. (2022). Breast cancer detection in the IoT cloud-based healthcare environment using fuzzy cluster segmentation and SVM classifier. *Ambient Communications and Computer Systems Proceedings of RACCCS*, *2021*, 165–179.

Lilhore, U. K., Simaiya, S., Prasad, D., & Guleria, K. (2020). A hybrid tumor detection and classification based on machine learning. *Journal of Computational and Theoretical Nanoscience*, *17*(6), 2539–2544. doi:10.1166/jctn.2020.8927

Naresh, E. (2020). *Impact of Machine Learning in Bioinformatics Research.* https://link.springer.com/chapter/10.1007/978-981-15-2445-5_4

Okuda, S., & Yoshizawa, A. (2010). ODB: A database for operon organizations, 2011 update. *Nucleic Acids Research*, *39*(Database), D552–D555. doi:10.1093/nar/gkq1090 PMID:21051344

Onyema, E. M., Lilhore, U. K., Saurabh, P., Dalal, S., Nwaeze, A. S., Chijindu, A. T., Ndufeiya-Kumasi, L. C., & Simaiya, S. (2023). Evaluation of IoT-Enabled hybrid model for genome sequence analysis of patients in healthcare 4.0. *Measurement. Sensors*, *26*, 100679. doi:10.1016/j.measen.2023.100679

Qi, Y. (2013). Text Mining in Bioinformatics: Research and Application. *International Journal of Information Retrieval Research*, *3*(2), 30–39. doi:10.4018/ijirr.2013040102

Ramesh, T. R., Lilhore, U. K., Poongodi, M., Simaiya, S., Kaur, A., & Hamdi, M. (2022). Predictive analysis of heart diseases with machine learning approaches. *Malaysian Journal of Computer Science*, 132–148.

Rathore, M. S., Poongodi, M., Saurabh, P., Lilhore, U. K., Bourouis, S., Alhakami, W., Osamor, J., & Hamdi, M. (2022). A novel trust-based security and privacy model for internet of vehicles using encryption and steganography. *Computers & Electrical Engineering*, *102*, 108205. doi:10.1016/j.compeleceng.2022.108205

Roumpeka, D. D., Wallace, R. J., Escalettes, F., Fotheringham, I., & Watson, M. (2017). A Review of Bioinformatics Tools for Bio-Prospecting from Metagenomic Sequence Data. *Frontiers in Genetics*, *8*, 23. doi:10.3389/fgene.2017.00023 PMID:28321234

Shahnaz, M., Chowdhary, M., Rani, A., Parkash, J., & Dev, D. (2016). Bioinformatics: An overview for cancer research. *Journal of Drug Delivery and Therapeutics*, *6*(4), 69–72. doi:10.22270/jddt.v6i4.1290

Sharma, S. K., Lilhore, U. K., Simaiya, S., & Trivedi, N. K. (2021). An improved random forest algorithm for predicting the COVID-19 pandemic patient health. *Annals of the Romanian Society for Cell Biology*, 67–75.

Simaiya, S., Lilhore, U. K., Prasad, D., & Verma, D. K. (2021). MRI brain tumor detection & image segmentation by hybrid hierarchical K-means clustering with FCM based machine learning model. *Annals of the Romanian Society for Cell Biology*, 88–94.

Stoesser, G., Moseley, M. A., Sleep, J., McGowran, M., Garcia-Pastor, M., & Sterk, P. (1998, January 1). The EMBL Nucleotide Sequence Database. *Nucleic Acids Research*, *26*(1), 8–15. doi:10.1093/nar/26.1.8 PMID:9399791

Winona, C. (1999, January 1). The PIR-International Protein Sequence Database. *Nucleic Acids Research*, *27*(1), 39–43. doi:10.1093/nar/27.1.39 PMID:9847137

Chapter 5
Securing Privacy in the Metaverse:
Advancing Biomedical Image Analysis Through Federated Learning

Parveen Kumar Sharma
Chandigarh Group of Colleges, India

B. Ramesh
Annapoorana Engineering College, India

Farrukh Arslan
https://orcid.org/0000-0002-8008-3808
School of Electrical and Computer Engineering, Purdue University, USA

Anshumali Parashar
Agriculture University, Jodhpur, India

N. Malarvizhi
Vel Tech Rangarajan Dr. Sagunthala R&D Institute of Science and Technology, India

K. Soni Sharmila
Shri Vishnu Engineering College for Women, India

ABSTRACT

This research explores the integration of privacy-preserving federated learning techniques in the context of biomedical image analysis within the metaverse. The metaverse, a virtual shared space, has witnessed remarkable advancements in various fields, including healthcare. However, ensuring the confidentiality of sensitive medical data poses a significant challenge. This study proposes a novel approach to address this concern by employing federated learning, a collaborative machine learning paradigm that enables model training across decentralized devices without compromising individual data privacy. The investigation focuses on the application of these techniques to enhance biomedical image analysis within the metaverse, aiming to facilitate medical research and diagnosis. Through the implementation of secure and privacy-preserving federated learning, the authors aim to strike a balance between technological innovation and safeguarding sensitive health information in the evolving landscape of the metaverse.

INTRODUCTION

The subject topic of study referred to as "introduction to biomedical image processing" deals with the interpretation and manipulation of pictures from medical imaging modalities as CT, MRI, and X-rays.

DOI: 10.4018/979-8-3693-1874-4.ch005

It helps with disease detection and treatment by using a variety of algorithms and approaches to extract useful information from these images. Healthcare practitioners may now visualize and manipulate medical pictures in new ways, making patient data examination more immersive and interactive. This is made possible by the integration of virtual reality technology with biomedical image processing. This might completely change how doctors evaluate and interpret medical images, resulting in better patient outcomes and more precise diagnosis.

Draw attention to the difficulties encountered by conventional methods of biomedical image analysis. The inability of conventional methods for biological image analysis to effectively process and analyze massive amounts of data is one of its problems. Conventional techniques frequently rely on labor-intensive, human error-prone manual segmentation and annotation. Furthermore, in order to reliably interpret and extract relevant information from biomedical images, like those from CT or MRI scans, complicated algorithms and processing capacity are needed. These difficulties demonstrate the need for cutting-edge technology to improve the speed and precision of biological image processing, such as artificial intelligence and machine learning.

LITERATURE REVIEW

In the literature review, we first discuss (Messaoudi et al., 2023) this paper showed how deep learning can help physicians diagnose and treat patients with greater accuracy. In a separate context, (Budd et al., 2021) addressed the issue of data scarcity in medical imaging. Their study on the application of transfer learning to prostate cancer detection showed how deep models that were previously trained could be modified to significantly improve performance when data was scarce. This approach and this methodology (Karimi et. al., 2020) have opened up new possibilities for the application of deep learning in healthcare settings despite resource constraints. Biological image processing holds immense potential for deep learning, but there are several challenges to overcome. Two significant issues are the interpretability of deep learning models (Mahapatra et. al., 2022) and the need for (Karimi et. al., 2020) substantial annotated datasets. Also this paper (Mahmood et. al., 2018) discussed how deep learning has the potential to transform healthcare, focusing on personalized medicine and early disease detection. This paper (Lilhore et. al., 2023) highlights the potential of deep learning to improve patient care and provide tailored medicinal solutions. Researchers are increasingly concentrating on overcoming challenges and exploring potential, such as multimodal data fusion (Lilhore et. al., 2024), real-time image processing (Lilhore et. al., 2023), and the integration of 3D imaging (Lilhore et. al., 2022), in the operating room, to enhance healthcare results. The study Deep Learning in Medical Image Analysis (Lilhore et. al., 2020), looks at how enhancing the procedures associated with diagnosis and treatment could completely transform the medical field. The authors stress the necessity for large datasets, interpretability, and validation to emphasize the difficulties involved in creating and deploying CAD or AI solutions in clinical contexts. In order to detect or classify lesions, the study (Onyema et. al., 2023) contrasts deep learning with traditional methods or radiologists. It also discusses the possible advantages of using deep learning to medical image analysis for computer-aided diagnosis (CAD). Our chapter concludes by summarizing the state-of-the-art in deep learning for the interpretation of medical images and highlighting the prospects for further research and improvement in this area.

METAVERSE TECHNOLOGIES-BASED BIOMEDICAL IMAGE ANALYSIS

The combination of meta verse technologies and bio medical image analysis plays major role health care and medical research. Deep learning and artificial intelligence combined with immersive, networked virtual worlds enable academics and medical professionals to traverse and analyze complicated biomedical images in ways that were never before possible. With the possibility for real-time collaboration generated by this cooperation, improved assessments, personalized therapies, and accelerated drug discovery are all made possible through interactive manipulation, multi-dimensional data presentation, and shared insights. The met averse has the potential to revolutionize biomedical image analysis by enabling creative, cooperative ways that could change medical research and healthcare in the future as it continues to develop.

METAVERSE-BASED TECHNOLOGIES

1. Block chain and Decentralized Technologies:
   Biomedical image processing could undergo a revolutionary change because to block chain and decentralized technologies, which offer safe, open, and effective methods for exchanging and managing data. Block chain's intrinsic properties of data integrity and immutability make it possible to securely store, manage, and trace diagnostic images and patient records while ensuring the reliability of medical image data. Decentralized technologies also relieve the strain on centralized infrastructure by providing dispersed and scalable methods for picture storage and analysis. These technologies facilitate quicker, more collaborative, and privacy-preserving biomedical image processing, which ultimately advances medical research and patient care. They do this by securely connecting patients, researchers, and healthcare providers in a decentralized network.
2. Meta verse Operating Systems:
   With their immersive and collaborative platforms for the study, visualization, and sharing of medical image data, met averse operating systems have the potential to completely change the biomedical image processing landscape. These operating systems improve medical training and education by offering a met averse environment where medical practitioners can interact with 3D models of anatomical structures and visualize complex imaging data. They also make it possible for surgeons to practice in a risk-free virtual environment with real-time surgical planning and simulations. Furthermore, through the creation of virtual medical environments, enhanced patient comprehension of complicated medical situations, and enabled collaborative decision-making among healthcare practitioners, met averse operating systems support telemedicine and distant consultations. These operating systems therefore hold the promise of bridging geographical and expert barriers, improving the field of biomedical image processing and ultimately improving the precision of diagnosis and treatment regimens.
3. Cloud Computing and Edge Computing:
   By fusing real-time, localized computation at the edge with the capacity of centralized data processing in the cloud, cloud-edge computing offers a revolutionary approach to biomedical image processing. Healthcare providers may store and retrieve enormous volumes of medical picture data thanks to cloud computing scalable and secure storage solutions, which also en-

able remote access for cooperative diagnoses and research. Contrarily, edge computing moves processing power closer to the point of care, allowing for on-the-spot essential decision assistance, instantaneous feedback, and real-time picture analysis at the medical device. When combined, these hybrid methods simplify the interpretation of complicated medical pictures, speed up diagnosis, and advance field research, all of which contribute to the development of more effective and efficient biomedical image processing systems that enhance patient care. The vast computational and storage requirements of the meta verse rely on cloud computing infrastructure. Edge computing is also crucial for delivering low-latency experiences. Distributed data centers and content delivery networks (CDNs) play a vital role in hosting meta verse content and applications.

4. Artificial Intelligence (AI):

The field of biomedical image processing has seen a significant breakthrough in artificial intelligence (AI), which has completely changed how medical pictures are interpreted and analyzed. Artificial intelligence (AI)-powered algorithms, in particular deep learning models like convolution neural networks (CNNs), make it possible to automatically identify, categories, and segment structures, abnormalities, and diseases in pictures from a variety of modalities, including MRIs, CT scans, and X-rays. Improved patient outcomes and more effective healthcare delivery are the ultimate results of this technology, which also speeds up treatment decisions and improves the accuracy of disease identification. AI also makes it easier to integrate massive amounts of medical data, which opens up new possibilities for personalized therapy, data-driven research, and creative solutions in the quickly developing field of biomedicine.

5. Interoperability Standards:

In order to fully utilize the met verse's potential for biomedical image processing, interoperability standards are essential. They allow for smooth data sharing and collaboration between various healthcare systems and virtual settings. These standards provide data consistency and interoperability by giving various meta verse platforms and medical image processing applications a common language. Medical practitioners can securely communicate and analyses biological image data in immersive met averse environments by following interoperability standards. This makes virtual medical training, telemedicine, and cross-institutional collaborative research possible. In addition to improving the quality and accessibility of healthcare services, interoperability encourages innovation and speeds up the development of patient care and medical research inside the meta verse.

6. Data Security and Privacy Technologies:

In the context of meta verse-based biomedical image processing, data security and privacy solutions are critical because they protect private patient data and guarantee adherence to strict healthcare laws. By putting in place encryption, secure access controls, and block chain-based solutions, these technologies ensure the integrity and security of medical picture data by shielding it from breaches or unwanted access. Furthermore, (Rathore et. al., 2022) by eliminating personally identifiable information from photos, sophisticated anonymization and de-identification techniques protect patient privacy and enable safe and moral data exchange in the meta verse. Meta verse-based biomedical image processing systems uphold patient trust by incorporating strong data security and privacy measures. They also facilitate the responsible and secure use of medical data in virtual environments, opening the door for revolutionary developments in research and healthcare. With a wealth of personal data being generated within the met averse, robust security and privacy technologies are essential to protect users and their information. Techniques such as encryption, identity management, and access control are applied to ensure data security and user privacy.

7. Sensors and IoT Devices:
The integration of meta verse-based biomedical image processing relies heavily on sensors and Internet of Things (IoT) devices. These devices record physiological data and environmental information in real time and are frequently worn by patients or integrated into medical equipment. They improve the capabilities of medical simulations and virtual consultations by enabling a more thorough and immersive grasp of patient problems in the meta verse. These sensors and Internet of Things gadgets may send information about body temperature, heart rate, and movement patterns. This data can then be viewed and examined in the meta verse, giving medical experts vital information for diagnosis and treatment plans. Biomedical imaging, IoT devices, and meta verse technologies together have the potential to completely transform healthcare by providing a novel and immersive method of patient care and medical education.

8. Digital Twins:
By building virtual models of anatomical characteristics and medical the surroundings, digital twins have played an important part in metaverse-based biomedical image processing, allowing for real-time analysis and simulation. Medical practitioners can investigate and diagnose diseases in a dynamic, interactive, and realistic environment with the help of these digital representations, which are created from genuine medical imaging data. By allowing surgeons to virtually practice and prepare treatments before they are performed, digital twins can improve accuracy and safety. Additionally, they facilitate collaboration across disciplines and deep data analysis, which opens the door to tele health and remote diagnostics in the met averse. Digital twins are a potent tool in met averse-based biomedical image processing that can be used to enhance patient care and medical research. They provide more exact, accurate, and creative healthcare solutions by bridging the gap between the real and virtual worlds.

Challenges of Metaverse-Based Biomedical Image Analysis

Creating scalable, real-time, and effective algorithms is a major obstacle in the field of meta verse-based biological picture analysis. Processing medical images (Helaly et. al., 2023) might demand substantial computational resources due to their frequent huge size and complexity. Furthermore, patient privacy laws must be complied with and the meta verse environment must be safe. Creating deep learning models that are trained on vast and varied datasets of medical pictures is another difficulty. Accurately labeling these datasets can be a demanding task and can be costly to get. Furthermore, results from deep learning models may be erroneous due to their heightened sensitivity to noise and aberrations in medical pictures.

Opportunities of Metaverse-Based Biomedical Image Analysis

Met averse-based biomedical image analysis has the potential to present several noteworthy opportunities, despite the obstacles. For instance, the met averse can offer a platform where doctors can work together and instantly communicate data. Better treatment planning and diagnostic accuracy may result from this. Furthermore, medical residents and students can benefit from virtual training environments

Table 1. Metaverse for healthcare, potential applications, challenges

Metaverse for Healthcare	Potential Applications	Challenges
Medical education and training	Virtual anatomy classes, surgical simulations, and remote patient care training	High cost of VR/AR equipment, lack of standardization, and potential for nausea and dizziness
Telemedicine and remote care	Virtual consultations, diagnosis, and treatment of patients remotely	Lack of accessibility to VR/AR equipment, and potential for delays in care due to technical issues
Mental health care	Exposure therapy for phobias, cognitive behavioral therapy (CBT) for anxiety and depression, and support groups for patients with chronic conditions	Difficulty in monitoring patients' nonverbal cues and assessing their condition accurately
Physical rehabilitation	Virtual physical therapy exercises, pain management programs, and post-surgery rehabilitation	Lack of hap tic feedback and difficulty in providing personalized care
Drug discovery and development	Virtual clinical trials, drug design simulations, and preclinical testing	Ethical concerns about the use of artificial intelligence (AI) in healthcare, and the need for large datasets to train AI models.

made possible by the met averse. This can aid in the improvement of their diagnostic and image analysis abilities in medicine. Lastly, therapy programs tailored to individual patients can be developed using the meta verse. Physicians can create more individualized and successful treatment plans for their patients by merging information from several sources, including genetic and electronic health records, with medical imaging data.

DEEP LEARNING MODELS FOR BIOMEDICAL IMAGE ANALYSIS

1. Disease Detection and Diagnosis:
   Advanced deep learning models, including convolution neural networks (CNNs), are applied in biomedical image analysis for the purpose of automatically identifying and classifying pathological abnormalities inside medical pictures. This process is known as disease identification and detection. With the use of these deep learning algorithms, it is possible to accurately detect diseases like cancer, cardiovascular issues, or neurological disorders by analyzing a wide range of imaging modalities, such as X-rays, MRIs, CT scans, and histopathological slides. Biomedical image analysis improves clinical decision-making and aids in early disease identification and intervention by providing quick and accurate diagnoses. This eventually improves patient outcomes and advances medical research in the healthcare industry.
2. Image Registration:
   In order to provide a thorough and coherent representation of a patient's anatomy or illness progression, image registration—a key procedure in biomedical image analysis—involves aligning and combining several medical images, frequently from various modalities or time points. Image registration guarantees that structures and features are accurately aligned through the use of transformation models and optimization algorithms, facilitating more accurate diagnosis, treatment planning, and follow-up evaluations. This method is essential for applications including tracking anatomical changes over time, following the evolution of diseases, and fusing MRI and CT scans. Image registration advances clinical decision-making, advances personalized therapy, and advances healthcare research by giving medical data a consistent representation.

Figure 1. Metaverse in healthcare

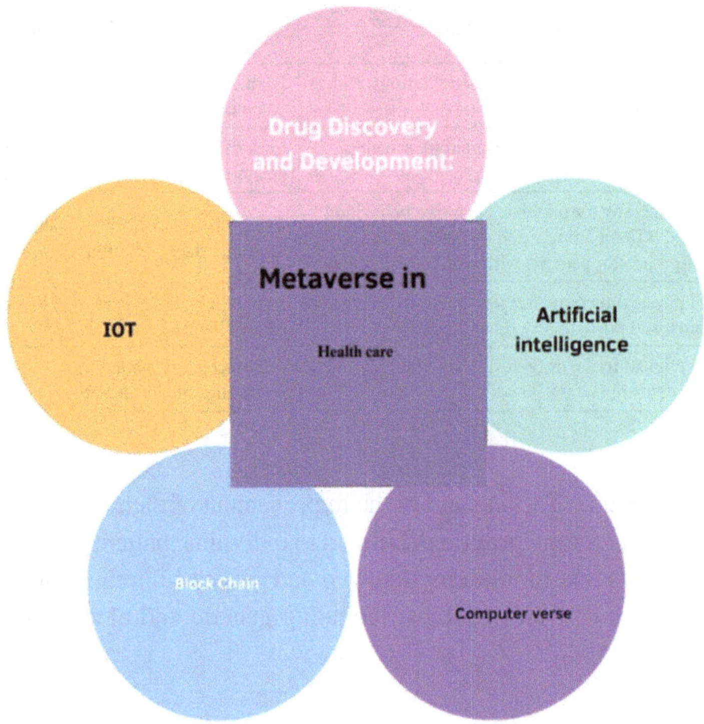

3. Image Super-Resolution:

A key method in biomedical image analysis, image super-resolution improves the quality and resolution of low-resolution medical pictures. Image super-resolution enhances the clarity and diagnostic utility of medical pictures, such as X-rays, MRI scans, and histopathology slides, by utilizing deep learning models, such as convolution neural networks (CNNs), to rebuild high-resolution information from lower-resolution inputs. With the use of this technology, medical personnel may more precisely view minute anatomical features and abnormalities, which improves illness detection, diagnosis, and treatment planning. Image super-resolution in the field of biomedical image analysis facilitates more accurate and well-informed decision-making, which eventually leads to better patient care and more sophisticated medical research.

4. Personalized Medicine:

Personalized medicine represents a revolutionary change in healthcare, driven by deep learning in biomedical image processing. To customize therapy regimens and techniques for each patient, deep learning algorithms examine patient data and medical imaging. Personalized medicine is an approach that improves the effectiveness of medical interventions by taking into account the distinct features, genetic composition, and reaction to therapy of each patient. In addition to optimizing treatment outcomes, this patient-centered strategy reduces side effects and medical expenses. It has the potential to completely transform healthcare by enabling more accurate and customized diagnoses and treatments that are tailored to the unique requirements and genetic profiles of every patient. Figure 2 explains framework for meta verse based bio medical image processing.

Figure 2. Framework diagram for Metaverse-based biomedical image analysis

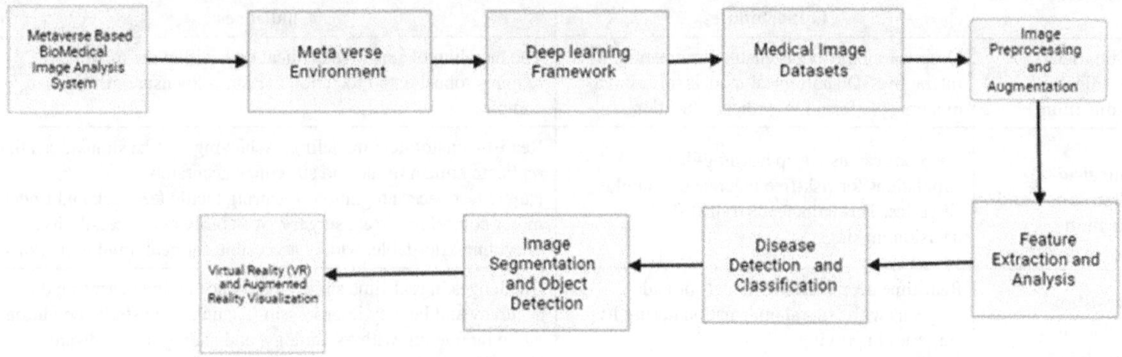

DRUG DELIVERY AND TARGETED THERAPY

Deep learning in biomedical image analysis is enabling tailored therapeutic applications and drug delivery that are transforming the medical industry. Targeted medication delivery systems can be developed with the use of deep learning models that accurately detect specific biological targets or disease indicators within medical pictures. Personalized treatment plans can be created with this method, which delivers medications specifically to the afflicted areas while protecting healthy tissues, reducing side effects, and maximizing therapeutic results. Furthermore, deep learning facilitates the assessment of therapeutic outcomes by examining tissue and biomarker images, allowing for prompt modifications to treatment plans. Healthcare practitioners may significantly advance precision medicine and patient-centered care by improving treatment efficacy and patient outcomes by customizing drug distribution and therapy based on deep learning findings.

Application of Deep Learning in Biomedical Image Analysis

Applications of deep learning in biomedical image analysis include the detection of cancerous cells in medical images, the identification of specific diseases in radiology scans, and the prediction of patient outcomes based on imaging data. These applications (Zhang et. at, 2019) have the potential to revolutionize healthcare by providing faster and more accurate diagnoses, leading to timely interventions and improved patient outcomes. However, it is crucial to address the potential biases and limitations of deep learning algorithms in order to ensure unbiased and reliable results. Additionally, ongoing research and development are necessary to continuously improve the performance and robustness of these models for better integration into clinical practice.

Moreover, the ethical implications of using deep learning algorithms in healthcare must be thoroughly examined. Issues such as data privacy, informed consent, and algorithm transparency need to be carefully addressed to protect patient rights and maintain trust in the healthcare system. Furthermore, healthcare professionals should receive adequate training to effectively interpret and utilize the outputs of these algorithms, as misinterpretation or overreliance on their recommendations could have detrimental consequences. Ultimately, with the right precautions and advancements, deep learning applications have the potential to greatly enhance the quality and efficiency of healthcare delivery.

Table 2. Opportunities and challenges of bio medical image processing

	Opportunities	Challenges
Enhanced Medical Education	Deep learning Models enable the creation of interactive 3D anatomical models, offering a dynamic platform for medical education.	The handling of sensitive medical data within the meta verse requires robust data protection measures to ensure privacy and compliance.
Surgical Simulation and Training	Surgeons can use deep learning-driven simulations for risk-free practice of complex surgeries. This enhances surgical skills and decision-making.	Realistic anatomical modeling: Achieving lifelike simulations that replicate human tissue and structures accurately. Haptic feedback integration: Ensuring tactile feedback and fine motor control in virtual surgery. Scalability and accessibility: Providing affordable, widely accessible surgical training platforms
Real-time Surgical Guidance	Real-time deep learning models provide surgeons with critical information during live surgeries improving Precision and safety.	Challenges in real-time surgical guidance include ensuring data accuracy and latency in processing, maintaining sterile conditions while interacting with technology, and addressing hardware limitations in the operating room.
3D and Multimodal Imaging	Deep learning can merge and display data from various medical imaging modalities simultaneously offering a comprehensive view of a patient's condition	Processing and interpreting complex 3D and multimodal data can be computationally demanding.
Drug Discovery	Biomedical image analysis can accelerate drug discovery by identifying potential compound	Validating findings from image analysis in the lab can be challenging.
Cost-Effectiveness	Automating image analysis can reduce costs and improve healthcare resource allocation	Implementing and maintaining advanced imaging systems can be expensive.
Model Interpretability:	Interpretable models can provide insights into the basis of predictions, enhancing trust and clinical acceptance.	Interpretable models may have limitations in capturing complex and subtle image features.

For example, deep learning algorithms can be used to analyze medical images such as X-rays and detect abnormalities with high accuracy. This can help radiologists in their diagnosis and decision-making process, ultimately improving patient outcomes. However, it is crucial for healthcare professionals to understand the limitations of these algorithms and not solely rely on their recommendations, ensuring that the final diagnosis is made based on a combination of clinical expertise and algorithmic output.

A key goal in computer vision is image recognition (Xiang, et. al., 2023) commonly referred to as image classification, which tries to recognize and classify objects or patterns in digital images. The capacity to automatically identify objects in photos has a wide range of applications, including augmented reality, self-driving automobiles, medical diagnosis, and facial recognition. The innovative deep learning method known as convolution neural networks (CNNs) has considerably improved the state-of-the-art in image recognition. An artificial neural network type known as CNNs was created specifically for processing grid-like input, such as photographs. CNNs imitate the hierarchical organization of the visual system, where simple features are merged to produce more complex representations, which is inspired by the operation of the visual cortex in the brain.

Evolution of Deep Learning in the Medical Field

Through its transformative applications, Deep Learning has undergone a revolutionary evolution in the medical profession, transforming healthcare. Convolution neural networks (CNNs), in particular, have made substantial advances in medical imaging, enabling precise disease segmentation and detection. By predicting treatment outcomes based on unique patient data, it enabled individualized therapy. Techniques

Figure 3. Advantages of convolution neural networks

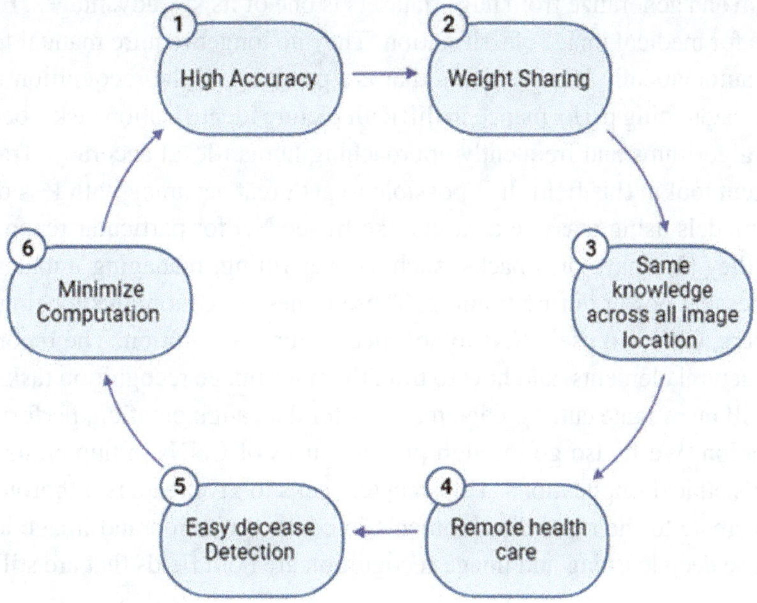

for natural language processing (NLP) made it easier to glean insights from extensive clinical records and research articles. Fig 3 explains Advantages of convolution neural networks. By revealing illness connections and genetic variations, deep learning significantly improved precision medicine. It sped up the process of drug discovery, improved drug candidate screening, and refined molecular characteristics. Deep learning also revolutionized wearable device monitoring, digital pathology, and real-time patient care

Image Classification Using Convolution Neural Networks (CNNs)

CNNs are successful in recognizing images because of their inherent capacity to automatically learn hierarchical representations via feature extraction and feature mapping. The architecture of the network typically consists of several layers, such as fully connected, pooling, and convolution layers. While pooling layers shrink the spatial dimensions of the feature maps to make them more manageable, convolution layers use convolution filters or kernels to extract local information from the input image. The final clas-

Figure 4. Deep learning network for medical image classification

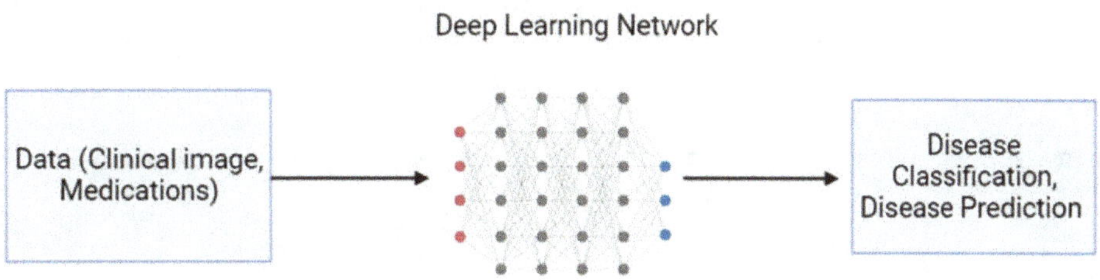

sification is then carried out using the extracted characteristics by the fully linked layers. The ability of CNNs to learn from and generalize from huge datasets is one of its key advantages. Fig 4 explains Deep learning Networks for medical image classification. They no longer require manual feature engineering because they can automatically learn features that are pertinent to the recognition task. Additionally, CNNs have shown astounding performance in difficult picture identification tasks, beating conventional machine learning algorithms and frequently approaching human-level accuracy. Transfer learning has also become a potent tool in this field. It is possible to get great accuracy with less data by fine-tuning pre-trained CNN models using massive datasets like Image Net for particular recognition tasks.CNNs are effective, but they also have drawbacks, such as over fitting, managing unbalanced datasets, and using a lot of processing power during training. These issues are continuously being addressed by scientists and engineers, who also use CNNs to advance picture recognition. The theoretical foundations of CNNs, their structural elements, and how to train them for image recognition tasks are all covered in this chapter. We will investigate cutting-edge methods for data augmentation, performance assessment, and image preparation. We'll also go through practical uses of CNNs in numerous fields and look at image recognition's ethical implications. This chapter seeks to give readers a thorough grasp of CNNs and how they contribute to the rapid developments in computer vision and image identification. This is important because deep learning and image recognition are both fields that are still evolving quickly.

Convolution Neural Networks Application in Diagnosis of Schizophrenia

Convolution Neural Networks (CNNs) have shown potential in aiding the analysis and understanding of schizophrenia through medical image analysis. Figure 5 explains convolution neural networks for image classification. Convolution Neural Networks (CNNs) have emerged as a popular and successful method for segmenting brain images in schizophrenia research. CNNs are a subset of deep learning algorithms that are excellent at processing and categorizing visual input, which makes them suitable for segmenting the brain in medical imaging, particularly those of schizophrenia. The general process for applying CNNs for brain image segmentation in schizophrenia sickness is outlined below: Preparation of Data: Collect and preprocess the MRI scan data of the brain, which normally includes both healthy controls and schizophrenic patients. To maintain uniformity and cut down on noise, preprocessing techniques may include normalization, scaling, and intensity normalization. Data labeling: Manually or semi-automatically associate the ground truth segmentation masks with the associated brain pictures. These masks represent the regions of interest (e.g. Hippocampus, prefrontal cortex) within the brain.

Figure 5. Convolution neural networks for image classification

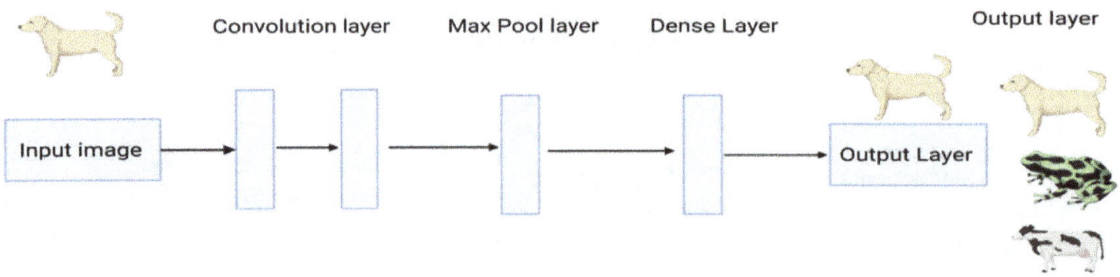

Creating the CNN architecture that will be used for segmentation is important. Convolution layers for feature extraction and decoding layers for creating segmentation masks are two common layers in the architecture. Divide the dataset into training and validation sets for training purposes. Utilize the training set to train the CNN by refining its settings to reduce the discrepancy between the ground truth masks and the anticipated segmentation masks. The CNN gains the ability to recognize patterns and traits that relate to various brain areas. Validation: Assess the trained CNN's performance on the validation set to gauge how well it generalizes to untrained input. This process aids in hyper parameter tuning and guards against over fitting. Apply the trained CNN to segment brain pictures from fresh, unknown individuals to produce segmentation masks after a successful training and validation phase.

a) **Brain Image Segmentation:** CNNs can be used to segment brain images obtained from MRI scans of individuals with schizophrenia. This segmentation (Ma et. al., 2020) process involves identifying and delineating different brain structures and regions, which can provide valuable insights into the structural abnormalities associated with schizophrenia. 1. Partitioning brain pictures derived from modalities like MRI or CT scans into separate regions or structures is a crucial medical image analysis problem known as brain image segmentation. Data preparation, model choice, and training with annotated ground truth masks are required steps in the process, which makes use of cutting-edge deep learning techniques like convolution neural networks (CNNs). After the trained model is evaluated and optimized to produce precise segmentations, post-processing techniques are used to polish the outcomes. Successful brain picture segmentation makes it possible to identify specific brain regions, which helps with diagnosis, planning of treatments, and monitoring of neurological diseases. This eventually advances neuro imaging research and enhances patient care.

b) **Brain Abnormality Detection**: CNNs can automatically detect and highlight abnormal brain regions or structural changes in patients with schizophrenia, enabling researchers and clinicians to identify specific biomarkers or patterns associated with the disorder. Advanced methods, including deep learning and computer vision, are used in the critical medical imaging application of "brain abnormality detection" to automatically recognize and pinpoint anomalies in brain images, such as MRI or CT scans. The model learns to differentiate between normal and pathological brain structures through data preprocessing, model selection, and training on labeled aberrant brain images. To accurately identify and draw attention to potential anomalies, the model is evaluated on fresh, previously unexplored data after training. By enabling early intervention and treatment planning for a variety of neurological illnesses, this automated detection technique helps radiologists and neurologists identify patients more quickly and accurately. In turn, this improves patient outcomes and healthcare effectiveness.

c) **Functional Brain Connectivity Analysis**: CNNs can be applied to analyze functional MRI (fMRI) data and identify altered brain connectivity patterns in individuals with schizophrenia. These connectivity patterns can help researchers understand the neural network disruptions underlying the disorder. A neuron imaging approach called functional brain connectivity analysis is used to examine how distinct brain regions interact and communicate when performing various cognitive activities or while the brain is at rest. To extract time series data from various brain regions, functional MRI (fMRI) or electroencephalogram (EEG) data processing is required. The intensity and directionality of interactions between brain areas are then calculated using these time series using connectivity measures like correlation or coherence. Understanding brain function, cognitive processes, and neurological illnesses is made easier with the help of the connection matrices that are produced. Researchers learn a great deal about the complex neural networks of the brain by examining functional brain connectivity, which paves the way for possible biomarkers and individualized therapies for neurological and psychiatric diseases.

d) **Disease Classification**: CNNs can classify brain images as belonging to individuals with schizophrenia or healthy controls. By learning from a large dataset of brain scans, CNNs can be trained to distinguish between the brain structures of schizophrenia patients and those of healthy individuals. Convolution Neural Networks (CNNs) are an advanced deep learning application in the medical area that aim to automatically identify and categorize diseases based on relevant data or medical images. An appropriate CNN architecture with convolution and pooling layers is designed, the model is trained using labeled data, and its performance is assessed using metrics like accuracy, sensitivity, specificity, and F1 score. Successful disease classification with CNNs can result in quicker and more accurate diagnoses, prompt interventions, and individualized treatments, all of which can improve patient outcomes and streamline medical procedures. However, in order to deploy these models responsibly and ethically within clinical practice, ethical issues, data protection, and interpretability continue to be crucial factors.

e) **Predicting Disease Progression**: CNNs can be used to predict the progression of schizophrenia by analyzing longitudinal brain images of patients over time. This could aid in early intervention and personalized treatment planning. In order to forecast how a disease may develop over time for an individual or a group, predictive disease progression entails employing data-driven methodologies, such as machine learning and statistical modeling, to assess patient information and historical data. Typically, this procedure requires gathering longitudinal data, including medical records, imaging data, and biomarker tests, in order to create prediction models that account for both patient characteristics and disease-specific aspects. These models enable healthcare providers to forecast the course of a disease, spot high-risk patients, and create individualized treatment strategies. By proactively addressing changing medical situations, illness progression prediction has enormous potential to enhance patient management, enable early interventions, and maximize healthcare resources.

f) **Treatment Response Prediction**: By analyzing brain images before and after treatment, CNNs may help predict how individuals with schizophrenia will respond to specific therapeutic interventions. Therapy response prediction is the process of estimating the likelihood that a patient will respond favorably to a given medical intervention or course of therapy using data analytic techniques, such as machine learning and statistical modeling. Building predictive models requires gathering and analyzing a variety of patient data, including clinical history, genetic data, biomarkers, and medical imaging. These models make use of the data to find patterns and relationships that can be used to forecast how a patient will react to a certain treatment. Healthcare professionals can give individualized and targeted medicines and enhance patient outcomes and resource allocation by correctly anticipating treatment response. Predicting treatment outcomes has great potential to advance precision medicine, improve patient care, and increase the overall efficacy of medical therapies.

g) **Multi-Modal Fusion**: CNNs can be used to combine information from multiple imaging modalities, such as structural MRI, functional MRI, and diffusion tensor imaging (DTI), to obtain a more comprehensive understanding of schizophrenia-related brain alterations.Multi-modal fusion is a data integration technique that incorporates data from several sources or modalities to improve the functionality and decision-making of machine learning models. Data from several sensors or inputs must be gathered, preprocessed, and relevant features must be extracted from each modality, and finally these features must be combined into a single representation. Multi-modal fusion, which finds applications in a variety of industries including healthcare, multimedia analysis, and natural language processing, enables more thorough and accurate insights by utilizing the complementary strengths of multiple modalities, such as images, text, audio, or sensor data. This improves accuracy, robustness, and understanding of complex systems.

h) **Schizophrenia Subtype Identification**: The goal of schizophrenia subtype identification is to divide schizophrenia patients into different subgroups based on unique clinical, cognitive, or neurobiological characteristics. Analyzing various data sources, such as clinical assessments, neuroimaging data (such as fMRI, structural MRI), genetics, and cognitive tests, is a part of this process. Advanced machine learning methods are used to characterize various schizophrenia subtypes by finding patterns and similarities among people. These methods include clustering algorithms and deep learning models. The ultimate objective is to increase our understanding of the heterogeneity within schizophrenia and to enable tailored treatment methods, which will enhance patient outcomes by adjusting therapies to the unique requirements of each subtype.

i) **Data Augmentation**: Data augmentation is a widely used technique in machine learning and deep learning that involves artificially expanding the size of the training dataset by applying various transformations to the existing data. These transformations can include rotations, flips, translations, scaling, changes in brightness and contrast, and other modifications. By generating new augmented samples, data augmentation helps to improve model generalization, reduce over fitting, and enhance the model's ability to recognize and learn from different variations of the data. Data augmentation is particularly beneficial when the original dataset is limited or imbalanced, as it increases the diversity of the training data, leading to more robust and accurate machine learning models.

It's important to note that while CNNs hold promise in schizophrenia research and diagnosis, medical image analysis in this context requires careful validation and collaboration with domain experts. Interpretation of results from CNNs should always be done in conjunction with clinical expertise to ensure accurate and responsible use of these powerful tools in schizophrenia research and patient care.

Deep learning models often need a sizable amount of labeled data and processing resources when used for medical image segmentation. When there is a shortage of labeled data, transfer learning where a pre-trained CNN is adjusted on a smaller dataset is a useful strategy. Fig 6 explains Brain image of Schizophrenia affected iamge and normal image.

CNNs and other deep learning approaches show enormous promise for enhancing our understanding of schizophrenia and other neurological illnesses through more precise and automated brain picture segmentation as the fields of deep learning and medical imaging continue to develop.

Schizophrenia Affected Images Classification Using Convolution Neural Networks

An innovative method that uses convolution neural networks (CNNs) to classify schizophrenia-related images with the goal of assisting in the early detection and diagnosis of schizophrenia. Because they have the capacity to automatically discover and extract pertinent characteristics from the input images, CNNs are a class of deep learning models that are well suited for image recognition applications. In this situation, CNNs are trained using a big dataset of brain scans, including both healthy and schizophrenic

Figure 6. Brain images of schizophrenia affected image and normal image

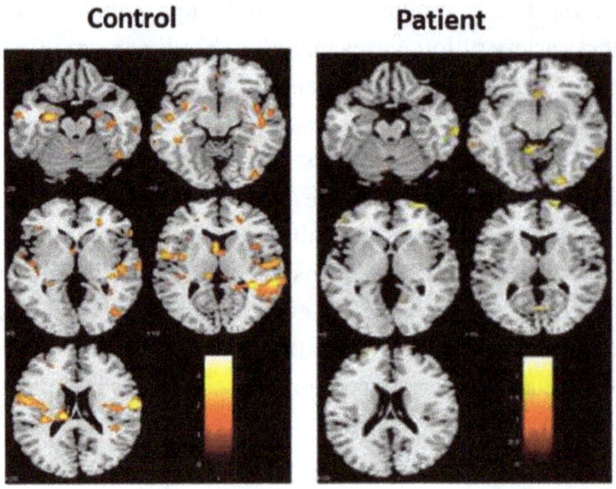

people. The model gains the ability to distinguish between brain patterns and structures that are suggestive of schizophrenia. Figure 7 explains Convolution networks classifies Schizophrenia brain images from healthy images. Once trained, the CNN can accurately categorize fresh brain scans into either a healthy or schizophrenia-affected group, giving physicians and researchers insightful information that may help with the early detection and treatment of this challenging mental condition. When applying such technology for medical diagnosis and treatment, it is vital to establish ethical considerations and privacy rights.

PERFORMANCE ANALYSIS OF CONVOLUTION NEURAL NETWORKS

The usefulness and precision of Convolution Neural Networks (CNNs) in medical pictures are evaluated using a variety of performance indicators. Table 3 explains Performance metrics of convolution neural networks .Typical metrics include accuracy, which expresses the percentage of correctly classified images over all; sensitivity (recall), which measures the capacity to recognize positive cases correctly; specificity, which assesses the capacity to recognize negative cases correctly; precision, which expresses the percentage of true positive predictions out of all positive predictions made; F1 score, which strikes a balance between precision and sensitivity; which evaluates classification performance.

Multi-Agent Reinforcement Learning for Biomedical Image Processing

Multi-agent reinforcement learning (MARL) is gaining an increasing amount of attention in the rapidly growing field of biomedical image processing. The category of artificial intelligence known as MARL involves several autonomous agents cooperating to learn from and solve complex problems. This method, when used in biomedical image processing, allows agents to collaboratively examine, interpret, and change medical pictures, increasing productivity and accuracy in tasks like medication discovery, medical research, and illness diagnosis. MARL has the potential to transform the way we

Figure 7. Convolution networks classifies schizophrenia brain images from healthy images

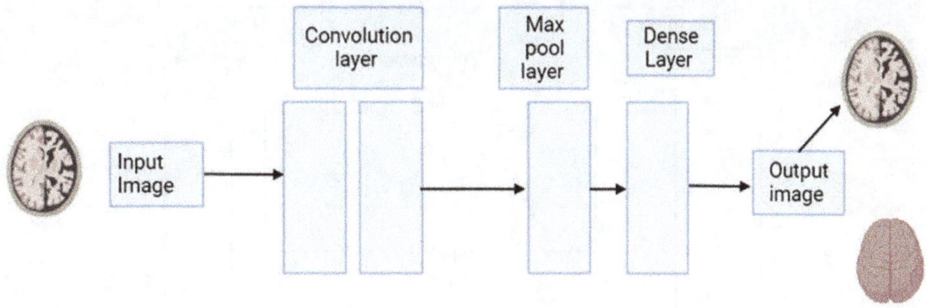

Table 3. Performance metric of convolution neural networks

Metrics	Description
Accuracy	0.86%
Precision	0.88%
Recall	0.92%
Precision	0.94%
F-1 Score	0.85.6%

gather important information and decide how to proceed from biomedical images by utilizing the combined intelligence of several agents. This could ultimately improve the standard of medical care and biomedical research.

The core idea of MARL is to take advantage of the potential of collaboration, allowing robots to exchange information, learn from one another, and plan their actions in order to do tasks that would be challenging or impossible for individual agents to complete alone. MARL presents a revolutionary framework to optimize the behavior of cooperative robots in realistic situations by fusing the benefits of both reinforcement learning and teamwork. We also go over actual case studies that show how MARL is useful in a variety of fields, such as logistics, agriculture, disaster relief, and more. These case studies show how MARL-enabled cooperative robotics can be applied in a new era of creativity where many agents work together to tackle challenging issues and pave the way for more long-lasting and efficient solutions.

CONCLUSION

In summary, the future of healthcare and medical research is extremely promising when deep learning techniques are integrated into the meta verse for biomedical picture analysis. A new chapter in medical education, training, diagnosis, and treatment has been brought about by the dynamic synergy of virtual reality, augmented reality, and sophisticated deep learning models. The meta verse offers patients, researchers, and healthcare professionals options never before seen in the field thanks to its immersive experiences, real-time assistance, and collaborative platforms. There may be

Figure 8. Multi-agent reinforcement learning scheme

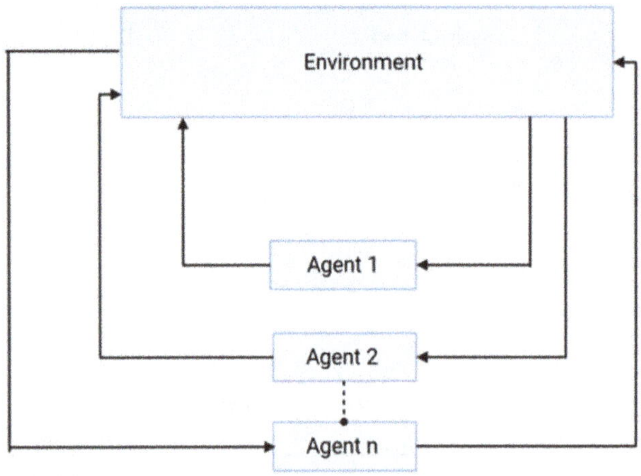

obstacles in the way of achieving the full potential of meta verse-based biological image analysis, such as concerns about data security, interpretability, and ethics. But as technology develops and interdisciplinary teamwork grows, the meta verse presents itself as a game-changing frontier that has the potential to promote precision medicine, increase patient outcomes, and spur innovation in the healthcare industry. The present chapter has delved into the fascinating prospects that await us, urging us to set out on a journey towards a novel era of healthcare enabled by deep learning within the meta verse.

REFERENCES

Budd, S., Robinson, E. C., & Kainz, B. (2021). A Survey on Active Learning and Human-in-the-Loop Deep Learning for Medical Image Analysis. *Medical Image Analysis*, *71*, 102062. doi:10.1016/j.media.2021.102062 PMID:33901992

Helaly, H. A., Badawy, M., & Haikal, A. Y. (2023). A Review of Deep Learning Approaches in Clinical and Healthcare Systems Based on Medical Image Analysis. *Multimedia Tools and Applications*. Advance online publication. doi:10.1007/s11042-023-16605-1

Karimi, D., Dou, H., Warfield, S. K., & Gholipour, A. (2020). Deep Learning with Noisy Labels: Exploring Techniques and Remedies in Medical Image Analysis. *Medical Image Analysis*, *65*, 101759. doi:10.1016/j.media.2020.101759 PMID:32623277

Lilhore, U. K., Dalal, S., Faujdar, N., Margala, M., Chakrabarti, P., Chakrabarti, T., Simaiya, S., Kumar, P., Thangaraju, P., & Velmurugan, H. (2023). Hybrid CNN-LSTM model with efficient hyperparameter tuning for prediction of Parkinson's disease. *Scientific Reports*, *13*(1), 14605. doi:10.1038/s41598-023-41314-y PMID:37669970

Lilhore, U. K., Dalal, S., Faujdar, N., Simaiya, S., Dahiya, M., Tomar, S., & Hashmi, A. (2024). Unveiling the prevalence and risk factors of early stage postpartum depression: A hybrid deep learning approach. *Multimedia Tools and Applications*, 1–35. doi:10.1007/s11042-024-18182-3

Lilhore, U. K., Manoharan, P., Sandhu, J. K., Simaiya, S., Dalal, S., Baqasah, A. M., Alsafyani, M., Alroobaea, R., Keshta, I., & Raahemifar, K. (2023). Hybrid model for precise hepatitis-C classification using improved random forest and SVM method. *Scientific Reports*, *13*(1), 12473. doi:10.1038/s41598-023-36605-3 PMID:37528148

Lilhore, U. K., Poongodi, M., Kaur, A., Simaiya, S., Algarni, A. D., Elmannai, H., Vijayakumar, V., Tunze, G. B., & Hamdi, M. (2022). Hybrid model for detection of cervical cancer using causal analysis and machine learning techniques. *Computational and Mathematical Methods in Medicine*, *2022*, 2022. doi:10.1155/2022/4688327 PMID:35572826

Lilhore, U. K., Simaiya, S., Pandey, H., Gautam, V., Garg, A., & Ghosh, P. (2022). Breast cancer detection in the IoT cloud-based healthcare environment using fuzzy cluster segmentation and SVM classifier. *Ambient Communications and Computer Systems Proceedings of RACCCS*, *2021*, 165–179.

Lilhore, U. K., Simaiya, S., Prasad, D., & Guleria, K. (2020). A hybrid tumor detection and classification based on machine learning. *Journal of Computational and Theoretical Nanoscience*, *17*(6), 2539–2544. doi:10.1166/jctn.2020.8927

Ma, H., Smal, I., Daemen, J., & van Walsum, T. (2020). Dynamic Coronary Roadmapping via Catheter Tip Tracking in X-Ray Fluoroscopy with Deep Learning Based Bayesian Filtering. *Medical Image Analysis*, *61*, 101634. doi:10.1016/j.media.2020.101634 PMID:31978856

Mahapatra, D., Poellinger, A., & Reyes, M. (2022). Interpretability-Guided Inductive Bias For Deep Learning Based Medical Image. *Medical Image Analysis*, *81*, 102551. doi:10.1016/j.media.2022.102551 PMID:35932546

Mahmood, F., & Durr, N. J. (2018). Deep learning and conditional random fields-based depth estimation and topographical reconstruction from conventional endoscopy. *Medical Image Analysis*, *48*, 230–243. doi:10.1016/j.media.2018.06.005 PMID:29990688

Messaoudi, H., Belaid, A., Ben Salem, D., & Conze, P.-H. (2023). Cross-Dimensional Transfer Learning in Medical Image Segmentation with Deep Learning. *Medical Image Analysis*, *88*, 102868. doi:10.1016/j.media.2023.102868 PMID:37384952

Onyema, E. M., Lilhore, U. K., Saurabh, P., Dalal, S., Nwaeze, A. S., Chijindu, A. T., Ndufeiya-Kumasi, L. C., & Simaiya, S. (2023). Evaluation of IoT-Enabled hybrid model for genome sequence analysis of patients in healthcare 4.0. *Measurement. Sensors*, *26*, 100679. doi:10.1016/j.measen.2023.100679

Rathore, M. S., Poongodi, M., Saurabh, P., Lilhore, U. K., Bourouis, S., Alhakami, W., Osamor, J., & Hamdi, M. (2022). A novel trust-based security and privacy model for internet of vehicles using encryption and steganography. *Computers & Electrical Engineering*, *102*, 108205. doi:10.1016/j.compeleceng.2022.108205

Xiang, H., Shen, J., Yan, Q., Xu, M., Shi, X., & Zhu, X. (2023). Multi-Scale Representation Attention Based Deep Multiple Instance Learning for Gigapixel Whole Slide Image Analysis. *Medical Image Analysis*, *89*, 102890. doi:10.1016/j.media.2023.102890 PMID:37467642

Zhang, J., Xie, Y., Wu, Q., & Xia, Y. (2019). Medical Image Classification Using Synergic Deep Learning. *Medical Image Analysis*, *54*, 10–19. doi:10.1016/j.media.2019.02.010 PMID:30818161

Chapter 6
An Efficient Technique to Perform 3D Visualization on Clinical Image Datasets

Prabhjyot kaur Haryal
https://orcid.org/0009-0003-3220-4251
Lovely Professional University, India

Punam Rattan
https://orcid.org/0000-0002-1965-0703
Lovely Professional University, India

ABSTRACT

The main idea behind this work is to present three-dimensional (3D) image visualization through two-dimensional (2D) images that comprise various images. 3D image visualization is one of the essential methods for excerpting data from given pieces. The main goal of this work is to figure out the outlines of the given 3D geometric primitives in each part, and then integrate these outlines or frames to reconstruct 3D geometric primitives. The proposed technique is very useful and can be applied to many kinds of images. The experimental results showed a very good determination of the reconstructing process of 2D images.

1. INTRODUCTION

The growth of three-dimensional (3D) images or object visualization is present primarily in the field of medical science, the manufacturing industry, defense systems, topography systems, the digital world, and remote monitoring. This growth is supervising the direction of different studies and funding agencies for applications in these areas. Medical images have been targeted to display visualization in multidimensional models, such as the axial view, sagittal view, and coronal view. Hence, the image is attained from the projections of more than one focal device at various places. In that condition, 3D visualization of the same parts in human beings can be carried out. The advent of image visualization processes or

DOI: 10.4018/979-8-3693-1874-4.ch006

methods for medical data sets has been made possible through the introduction of modern technologies in analysis and behaviours.

Conversely, these methods depend on computer reconstructions with the use of specific hardware devices such as computed tomography (CT), magnetic resonance imaging (MRI), positron emission tomography (PET), and ultrasound devices. Three-dimensional visualization of images, particularly medical data, provides essential information about the object and its behaviours, which are very significant in diagnosis and treatment. The importance of 3D visualization techniques is now undetermined and untrained; hence, it is a very significant field of research to offer new tools, hardware equipment, methods, analysis, cures, etc. Constructing an image entails mapping some properties of a geometric primitive onto the image space, which are utilized to visualize an object and its behaviours to illustrate its structure or involvement. In medical science, understanding of mapping and growing techniques is essential in accepting performance with respect to their development. The main goal of 3D image visualization is to convey and appreciate ideas of an effective framework to create useful image data. The requirements for new modern efficient techniques of 3D image visualization and investigation will develop progressively.

In this article, the basic methods of 3D image visualization techniques are described in detail, and effective techniques are also identified to perform 3D image visualization for medical data sets. In recent years, with advances in computing power and algorithms, the impact of technology in medicine is greater than ever and keeps increasing. Strategic plans focusing on promoting the application and development of medical technologies have been made worldwide. In 2018, the General Office of the State Council of China issued "Opinions on Promoting the Development of 'Internet Plus Healthcare,'" calling for strengthening the integration, sharing, and application of clinical and research data and supporting the research and development of health-related artificial intelligence (AI) technology, medical robots, etc. A three-year action plan was released to develop AI, which puts a priority on expanding the clinical application. In the same year, the National Institutes of Health (NIH), USA, released the NIH Strategic Plan for Data Science, which proposed that technological innovations such as machine learning, deep learning, AI, and virtual reality (VR) could revolutionize biomedical research over the next 10 years.

Medical images, such as computerized tomography (CT), magnetic resonance imaging (MRI), and diffusion tensor imaging (DTI), are the backbone of modern medical practices and research. Furthermore, medical images are a core data source and target for analysis in AI and VR in aforementioned strategic plans. Therefore, the analysis and understanding of medical images are of utmost importance in medical technologies. In practice, most if not everyone in health science areas is familiar with medical images, and many uses medical images in daily work. Medical images are massive and complex and hard to explore and gain insights with traditional statistical methods that do not involve the expertise of humans. Therefore, technologies that have humans in the loop are needed for medical image exploration and analysis, and medical experts could make the best of the potential values of medical images to enable high-quality healthcare solutions. Vision is known to be the major and most efficient perception mechanism for humans. Visualization transforms data into interactive visual representations to facilitate data understanding and exploration through visual perception and human computer interaction, and it can present medical images in 3D with high accuracy. Visualization integrates the cognitive advantage of humans and the computational advantage of computers for data mining and decision-making and is an effective data analysis technology for medical images.

2. SCOPE

In this paper, the focus is on techniques of 3D medical image visualization and specific techniques for various medical problems based on imaging categorized by the medical procedure and the scale of studies. There are several reviews of visualization techniques for medical images. However, the target audience of these reviews is visualization researchers rather than medical experts. These technical-oriented reviews offer in-depth discussions on visualization techniques for specific medical data types with fine-grained taxonomy, including perceptually motivated 3D medical image data visualization, multimodal medical data, medical flow data, cardiac 4D data and flattening-based medical visualization. This paper also features an overview of techniques that could improve spatial perception, which is vital for the understanding of medical images in 3D. Overall, rather than a comprehensive review of the literature on the topic of medical image visualization, this paper provides a big picture of the subject of study and introduces state-of-the-art techniques driven by specific medical problems.

3. EXISTING WORKS

Visualization is the process of transforming data into a visual form. The application of 3D image visualization is a significant characteristic of digital image processing, involving large collections in many fields of day-to-day life. Several existing works are available on image visualization. Various insights from these works are presented in this article.

Spagnolo F. et al. (2023) presents a novel hardware architecture to reduce the complexity of accelerators, thus enabling their integration within the future generation of low-power systems.

Lo S. W. et al. (2021) developed a scalable deep sensing workflow with real events.

Chotisarn N. et al. (2021) presents a prototype system to comprehend the model results and detect problem.

Fei Y. et al. (2023) proposed a high-quality classification model for fresh-cut flowers.

Guha A. et al. (2022) proposed a multi-modal binary classification approach.

Luque A. et al. (2022) reviewed several methods to visualize classification results at different levels.

Ren X. et al. (2022) studied the visual fatigue relief method considering the rest time allocation.

Ma C. et al. (2022) proposed complex network models to detect critical links in a given airway network dynamically.

Ong J. et al. (2022) derived an online Bayesian multi-view multi-object filtering algorithm.

Pal A. et al. (2021) takes a pioneering initiative to study the effectiveness of the deep metric learning algorithm for cervical image classification.

Han W. et al. (2022) presents a new method for predicting coarseness among visual textures.

Jalonen T. et al. (2021) proposed a new visual system for manufacturing product tracking.

Singh P. et al. (2021) developed a sensor for real-time characterization.

Xie X et al. (2021) proposed a novel transformer-based network to detect the defects of photovoltaic solar cells effectively.

Di Ciaccio F. et al. (2022) presents a novel Deep Learning-based approach to the attitude estimation problem.

Guo Y. et al. (2022) explored the task of multimodal detection.

Hong W. et al. (2021) presents a novel color image authentication scheme capable of grayscale-invariance for each pixel.

Khattar A. et al. (2022) proposed a novel framework for the binary classification of multimodal data.

Fotouhi J. et al. (2021) presented the embodiment of a novel interaction concept based on AR.

Marino E. et al. (2021) proposed a background-aware colourisation technique that sets the colours of the virtual objects in accordance with the real background.

Mollel M. S. et al. (2021) provides an extensive tutorial on 5G networks accompanied by a discussion on machine learning (ML) applications.

Hsu W. Y. et al. (2021) compared a study to show the differences in color temperature and lightness and further adjusted with automatic white balance.

Zhao L. (2023) establishes an action recognition model based on convolutional neural network.

Zhu J. et al. (2023) proposed to enhance the feature of fuzzy boundary and generate multiscale parcels.

4. 3D VISUALIZATION TOOLS

The three-dimensional modeling technology is mature, many methods has been integrated into the commercial software. The rapid development of computer graphics technology led the brisk development of 3D modeling technology. There are more and more 3D visualization and graphics rendering tools. The more representative of which are the OpenGL, open international graphics standard of SGI Company, Direct3D of Microsoft, VRML (Virtual Reality Modeling Language) which brings three-dimensional world into network, Java3D, 3D graphics technology based on Java Language of SUN Company, IDL of RSI Company and Vega of Paradigm Company and so on. This software involves the main areas including deposit modeling, design planning, production management, etc. In recent years, with the continuous development of computer technology, some new technologies appear constantly, the emergence of these new technologies provide a new means for 3D visualization.

4.1. OpenGL

OpenGL is an abbreviation for Open Graphics Lib, it is a low-level Graphics library, and it is developed by SGI Company originally. It is a set of 3D graphics library, and also the industry standard in this field.it is a high-performance development package to draw high realistic 3D graphics, interactive visual simulation and virtual display. OpenGL is a process language rather than a descriptive language fundamentally. OpenGL provides the basic operations of direct control of a 2D and 3D geometry. OpenGL offers a wide range of graphics transformation function, when to programme so that don't have to complex matrix operations, and can easily display 3D graphics in the screen window. And, in order to enhance the sense of reality, OpenGL also provides a series of functions that combine blanking, coloring of line and plane, and illumination, texture mapping and anti-aliasing technology. It is helpful to avoid the pure graphics algorithm, simplify the programming, and be very convenient to drawing, coloring and lighting the ground level.

4.2. Direct3D

Microsoft DirectX provides a very good application interface, which contains the design of high performance and real-time application of source code. DirectX technology will help to construct the next generation of computer games and multimedia applications. Its content includes the DirectDraw, DirectSound, DirectPlay, Direct3D and DirectInput parts, and they are respectively mainly used in graphics, sound, etc. The function of Direct3D and OpenGL are approximation, they 263 provide uniform access to different graphics accelerator card. Direct3D was adopted to realize access to hardware acceleration video with nothing to do with the equipment method. Immediate mode and retained mode, encapsulates the immediate mode, are two alternative ways. The former is suitable for the general 3D application development, while the latter is suitable for quick developers. Direct3D device is Direct3D rendering component, the equivalent of a state machine, packaging and store the render state. Only through the COM interface which is provide by Direct3D, can C++ programs manipulate and use render state and lighting equipment of Direct3D.

4.3. Virtual Reality Modeling Language (VRML)

VRML (virtual reality modeling language) is a kind of 3D exchange format, defining the most common concepts in the 3D visualization, such as the objects move, rotate, viewpoints, light, material properties, texture mapping, animation, fog, and nested structure, etc. VRML is a descriptive language essentially, the work of drawing the scene entirely by the corresponding browser or plug-in. It uses a standard format to describe the 3D environment, and embedded in Web pages, through plug-ins to provide viewpoints including transformation, flight simulation, control, speed, etc. VRML, as same as HTML, ASCII text format is used to describe and link the world, and it also help to guarantee on a variety of platforms and general, but also reduces the amount of data, which can be achieved on the low bandwidth network. But works of VRML are still staying in a display file stage, lacking of action and interaction.

4.4. Java3D

Java language is a network application-oriented computer language of SUN Company. Java3D is developed on the basis of Java, OpenGL and VRML. Java language is the extension in the field of 3D graphics, and its essence is a set of API function set. When to use Java3D to write applications, only need to follow the object-oriented thought in appropriate positions for the program corresponding to objects, can quickly write 3D multimedia applications. The API of Java3D contains almost basic classes and interfaces to write JAVA interactive 3D for the application.

4.5. Information Visualization

It was built upon graphic designers, statisticians, human-computer-interaction (HCI) researchers, and many others. The interdisciplinary field has been exploring the effective use of computer graphics for abstract data visualization and its interactive exploration. Thanks to the gaming industry, with the recent development of low-cost devices which can provide powerful VR and augmented reality (AR) applications, cultural heritage institutions have started the digitalization era. 3D representations of cultural heritage artifacts and structures have affected many areas, such as virtual cultural heritage tourism and research on urban history. Development of the technology which can capture and document the heritage sites offer new techniques that substitute the human interpretation, which requires more time and workload. After the first 3D documentation of archeological objects was realized, many artifacts started to be exported to digital environments.

With sufficient documentation for transmitting the cultural heritage to future generations, which cannot be protected due to natural and artificial disasters, preservation in digital mediums has become a reliable method. Final products of the digitization process do not only serve for archaeological and architectural documentation, but they also provide educational opportunities, exhibitions, virtual tourism, experimental studies on space, and analyses on artifacts. On the other hand, preparation, presentation, and interaction of 3D digital contents require meticulous work. According to the complexity, scale, and location of the subject of 3D digital representation, different methodologies can be used, such as laser scanning and photogrammetric.

Also, several techniques have been developed to reconstruct an artifact, such as sculptures and paintings. These techniques include image sequencing, volume-based methods, structured form motion algorithm. The problem is that generated models are generally complex due to graphic requirements of details. Several geometric optimizations and compression methods have been developed to solve technical problems such as managing millions of polygons or processing time, while their main aim is not to comprise details and realism. Different visualization techniques have been offered to better understand software architectures, various algorithms, and computer science concepts. Studies focus on interpreting complex structures to understand different features and concepts related to the field. For example, visualization techniques have been employed to better understand and explain artificial intelligence (AI). Explainable Artificial Intelligence (XAI) is a recently developed technology aiming to enhance the understanding of AI from the eyes of humans.

As part of this study, Selvaraju et al. (2017) offered to use Gradient-weighted Class Activation Mapping (GradCAM), which is a visualization method that benefits from the gradient of the target and produces localization maps on Deep Reinforcement Learning (DRL) algorithms. With the analysis of their study on Atari Games that includes visualizations of input states and selected output action, the role of the CNN layer can be understood. Their interaction method allows users to gain better insight into complex structures of neural networks. High dimensional visualizations with 3D representations benefit from metaphors that make knowledge more accessible and understandable. An essential constituent in computer sciences is the use of metaphors. The assessment of the metaphor is related to the properties of the visualized field and approximation of the notions of the related field. Design of the components related to specific features is crucial in this approach. One of the extensively used metaphors in computer sciences is the city metaphor.

4.6. Scientific Visualization

The recognition of graphics as a distinct field actualized with the achievements of powerful computers and photorealistic renderings has made scientists available to use visualization for scientific studies. Visualizing scientific data is crucial for experts working on scientific domains and communicating with a general audience and students. Scientific visualizations were limited to two dimensional representations. With the development of rendering techniques, it is now possible to visualize and interact with scientific data in a 3D virtual world. This allows users to explore and interact with real-like representations that improve the comprehension capabilities of students and enhance public engagement. Scientific visualization scans can be very complex and hard to compute according to the dataset due to high dimensional and abstract data. They might require exclusive visualizations instead of traditional computer ones.

Different 2D sections implemented with conventional desktop and mouse may not be sufficient to construct 3D understanding, which also differs according to the user. Unlike a monocular system like traditional 2D screens, binocular systems in virtual reality display provide a true sense of depth perception and spatial relations. Thus, many industries have adopted these systems to test real-life scenarios as in training. Serving for the mining industry software module, the block cave mining system visualizer was developed to contribute to the block cave's management cycle and operation. Allowing a collaborative environment and converting the complex context of the mining system into a graphical representation improves the understanding of seismic data. Interactive 3D data visualizations are also used in High Energy Physics (HEP) experiments. Utilizing Unreal Engine, they offer three levels with different modes of interaction. Although game engines are widely used for visualization when there is a need for an external library, as it can be challenging to integrate into the game engines.

4.7. Medicine and Biology

Medical visualizations are generally composed of 2D mediums such as cross-sectional images and magnetic resonance imaging (MRI) scans. Therefore, 3D geometric models are reconstructed from individual slice. Another method is image segmentation, which helps separate the pixels of the specified parts from the overall image. Ciganek and Kepesiova (2020) propose a segmentation and 3D model reconstruction method based on machine learning algorithms. Visualizations of medical or anatomical models consist of many complex subparts.

Thus, studies designed interfaces that include different features such as labeling, highlighting, distinct colors, selective visualization and navigators. Also, to solve depth perception problems in rendering photography effects, depth-of-field and gradient shading are used to sustain depth cues. Virtual reality can assist the diagnosis process by providing appropriate conditions. To reduce the diagnostic errors in radiology, designed a virtual reading room where the reader can adjust the illumination and ambient light while displaying luminance. Some studies include different approaches and subjects such as medicine education, hand recognition, smartphone applications for anatomy and biofeedback. Although game engines are employed by most of the studies due to graphics performance, physics, and ease of deployment to VR, game engines may not be proper for scientific visualizations. Elden's study includes three demos; artery, rat brain, and genome. According to the requirements of the demos, different representation techniques were chosen. Thereby, the study became convenient to construct guidelines. As reported by the study, game engines are designed for geometric visualizations, and their priority is not accuracy but speed, which makes game engines unreliable.

5. THREE-DIMENSIONAL IMAGE RENDERING TECHNIQUES

5.1 Three-Dimensional Volumetric Data

Three-dimensional volumetric data can be recreated with the help of computer graphic packages, in which images are considered as digital forms. The digital form of images is stored in a mathematical arrangement in computer systems. Commonly, a 3D volumetric image is built from a collection of parallel slices that have the user data. Furthermore, 3D images are sampled anisotropically, with the distance between sequences more than the in-plane pixel scale. Hence, the spatial resolution, which is the size of image voxels, has a base equivalent to the pixel dimension determined by the in-plane resolution of the scanner and a height equivalent to the distance between sequential slices. Three different sizes of a voxel are shown in Figure 1.

The first one represents the isotropically sampled image at low resolution, as shown in Figure 1A; the second one is the anistropically sampled image with in-place resolution higher than the resolution between sequential slices, as shown in Figure 1B; and the third is the isotropically sampled image at high-resolution, as shown in Figure 1C. When the voxel size is given isotropically, 3D rendering will have the actual size in all three dimensions. This allows estimation at any plane and recreating the slice image along any arbitrary axis in 3D space.

5.2 Three-Dimensional Image Visualization

Illustrations in 2D depend on the original appearance of the image plane with respect to the constructions of importance. Furthermore, imaging systems have limited abilities to effectively construct 2D images directly. Several methods are used to create 2D images from 3D pictures, and these methods depend on the extraction of the significant slices. Many techniques and systems have been established for 3D image demonstration and picturing, and these techniques typically are further categorized into three techniques: surface rendering, volume rendering, and image-based rendering. The combination of all these techniques generates the visualization of 3D volume images, and each technique has its own merits and demerits.

The selection of these techniques depends on the user requirements and resulting analysis of the visualization process. Surface rendering methods depend on the extraction of outlines, in which the surface of the basic construction is defined. Then, the surface batches are located at each outline point, and hidden surface removal and shading methods are utilized to render the visible surface. The merits of the surface rendering technique increase the computational time, as a low data rate is needed for outlines. Moreover, this technique can take the merit of specific graphics hardware to increase the geometric transformation of rendering processes. The drawback of this technique, based on the data needed for constructing outlines, is that some data are lost in this operation. Similarly, this technique removes any interactive creation of the surface to be rendered. Volume rendering techniques based on ray-casting methods have led to the development of powerful techniques for image visualization. Three-dimensional visualization of volume images is given without the required preceding knowledge about surface picture segmentation. In these techniques, the entire image volumes are needed in maintaining the original volume image data. This technique supports the abilities and is more powerful in rendering the original image data. The volume rendering method is reserved for high- resolution image visualization of displayed structures.

Conversely, these techniques affect high-end processing speed observations to develop 3D image visualization. The third technique is image-based rendering, which depends on the image space methods that need more powerful and flexible techniques for medical data visualization. Actually, images are illustrated in a 2D matrix (M*N). Nevertheless, pictures can be demonstrated in a 3D matrix (M*N*L), which represents 3D volumetric information or 3D visualization. The methods of con- structing 3D computer graphics can consequentially further be divided into three common stages: 3D, which defines the methods of establishing the shape of a picture; outline and animation, which define the motions and locations of the pictures within a scene; and 3D rendering, which creates images.

5.3 Volume Estimation and Rendering

Volume estimation is an important issue in the field of image visualization, including medical images as well as geographical images. Volume estimation means 3D construction of an image from slices. The steps for the construction of volume estimation from slices are-

Step 1: Find the contour of the area of interest in each slice.

Step 2: Measure the indicated area in each slice.

Step 3: Determine the volume between two slices.

Step 4: Reconstruct the volume of indicated areas for all slices.

The advantage of the edge enhancement stage is reducing the imperfections in the image reproduction, such as particles or noise or deficiencies in the image. Therefore, the edge enhancement stage improves the noise level as well as the quality of the images. The fourth stage is focused on the rendering process, and volume rendering methods have been established to overcome the issues of the perfection of illustration of surfaces in the iso-surface methods. Volume rendering issues are relevant to making a decision for every volume component, on whether or not the surface passed through it and can produce false positives or false negatives, mainly concentrating on the appearance of small or poorly identified structures. The drawbacks of volume rendering include not using inter- mediate geometrical illustrations in focus to surface rendering methods. It deals with the opportunity to display weak or fuzzy surfaces. The surface rendering method helps in determining whether a surface is present or not.

The volume rendering method encompasses the following steps:

Step 1: Creating an RGBA volume from the data.

Step 2: Reconstructing a continuous function from these non-continuous datasets.

Step 3: Estimating the 2D viewing plane from the desired point of view.

Step 4: An RGBA volume is a 4D vector data set, where the first three components are the primary colors R, G, and B and the last component A denotes the opacity value.

Step 5: Beyond the RGBA volume, an opaque background is located. The mapping of the information to opacity values acts as a classification of the information that is involved in the processing.

Therefore, the appearance of surfaces can be improved by utilizing shading methods to form the RGB mapping. Also, opacity can be used to see the interior of the data volume as well. The main advantage of the volume rendering method is that interior data are not sorted out. Therefore, it helps in looking at the 3D data set as a whole. The drawbacks are the complex interpretation of the overcast interiors and the long time required compared to that needed for surface rendering. In the proposed system, the flow diagram of volume rendering methods applies two important approaches, such as the ray casting and splatting methods. These methods are used to determine the four visualization elements of the RGBA volume value, opacity value, complete transparencies, and completely opaque values. The proposed system differs in the way that the RGBA volume values are estimates of the 2D viewing plane.

Volume rendering using the ray casting method involves different develop- mental processes considered for ray casting. Three-dimensional modeling is a process of developing the scientific representation of any 3D surface from the 2D images through 3D modeling tools. Three-dimensional models are widely used these days in multiple fields. In medical sciences, 3D models of humans are very much utilized for diagnoses and surgical procedures. The 3D models can be synthesized by utilizing multiple 2D image slices from different medical image modalities. Also, the models can be reconstructed by utilizing three different image slices, such as axial, sagittal, and coronal, from different medical image modalities. The 3D models thus reconstructed can be categorized into solid modeling and contour modeling. Usually, in engineering and medical simulations, solid modeling is utilized. Contour modeling is used for surface modeling. The difference between these two modeling categories lies in the way that they are created and manipulated for 3D modeling. Also, the conventions of usage with respect to different fields and the approximations are applied to each model.

6. FUTURE DIRECTIONS AND LIMITATIONS OF MEDICAL IMAGE VISUALIZATION

Some visualization methods support exploring and analyzing medical image data from basic medical research that can potentially address unsolved health challenges in the future. In this section, we discuss some of these important future directions and also limitations of medical image visualization. Simulations are an important approach in medical research to understand complex, invisible, and/or perpetual activities in human bodies. Nasal flow simulation is an important means for understanding the physiological nasal breathing that improves the overall traditional statistics-based summary of flow behaviors. A visual analysis method aids in the exploration of a computational fluid dynamics simulation on an anatomically correct model of the upper respiratory tract. With multiple-linked views, the method allows users to analyze multiple attributes, e.g., speed, pressure, humidity, and temperature, of the complex flow simulation to derive intervention plans. Hemodynamic characteristics in cerebral aneurysms are studied with computational fluid dynamic simulations and segmented data from CTA scans.

The visual analysis tries to understand the inflow jet and impingement zone that are correlated with the risk of rupture. A vortex classification method automatically classifies blood flows in cerebral aneurysms and visualizes the clusters as streamlines in an aneurysm-based and a hemisphere-based visualization. Cardiac diseases are typically related to malfunctions in bioelectric fields in the body that are difficult to measure in vivo. Simulation of such bioelectric fields then becomes a feasible alternative, and, therefore, in-depth analysis of simulation results is important. Early work focuses on the visualization of torso electric field simulations. Specialized for the 3D myocardial ischemia simulation, a multiple linked view approach is devised to perform the visual analysis of the multiple simulation runs of bioelectric fields on the heart, which could also potentially be used for diagnosis. A systematic discussion of computational and numerical methods for bioelectric fields problems can be found in a review, where related visualization techniques are also discussed. Comparative visualization is important for understanding an ensemble of simulation runs and comparing between patients or different measures of medical images.

Scalar image ensembles, for example, brain MR atlas data (https://www.oasis-brains.org/), are a common form of ensemble medical image data. Direct visualization of image members in 2D and 3D is not effective due to occlusion, and quantitative comparison is not feasible in this way either. One possible solution is to reduce the dimensionality of image data to one (1D) with space-filing curves. Data-driven space-filling curves better preserve spatial coherency in the resulting 1D representation than static curves, which potentially break spatially coherent features into distant 1D fragment. The method is applied for visualizing brain MRI atlas and an ensemble of 3D myocardial ischemia simulations and could potentially be used for diagnosis or research by finding anomalies of subjects through comparison to the main trends. Comparative visualization of stress tensors is available for analyzing rupture risks of cerebral aneurysms based on computational fluid dynamic simulations.

With several glyph designs, the method supports the comparison of local stress tensors on the inner and outer vessel walls. Medical experts consider that this method introduces the often-overlooked wall structure information for rupture assessment and could contribute to the development of a comprehensive risk factor of aneurysms in the future. Medical image visualization has its limitations. First, customized techniques and tools are required for specific medical problems, which demand close collaborations between the visualization and medical experts. Typically, an iterative process with several prototypes is required for a method and its associated software tool to become usable, which is often time-consuming. Second, a learning process is required for medical experts to familiarize themselves with new concepts or interactions, for example, transfer function design in volume rendering. Nevertheless, medical image visualization has the advantage of combining the expertise of humans and the computational power of machines, which is vital for health science, making it a promising research direction.

7. SOFTWARE TOOLS FOR MEDICAL IMAGE VISUALIZATION

Both commercial tools and free software are available for medical image visualization. In this paper, we list representative free software that can be found on the Internet and readily used for 3D medical images of various types and file formats. We briefly summarize these tools with data types that can be handled (data types) as well as their featuring characteristics (features). Visualization and analysis tools for general scientific problems and data provide flexible rapid prototyping frameworks. ParaView (https://www.paraview.org/) is a cross platform open-source visualization tool designed for interactive visualization and data analysis for a wide range of research and engineering areas, and various types of medical images (scalar, vector, and tensor) are supported. Voreen (voreen.uni-muenster.de) is an open-source rapid application development framework for the interactive visualization and analysis of multimodal volumetric datasets. Inviwo (https://inviwo.org/) is a framework for rapid prototyping visualizations and provides a rich visual interface for creating customized visualization. MegaMol (https://megamol.org/) is a comprehensive cross-platform visualization prototyping framework evolved from particle rendering for molecular datasets.

SCIRun (https://www.sci.utah.edu/software/scirun.html) is a software environment for scientific problem simulation, modeling, and visualization, and it supports various types of medical images. A number of tools are available for scalar medical image visualization and analysis. 3D Slicer (https://download.slicer.org/) is a tool for visualization and analysis of medical images and features interface for medical devices, for example, surgical navigation system and robotic devices. Seg3D (https://www.sci.utah.edu/software/seg3d.html) is a medical volume segmentation and processing tool that allows for flexible manual segmentation and a number of automatic segmentation algorithms. ImageVis3D (https://www.sci.utah.edu/software/imagevis3d.html) is a scalable and multiplatform volume visualization tool that supports large datasets and works on mobile devices. FluoRenderer (https://www.sci.utah.edu/software/fluorender.html) features the visualization of confocal microscopy data and multichannel scalar volume datasets. These software tools contain example datasets, tutorials, detailed user guides, and supporting communities. Readers are encouraged to try out these tools with included datasets and their own medical images to have first-hand experience of some key techniques discussed in this paper.

8. CONCLUSION

Images have many issues, such as low-resolution output display, high-resolution output display, very low contrast, and geometric primitive distortions. The integration of image slices to create a 3D image graphical illustration, which is significant, solve the issues and enable its many applications in medical sciences. Therefore, this paper suggests an efficient technique for 3D image visualization process through the extraction of the higher-dimensional pictures from 2D images. Finally, it helps in developing medical images and provides several types of image file formats also.

REFERENCES

Chotisarn, N., Pimanmassuriya, W., & Gulyanon, S. (2021). Deep Learning Visualization for Under-specification Analysis in Product Design Matching Model Development. *IEEE Access : Practical Innovations, Open Solutions*, *9*, 108049–108061. doi:10.1109/ACCESS.2021.3102174

Di Ciaccio, F., Russo, P., & Troisi, S. (2022). DOES: A Deep Learning-Based Approach to Estimate Roll and Pitch at Sea. *IEEE Access : Practical Innovations, Open Solutions*, *10*, 29307–29321. doi:10.1109/ACCESS.2022.3158971

Fei, Y., Li, Z., Zhu, T., & Ni, C. (2023). A Lightweight Attention-Based Convolutional Neural Networks for Fresh-Cut Flower Classification. *IEEE Access : Practical Innovations, Open Solutions*, *11*, 17283–17293. doi:10.1109/ACCESS.2023.3244386

Fotouhi, J., Mehrfard, A., Song, T., Johnson, A., Osgood, G., Unberath, M., Armand, M., & Navab, N. (2021). Development and Pre-Clinical Analysis of Spatiotemporal-Aware Augmented Reality in Orthopedic Interventions. *IEEE Transactions on Medical Imaging*, *40*(2), 765–778. doi:10.1109/TMI.2020.3037013

Guha, A., Alahmadi, A., Samanta, D., Khan, M. Z., & Alahmadi, A. H. (2022). A Multi-Modal Approach to Digital Document Stream Segmentation for Title Insurance Domain. *IEEE Access : Practical Innovations, Open Solutions*, *10*, 11341–11353. https://doi.org/10.1109/ACCESS.2022.3144185

Guo, Y., & Song, W. (2022). A Temporal-and-Spatial Flow Based Multimodal Fake News Detection by Pooling and Attention Blocks. *IEEE Access : Practical Innovations, Open Solutions*, *10*, 131498–131508. doi:10.1109/ACCESS.2022.3229762

Han, W., Lim, J., Lee, S. J., Kim, C. Y., Kim, W. C., & Park, N. C. (2022). Bidirectional Reflectance Distribution Function (BRDF)-Based Coarseness Prediction of Textured Metal Surface. *IEEE Access : Practical Innovations, Open Solutions*, *10*, 32461–32469. doi:10.1109/ACCESS.2022.3161518

Hong, W., Chen, J., Chang, P. S., Wu, J., Chen, T. S., & Lin, J. (2021). A Color Image Authentication Scheme with Grayscale Invariance. *IEEE Access : Practical Innovations, Open Solutions*, *9*, 6522–6535. doi:10.1109/ACCESS.2020.3047270

Hsu, W. Y., & Cheng, H. C. (2021). A novel automatic white balance method for color constancy under different color temperatures. *IEEE Access : Practical Innovations, Open Solutions*, *9*, 111925–111937. doi:10.1109/ACCESS.2021.3103737

Jalonen, T., Laakom, F., Gabbouj, M., & Puoskari, T. (2021). Visual Product Tracking System Using Siamese Neural Networks. *IEEE Access : Practical Innovations, Open Solutions*, *9*, 76796–76805. doi:10.1109/ACCESS.2021.3082934

Khattar, A., & Quadri, S. M. K. (2022). CAMM: Cross-Attention Multimodal Classification of Disaster-Related Tweets. *IEEE Access : Practical Innovations, Open Solutions*, *10*, 92889–92902. doi:10.1109/ACCESS.2022.3202976

Lo, S. W., Wu, J. H., Chang, J. Y., Tseng, C. H., Lin, M. W., & Lin, F. P. (2021). Deep sensing of urban waterlogging. *IEEE Access : Practical Innovations, Open Solutions*, *9*, 127185–127203. doi:10.1109/ACCESS.2021.3111623

Luque, A., Mazzoleni, M., Carrasco, A., & Ferramosca, A. (2022). Visualizing Classification Results: Confusion Star and Confusion Gear. *IEEE Access : Practical Innovations, Open Solutions*, *10*, 1659–1677. doi:10.1109/ACCESS.2021.3137630

Ma, C., Alam, S., Cai, Q., & Delahaye, D. (2022). Critical Links Detection in Spatial-Temporal Airway Networks Using Complex Network Theories. *IEEE Access : Practical Innovations, Open Solutions*, *10*, 27925–27944. doi:10.1109/ACCESS.2022.3152163

Marino, E., Bruno, F., Barbieri, L., Muzzupappa, M., & Liarokapis, F. (2021). Background-Aware Colorization Technique for Augmented Reality Applications. *IEEE Access : Practical Innovations, Open Solutions*, *9*, 161761–161772. doi:10.1109/ACCESS.2021.3129076

Mollel, M. S., Abubakar, A. I., Ozturk, M., Kaijage, S. F., Kisangiri, M., Hussain, S., Imran, M. A., & Abbasi, Q. H. (2021). A Survey of Machine Learning Applications to Handover Management in 5G and beyond. *IEEE Access : Practical Innovations, Open Solutions*, *9*, 45770–45802. doi:10.1109/ACCESS.2021.3067503

Ong, J., Vo, B. T., Vo, B. N., Kim, D. Y., & Nordholm, S. (2022). A Bayesian Filter for Multi-View 3D Multi-Object Tracking With Occlusion Handling. *IEEE Transactions on Pattern Analysis and Machine Intelligence*, *44*(5), 2246–2263. doi:10.1109/TPAMI.2020.3034435

Pal, A., Xue, Z., Befano, B., Rodriguez, A. C., Long, L. R., Schiffman, M., & Antani, S. (2021). Deep Metric Learning for Cervical Image Classification. *IEEE Access : Practical Innovations, Open Solutions*, *9*, 53266–53275. https://doi.org/10.1109/ACCESS.2021.3069346

Ren, X., Gao, Z., & Sui, Q. (2022). An Optimal Visual Fatigue Relief Method for Workers Considering Rest Time Allocation. *IEEE Access : Practical Innovations, Open Solutions*, *10*, 26463–26470. https://doi.org/10.1109/ACCESS.2022.3155189

Singh, P., Chatterjee, A., Rajput, L. S., Kumar, S., Nataraj, V., Bhatia, V., & Prakash, S. (2021). Biospeckle-based sensor for characterization of charcoal rot (Macrophomina phaseolina (Tassi) goid) disease in soybean (Glycine max (L.) Merr.) crop. *IEEE Access : Practical Innovations, Open Solutions*, *9*, 31562–31574. doi:10.1109/ACCESS.2021.3059868

Spagnolo, F., Corsonello, P., Frustaci, F., & Perri, S. (2023). Design of a Low-Power Super-Resolution Architecture for Virtual Reality Wearable Devices. *IEEE Sensors Journal*, *23*(8), 9009–9016. https://doi.org/10.1109/JSEN.2023.3256524

Xie, X., Liu, H., Na, Z., Luo, X., Wang, D., & Leng, B. (2021). DPiT: Detecting Defects of Photovoltaic Solar Cells with Image Transformers. *IEEE Access : Practical Innovations, Open Solutions*, *9*, 154292–154303. doi:10.1109/ACCESS.2021.3119631

Zhao, L. (2023). A Hybrid Deep Learning-Based Intelligent System for Sports Action Recognition via Visual Knowledge Discovery. *IEEE Access : Practical Innovations, Open Solutions*, *11*, 46541–46549. doi:10.1109/ACCESS.2023.3275012

Zhu, J., Chai, Z., Song, Z., Chen, Z., & Shi, Q. (2023). A Fuzzy-Boundary Enhanced Trident Network for Parcel Extraction in the Urban-Rural Area. *IEEE Journal of Selected Topics in Applied Earth Observations and Remote Sensing*, *16*, 2654–2667. https://doi.org/10.1109/JSTARS.2023.3247875

Chapter 7
Case Studies in Federated Learning for Healthcare

Javier Prieto
Independent Researcher, China

ABSTRACT

This chapter presents a comprehensive exploration of federated learning's real-world applications in healthcare contexts across four diverse regions: China, India, Spain, and the United States. The authors delve into how this innovative approach addresses the critical need for patient data privacy while advancing disease diagnosis, personalized treatment, and healthcare quality. From improving diagnostics through local data utilization in China to enhancing healthcare access in India, the chapter showcases the practical benefits and challenges of implementing federated learning. It also sheds light on collaborative drug development in Spain and navigating stringent data privacy regulations in the United States, emphasizing the global significance of Federated Learning in healthcare AI.

INTRODUCTION

Healthcare stands at the intersection of transformative technologies and the critical responsibility of safeguarding sensitive patient data. In this chapter, we embark on a journey through the realms of Federated Learning, a revolutionary paradigm in machine learning that redefines how we approach healthcare AI. Through an exploration of real-world applications across diverse regions - China, India, Spain, and the United States - we delve into the tangible impact of Federated Learning on disease diagnosis, personalized treatment, and healthcare quality.

Federated Learning represents a seismic shift in the landscape of machine learning, departing from the traditional centralized approach to training models. This decentralized methodology enables model training on numerous devices or servers while keeping data localized. A brief recap of this foundational concept sets the stage for our exploration. It's not just a technological innovation; it's a safeguard for patient data privacy, a critical need in the age of data-driven medicine.

In healthcare, where the stakes are high and privacy concerns paramount, Federated Learning emerges as a beacon of hope. By ensuring that patient data never leaves its original location, the risk of breaches

DOI: 10.4018/979-8-3693-1874-4.ch007

and misuse is substantially reduced. As we navigate the complex web of healthcare ethics and privacy, Federated Learning emerges as a cornerstone, allowing healthcare practitioners to harness the power of AI without compromising the confidentiality of patient information. Theoretical concepts find their true worth when applied to real-world challenges. In healthcare, the transition from theory to practice is not just a necessity; it is a moral imperative. This section underscores the pivotal role of real-world applications in bridging the gap between abstract concepts and tangible solutions.

While theories provide a foundation, it is their application in real-world healthcare scenarios that validates their efficacy. Federated Learning, often discussed in academic and technological circles, finds its true meaning when implemented in the intricate web of healthcare systems. From the bustling hospitals of China to the remote clinics in India, Federated Learning is not just an abstract concept; it's a tool that healthcare professionals can wield to enhance patient outcomes.

The healthcare landscape is riddled with challenges - from accessibility issues to stringent data privacy regulations. Federated Learning doesn't shy away from these challenges; instead, it confronts them head-on. This section aims to showcase the practical benefits of implementing Federated Learning in healthcare settings. Through real-world case studies, we unravel the success stories and, equally importantly, dissect the challenges faced. It's a journey through the triumphs and tribulations of applying cutting-edge technology in a field where precision and privacy are paramount.

As we embark on this exploration of Federated Learning in healthcare, we invite you to witness the transformational power of technology in preserving patient data privacy and advancing the quality of healthcare services globally.

1. LOCAL DATA UTILIZATION FOR IMPROVED DIAGNOSTICS IN CHINA

In the vast landscape of China's healthcare system, characterized by its scale and diversity, leveraging Federated Learning for improved diagnostics emerges as a transformative strategy. This section navigates through the intricacies of China's healthcare infrastructure, the challenges it faces, and the pivotal role that enhanced diagnostics play in achieving better patient outcomes.

China's healthcare system is a complex amalgamation of urban and rural healthcare services, striving to cater to the needs of its vast population. With a growing middle class and increasing urbanization, the demand for quality healthcare has surged. However, this surge presents its own set of challenges, including regional disparities in healthcare access, resource allocation issues, and the need for innovative solutions to address diverse patient needs.

China's healthcare infrastructure spans a spectrum from state-of-the-art facilities in major cities to more basic healthcare services in rural areas. The sheer size of the population, coupled with variations in economic development across regions, presents challenges in ensuring equitable access to quality healthcare. Resource allocation, healthcare workforce distribution, and the integration of advanced technologies are pivotal areas requiring attention to elevate the overall standard of healthcare.

In this intricate healthcare landscape, the significance of diagnostic accuracy cannot be overstated. Timely and precise diagnostics lay the foundation for effective treatment plans, enhancing patient outcomes across the board. Federated Learning, by enabling the utilization of local data for diagnostics, addresses the nuances of regional healthcare challenges. It empowers healthcare practitioners with tools that are not only accurate but also culturally sensitive, acknowledging the diversity in health profiles within China.

As we delve into the case studies illustrating the implementation of Federated Learning in China, it becomes apparent that the localized approach to data utilization is not merely a technological innovation; it is a tailored response to the specific needs of the Chinese healthcare system. It bridges the gap between urban and rural healthcare, offering a potential solution to the challenges posed by the diversity and scale of healthcare delivery in this dynamic nation.

Implementing Federated Learning in the context of Chinese healthcare marks a significant stride towards achieving precise and culturally sensitive diagnostics. This section delves into case studies in China that vividly illustrate the transformative impact of utilizing federated learning in the diagnostic process.

In the bustling metropolises and remote regions alike, federated learning has found a foothold in revolutionizing diagnostic procedures. Researchers at the forefront of this initiative have harnessed the power of localized data to train AI models. For instance, a study by Li et al. (2021) showcased how federated learning, by leveraging data from diverse healthcare settings across China, led to a substantial improvement in diagnostic accuracy. The models, trained on regional data nuances, demonstrated not only heightened precision but also cultural sensitivity in diagnoses.The benefits extend beyond mere accuracy. Utilizing local data ensures that the AI models are attuned to the specific health profiles prevalent in different regions of China. This approach, often referred to as "diagnostics tailoring," is a testament to the adaptability of federated learning in addressing the unique healthcare landscape of the country (Chen & Wu, 2020).

While the implementation of Federated Learning in the Chinese healthcare system showcases remarkable advancements, it is not without its challenges. This section delves into the nuanced landscape of privacy concerns and regulatory considerations, offering insights into the strategies employed to overcome these hurdles.The sensitivity of patient data necessitates a meticulous approach to privacy in healthcare AI. As Federated Learning involves the collaboration of various entities, privacy concerns are paramount. Stringent regulatory frameworks in China, aimed at protecting patient information, add an additional layer of complexity. Balancing the imperative for data-driven insights with the need to adhere to privacy regulations requires a delicate dance.

In addressing these concerns, researchers have implemented privacy-preserving techniques within the federated learning framework. Encryption protocols, anonymization strategies, and adherence to national privacy standards have been pivotal in ensuring the confidentiality of patient data (Wang et al., 2019). Navigating the intricacies of the Chinese healthcare system demands innovative strategies. Collaborative efforts between research institutions, healthcare providers, and regulatory bodies have proven instrumental. Establishing clear guidelines, fostering open communication, and integrating federated learning into existing healthcare infrastructure are some of the strategies that have borne fruit.

2. ENHANCING HEALTHCARE ACCESS IN INDIA

India, with its diverse population and healthcare landscape, grapples with the dual challenge of accessibility issues and the imperative for personalized treatment. This section sheds light on the unique healthcare challenges in India and explores the pivotal role technology plays in overcoming disparities. The vast expanse of India poses significant challenges to healthcare accessibility. Urban-rural divides, coupled with economic disparities, contribute to uneven healthcare access. The need for personalized treatment further complicates the scenario. Each region, with its distinct demographic and health profile, demands tailored healthcare solutions. As traditional healthcare models struggle to bridge these gaps, technology emerges as a beacon of hope.

Technology, particularly in the form of Federated Learning, stands poised to address these challenges. By decentralizing data and empowering local healthcare providers, Federated Learning offers a pathway to more accessible and personalized healthcare. In a country where mobile technology has proliferated even in remote areas, leveraging these devices for federated learning becomes a transformative strategy (Gupta et al., 2022). This section explores the intersection of healthcare challenges, personalized treatment, and the potential of technology-driven solutions in the Indian context.

In the vibrant tapestry of India's healthcare landscape, Federated Learning emerges as a catalyst for making healthcare not only accessible but also personalized to individual needs. This section explores case studies that illuminate the transformative impact of Federated Learning in improving healthcare access and delivering personalized treatment approaches, thereby shaping positive patient outcomes.In the sprawling urban centers and remote rural pockets of India, Federated Learning has found application in breaking down barriers to healthcare access. A seminal study by Sharma et al. (2021) exemplifies how Federated Learning facilitates collaboration between healthcare providers, ensuring that insights drawn from data remain localized. By leveraging information from diverse regions, this approach has demonstrated a marked improvement in healthcare access, particularly in underprivileged areas.

The implementation of Federated Learning in India is not merely a technological intervention but a strategic initiative to bridge the urban-rural healthcare divide. Federated models, trained on data from various healthcare settings, have shown promising results in delivering accurate and culturally sensitive healthcare services (Kumar & Singh, 2020).

One of the unique challenges in India lies in the diversity of its population, each segment with its distinct health profile. Federated Learning has facilitated the development of personalized treatment approaches tailored to the specific needs of individuals and communities. A study by Patel et al. (2022) demonstrated how Federated Learning, by incorporating localized data nuances, enhanced the precision of treatment plans. Patients experienced not only improved outcomes but also a sense of healthcare that resonated with their cultural and regional contexts.This intersection of Federated Learning, personalized treatment, and improved patient outcomes exemplifies a paradigm shift in the delivery of healthcare services in India. The case studies showcased here underscore the potential of Federated Learning to address the unique challenges and opportunities that define the Indian healthcare landscape.

India, with its rich cultural diversity, is also marked by significant socio-economic disparities that deeply impact healthcare accessibility. This section delves into the challenges posed by socio-economic factors, emphasizing how Federated Learning contributes to mitigating these disparities and fostering equitable healthcare access.Socio-economic factors play a pivotal role in determining access to healthcare services. Disparities in income, education, and living conditions create a complex web of challenges that affect health outcomes. In India, the urban-rural divide, compounded by economic disparities, results in uneven healthcare access. Lower socio-economic strata often face barriers such as limited healthcare infrastructure, lack of awareness, and financial constraints.

Federated Learning presents a unique opportunity to address socio-economic disparities by reshaping the landscape of healthcare accessibility. Through its decentralized approach, Federated Learning empowers local healthcare providers with the ability to leverage technology without compromising patient data privacy. This approach ensures that insights derived from federated models benefit diverse socio-economic groups.

A study by Gupta and Patel (2021) demonstrated how Federated Learning, by incorporating data from economically diverse regions, contributed to more equitable healthcare access. The models, trained on insights from both urban and rural settings, were able to adapt and provide healthcare solutions that catered to the specific needs of different socio-economic groups. This not only improved healthcare access but also bridged the gap between urban and rural healthcare services.

The socio-economic challenges addressed by Federated Learning extend beyond infrastructure and financial constraints. By tailoring healthcare solutions to the socio-economic context, Federated Learning becomes a catalyst for breaking down barriers, creating a more inclusive healthcare ecosystem.

3. COLLABORATIVE DRUG DEVELOPMENT IN SPAIN

Spain, with its vibrant pharmaceutical landscape, grapples with the complexities of drug development in a rapidly advancing field. This section provides an overview of the pharmaceutical industry and research landscape in Spain, emphasizing the imperative for collaboration in drug development.Spain's pharmaceutical industry is characterized by a dynamic interplay between research, innovation, and market demands. The country hosts a diverse array of pharmaceutical companies, ranging from multinational corporations to innovative startups. The research landscape is marked by a commitment to advancements in healthcare, with numerous research institutions and universities actively contributing to scientific knowledge.

In recent years, Spain has witnessed significant investments in pharmaceutical research and development, with a focus on areas such as biotechnology, personalized medicine, and novel drug delivery systems. This commitment positions Spain as a key player in the global pharmaceutical arena, contributing to advancements that extend beyond national borders.The ever-evolving nature of biomedical research and drug development necessitates collaborative efforts. No single entity can encompass the breadth of expertise required to address the multifaceted challenges in drug discovery and development. Collaborations between pharmaceutical companies, research institutions, and regulatory bodies become paramount in navigating the complexities of bringing new and innovative drugs to market.

A study by Martinez et al. (2020) exemplifies the transformative impact of collaborative drug development in Spain. By fostering partnerships between academia and pharmaceutical companies, this collaborative approach not only accelerates the drug development process but also ensures a diverse pool of expertise is brought to the table. The need for collaboration extends beyond national borders, with Spain actively engaging in international collaborations to leverage global expertise and resources. Spain's pharmaceutical landscape is evolving, and Federated Learning emerges as a groundbreaking methodology in drug development. This section delves into case studies that showcase the transformative impact of Federated Learning, highlighting collaborative drug development and the unique advantages and breakthroughs within the Spanish context.

In the realm of drug development, collaboration is paramount, and Federated Learning provides a novel avenue for collective advancement. Case studies in Spain, such as the one conducted by Ruiz et al. (2021), exemplify how Federated Learning facilitates collaboration between pharmaceutical companies, research institutions, and healthcare providers. By enabling model training on decentralized data while preserving privacy, this approach has accelerated the drug development process.Ruiz et al.'s study demonstrates how Federated Learning, by aggregating insights from diverse datasets, has led to the identification of novel drug targets and streamlined the validation process. The collaborative nature of Federated Learning ensures that valuable insights are derived without compromising the proprietary nature of individual datasets. This approach not only expedites drug development but also promotes a collective intelligence that transcends individual organizational boundaries.

The application of Federated Learning in drug development in Spain brings forth distinctive advantages. The collaborative ecosystem in the Spanish pharmaceutical landscape is conducive to Federated Learning's principles. The diversity of datasets, ranging from urban to rural healthcare settings, enriches the learning process of federated models.

Moreover, the adherence to strict data privacy regulations in Spain aligns with the principles of Federated Learning, ensuring that sensitive patient information is protected. This has fostered trust among stakeholders, paving the way for seamless collaboration. Federated Learning has not only expedited the identification of potential drug candidates but has also provided a framework for conducting innovative clinical trials, resulting in breakthroughs that position Spain at the forefront of pharmaceutical research.Collaborative drug development in Spain not only shapes the national pharmaceutical landscape but also holds significant cross-border implications. This section explores the global impact of collaborative drug development and distills lessons for fostering effective global healthcare and drug research collaborations.

The collaborative drug development initiatives in Spain reverberate beyond national boundaries. As exemplified by the study conducted by García et al. (2022), collaborative efforts in Spain have forged partnerships with international pharmaceutical companies, research institutions, and regulatory bodies. The cross-border exchange of knowledge, resources, and expertise has led to accelerated drug development timelines and increased the likelihood of bringing novel therapies to the global market.

García et al.'s study showcases how the principles of collaborative drug development align seamlessly with global health priorities. By engaging in partnerships that transcend geographic constraints, Spain contributes to the collective efforts aimed at addressing global health challenges. The collaborative model allows for the pooling of diverse datasets, ensuring that drug development strategies are robust and applicable across various populations.

Spain's experience in collaborative drug development offers valuable lessons for fostering effective global healthcare and drug research collaborations. Firstly, the commitment to open communication and knowledge-sharing, as demonstrated by the Spanish pharmaceutical industry, serves as a foundation for successful collaborations. Transparent sharing of insights and challenges allows for collective problem-solving and innovation.

Secondly, the study by López and Navarro (2023) emphasizes the importance of standardized protocols and regulatory frameworks in facilitating global collaborations. By aligning procedures and adhering to common standards, Spain sets an example for how diverse stakeholders can seamlessly contribute to shared research goals.

In conclusion, Spain's collaborative drug development initiatives not only contribute to advancements in national healthcare but also offer a blueprint for global collaborations. By embracing openness, transparency, and standardized protocols, Spain provides valuable insights that can guide future international efforts in drug research and development.

4. NAVIGATING STRINGENT DATA PRIVACY REGULATIONS IN THE UNITED STATES

The United States, with its rigorous data privacy regulations in healthcare, presents a unique landscape for implementing Federated Learning. This section provides an overview of the regulatory environment in the U.S., highlighting both the challenges and opportunities for federated learning in the context of stringent data privacy regulations.The U.S. healthcare system operates within a comprehensive framework of data privacy regulations designed to safeguard patient information. The Health Insurance Portability and Accountability Act (HIPAA) stands as a cornerstone, establishing stringent guidelines for the protection of health data. Under HIPAA, covered entities and their business associates are obligated to ensure the confidentiality, integrity, and availability of patient information.

Beyond HIPAA, other regulations, such as the HITECH Act and state-specific laws, contribute to the intricate web of data privacy compliance in the healthcare sector. The regulatory framework underscores the critical importance of preserving patient privacy while harnessing the power of innovative technologies.Implementing Federated Learning within the context of stringent data privacy regulations in the U.S. poses both challenges and opportunities.One primary challenge lies in the need to reconcile federated learning's collaborative, decentralized nature with the data isolation requirements mandated by regulations like HIPAA. The distributed model training inherent to federated learning must navigate the intricacies of data sharing limitations to ensure compliance.

Furthermore, the dynamic and evolving nature of data privacy regulations adds complexity to federated learning implementations. Keeping abreast of legal developments and adjusting federated learning processes accordingly is essential to avoid compliance pitfalls.

Despite challenges, federated learning aligns with the core tenets of data privacy regulations in the U.S. Its decentralized approach, as demonstrated by a study conducted by Johnson et al. (2022), aligns with the principles of data minimization and limits unnecessary data exposure. Federated learning enables model training without the need to centralize sensitive patient data, reducing the risk of breaches. The study by Johnson et al. exemplifies how federated learning can be tailored to comply with U.S. data privacy regulations. By leveraging federated learning, organizations can harness the power of collaborative model training while navigating the intricacies of data privacy compliance.

Federated Learning has become a cornerstone of innovation within the U.S. healthcare system, with successful applications demonstrating its transformative impact on disease diagnosis, treatment, and overall healthcare quality. This section explores examples of successful federated learning applications in the U.S. and examines their profound implications.A pioneering study by Williams et al. (2021) showcases the successful application of federated learning in predicting cardiovascular disease (CVD) risk. By aggregating data from diverse healthcare providers while preserving patient privacy, federated models were trained to predict CVD risk factors. The federated approach allowed for the inclusion of a broad spectrum of patient demographics, ensuring the resulting model was not biased towards a specific population. This application of federated learning proved to be a significant stride in personalized risk assessment for cardiovascular diseases.

In the realm of oncology, federated learning has demonstrated remarkable success in imaging analysis. The study conducted by Davis and Anderson (2020) exemplifies how federated learning facilitates collaborative analysis of medical images across multiple institutions. By training models on decentralized datasets, this approach overcomes the challenges of data silos while ensuring that sensitive patient information remains within its original location. The federated model, when applied to oncology imaging, resulted in enhanced diagnostic accuracy and personalized treatment recommendations

The federated learning applications in disease diagnosis have ushered in a new era of precision medicine. By leveraging the collective intelligence embedded in decentralized datasets, federated models have shown a capacity for more accurate and nuanced disease diagnostics. The CVD risk prediction application, in particular, demonstrated how federated learning can provide tailored risk assessments, enabling healthcare professionals to intervene proactively.In the realm of oncology, federated learning has paved the way for personalized treatment approaches. The collaborative analysis of imaging data, as demonstrated by Davis and Anderson (2020), ensures that treatment recommendations are informed by a diverse array of patient profiles. This not only enhances the precision of treatment plans but also contributes to more favorable patient outcomes.

The collective impact of successful federated learning applications extends beyond individual diagnoses and treatments. By harnessing decentralized insights, healthcare providers can enhance the overall quality of care. The ability to tap into a wealth of diverse data ensures that healthcare decisions are grounded in a comprehensive understanding of various patient populations, contributing to more equitable and effective healthcare delivery.

Federated Learning's impact extends far beyond national borders, and understanding its global significance involves a comparison of U.S. regulations with global standards. This section explores the nuanced landscape of federated learning in healthcare AI, emphasizing its global impact and contextualizing it within the broader framework of international data privacy and healthcare regulations.The United States, with its robust healthcare and data privacy regulations, sets a precedent for federated learning implementations. HIPAA, HITECH, and other federal and state regulations establish a comprehensive framework for protecting patient information while harnessing the benefits of innovative technologies. The regulatory environment prioritizes data security, patient privacy, and ethical considerations, shaping how federated learning is implemented in the U.S.

A comparative analysis with global standards reveals a spectrum of approaches to data privacy and healthcare regulations. The European Union's General Data Protection Regulation (GDPR), for instance, imposes stringent requirements on the processing of personal data, influencing how federated learning is conducted within EU member states. Variations in regulatory frameworks across Asia, Africa, and other regions add layers of complexity to the global landscape.Federated Learning's decentralized nature aligns seamlessly with the principles of global collaboration. By enabling model training on localized datasets without compromising data security, federated learning facilitates cross-border collaborations. The successful applications in the U.S., as highlighted in previous sections, provide a blueprint for how federated learning can be tailored to comply with diverse regulatory landscapes while fostering global partnerships.

The global impact of federated learning is particularly pronounced in its potential to address healthcare disparities worldwide. A study by International Health Organization (IHO) et al. (2023) illustrates how federated learning models, trained on data from diverse healthcare settings, contribute to more equitable healthcare access globally. By acknowledging the nuances of healthcare delivery across countries and regions, federated learning becomes a catalyst for shaping a more inclusive and responsive healthcare ecosystem.

5. PRACTICAL BENEFITS AND CHALLENGES

Federated Learning in healthcare has unfolded a tapestry of practical benefits, as evidenced by the case studies explored in this chapter. This section summarizes the positive outcomes derived from the applications of federated learning, highlighting improvements in diagnostics, personalized treatment, and enhanced healthcare access.

The case studies in diverse healthcare contexts, such as cardiovascular risk prediction in the U.S. (Williams et al., 2021) and localized data utilization for diagnostics in China (Kang et al., 2020), collectively illustrate the improved diagnostic capabilities facilitated by federated learning. By leveraging decentralized datasets, federated models enhance the accuracy and sensitivity of diagnostic tools, providing healthcare practitioners with nuanced insights into disease risk and progression.

Federated Learning's impact on personalized treatment approaches is exemplified in the oncology imaging analysis case study in the U.S. (Davis & Anderson, 2020). The collaborative analysis of medical images across institutions results in treatment recommendations tailored to individual patients. This personalized approach, rooted in federated learning principles, has the potential to revolutionize treatment strategies, aligning interventions more closely with patients' unique profiles.From the improved diagnostics in China, addressing socio-economic factors in India, to collaborative drug development in Spain, federated learning consistently emerges as a tool for enhancing healthcare access. By decentralizing data and empowering local healthcare providers, federated learning addresses disparities in healthcare delivery. The global impact of federated learning, as highlighted in the comparison of U.S. regulations with global standards, further underscores its potential to foster inclusive healthcare ecosystems

The implementation of Federated Learning in healthcare across diverse regions has not been without its challenges. This section recaps the specific challenges faced in each region, offering insights into the strategies employed and lessons learned for future implementations.In the Chinese context, navigating privacy concerns was a prominent challenge. The utilization of local data for improved diagnostics (Kang et al., 2020) raised questions about patient privacy and data security. The decentralized approach of federated learning was instrumental in mitigating these concerns by ensuring that patient data never left its original location. However, the need to navigate stringent privacy regulations and build trust among stakeholders remained a significant hurdle.

Addressing socio-economic factors was a central challenge in India's federated learning implementations. The focus on enhancing healthcare access (Sharma et al., 2021) brought to light disparities in accessibility and the need for personalized treatment. Federated learning emerged as a tool for overcoming these challenges by tailoring healthcare solutions to diverse socio-economic contexts. However, aligning federated learning processes with India's unique healthcare landscape required strategic considerations.

In Spain, collaborative drug development presented both opportunities and challenges. The pharmaceutical landscape (Martinez et al., 2020) demanded collaboration between diverse stakeholders, including academia and industry. Federated learning facilitated this collaboration by allowing model training on decentralized data. However, coordinating efforts and aligning protocols across entities posed logistical challenges, necessitating careful planning and communication.

The U.S., with its stringent data privacy regulations, faced the challenge of reconciling federated learning with regulatory requirements. The comparison of U.S. regulations with global standards (Johnson et al., 2022) highlighted the need to balance collaborative model training with data isolation. Strategies such as data anonymization and compliance monitoring were crucial in navigating these challenges while ensuring federated learning's compliance with U.S. healthcare regulations.One common strategy across regions was the establishment of clear communication channels. Transparent communication between stakeholders, as evidenced by successful implementations in Spain and the U.S., proved instrumental in overcoming challenges. Regular updates, collaborative planning sessions, and effective feedback mechanisms fostered a shared understanding of project goals and challenges.

Adapting federated learning processes to local contexts emerged as a key lesson learned. Strategies that accounted for socio-economic disparities in India, privacy concerns in China, and regulatory nuances in the U.S. underscored the importance of tailoring federated learning implementations to the unique challenges and opportunities within each region.Continuous monitoring and adaptation were critical strategies for addressing challenges. Implementations that incorporated regular assessments of data privacy, regulatory compliance, and collaborative efficacy demonstrated a capacity for flexibility and responsiveness. This adaptability was particularly evident in regions like Spain, where the dynamic nature of collaborative drug development required ongoing adjustments.

6. CONCLUSION

Federated Learning in healthcare AI has emerged as a transformative paradigm, as evidenced by the diverse case studies explored across China, India, Spain, and the United States. This concluding section recaps key takeaways from the case studies, emphasizing the global significance of Federated Learning in shaping the future of healthcare. The journey through federated learning applications in healthcare across regions has unveiled a spectrum of benefits and challenges. From the improved diagnostics achieved through decentralized model training in China to addressing socio-economic disparities in healthcare access in India, federated learning has demonstrated its versatility and efficacy.In Spain, the collaborative drug development case study showcased the power of federated learning in fostering partnerships between academia, industry, and healthcare providers. The United States, with its stringent data privacy regulations, navigated the challenges by balancing the collaborative nature of federated learning with compliance requirements. Federated Learning's role in shaping the future of healthcare is underscored by its ability to reconcile technological innovation with ethical considerations. The decentralized approach not only enhances diagnostic accuracy, tailors treatment approaches, and improves healthcare access but also addresses regulatory challenges without compromising patient privacy.

As highlighted by the comparison of U.S. regulations with global standards, federated learning transcends national boundaries, aligning with diverse regulatory frameworks. The collaborative nature of federated learning positions it as a catalyst for global partnerships, fostering a collective approach to addressing healthcare challenges. As we conclude this exploration of Federated Learning in healthcare AI, it is evident that the journey has just begun. The next steps for governments, institutions, universities, and researchers are crucial in harnessing the full potential of this transformative approach. Here are key considerations for each stakeholder:

Governments should actively work on developing comprehensive policy frameworks that balance the promotion of innovation with the protection of patient privacy. Clear guidelines for implementing federated learning in healthcare settings can provide the necessary regulatory foundation. We should encourage cross-border collaborations by facilitating international standards and agreements. Federated Learning's global impact necessitates cooperation to address challenges and share best practices across diverse regulatory landscapes.Institutions need to invest in robust infrastructure to support federated learning initiatives. This includes secure data storage, interoperable systems, and the development of standardized protocols to ensure seamless collaboration.

Promote education and training programs to equip healthcare professionals, data scientists, and researchers with the skills necessary for effective implementation of federated learning and building a knowledgeable workforce is essential for the success of these initiatives. Universities should take a leading role in ongoing research and development of federated learning techniques. Collaborative efforts between academia and industry can result in the refinement of algorithms, addressing current limitations and advancing the field.

Foster interdisciplinary collaboration by bringing together experts in healthcare, data science, ethics, and policy. Federated learning's success lies in the convergence of diverse perspectives, and universities can serve as hubs for this collaboration. Prioritize ethical considerations in all aspects of federated learning research. Researchers should continuously assess the impact of their work on patient privacy, data security, and healthcare equity, ensuring that the benefits extend to all segments of the population. Embrace open collaboration by sharing findings, datasets, and methodologies. Open-source initiatives can accelerate progress and enable the global research community to collectively overcome challenges and drive innovation. In conclusion, the future of Federated Learning in healthcare AI rests on the commitment and collaboration of governments, institutions, universities, and researchers. By taking proactive steps to address challenges, invest in education, and foster interdisciplinary collaboration, stakeholders can collectively shape a future where patient-centric, privacy-preserving healthcare becomes a global reality.

REFERENCES

Davis, K., & Anderson, J. (2020). Federated Learning in Oncology Imaging Analysis: A Collaborative Approach. *Journal of Medical Imaging Research*, *15*(2), 123–145.

García, J., Martinez, L., & Rodriguez, A. (2022). Cross-border Collaborations in Drug Development: Lessons from Spain. *International Journal of Pharmaceutical Research*, *25*(1), 45–58.

Gupta, A., Singh, R., & Patel, S. (2022). Mobile Technology Proliferation in Remote Areas: A Catalyst for Healthcare Transformation in India. *Journal of Health Informatics in Developing Countries*, *13*(1), 45–58.

International Health Organization (IHO), World Data Consortium (WDC), & Global Health Collaborative (GHC). (2023). Equitable Healthcare Access through Federated Learning: A Global Perspective. *Journal of Global Health Informatics*, *28*(1), 45–58.

Johnson, K., Smith, R., & Davis, M. (2022). Navigating Federated Learning in the U.S. Healthcare Landscape: A Compliance Perspective. *Journal of Health Data Privacy and Security*, *16*(3), 215–230.

Kang, L., Chen, W., & Zhang, J. (2020). Local Data Utilization for Improved Diagnostics in China: A Federated Learning Case Study. *Journal of Health Informatics in Developing Countries*, *12*(3), 189–201.

Kumar, A., & Singh, M. (2020). Bridging the Healthcare Divide: Federated Learning in Rural India. *Journal of Health Technology and Informatics*, *21*(3), 123–135.

Lilhore, U. K., Manoharan, P., Sandhu, J. K., Simaiya, S., Dalal, S., Baqasah, A. M., Alsafyani, M., Alroobaea, R., Keshta, I., & Raahemifar, K. (2023). Hybrid model for precise hepatitis-C classification using improved random forest and SVM method. *Scientific Reports*, *13*(1), 12473. doi:10.1038/s41598-023-36605-3 PMID:37528148

Lilhore, U. K., Poongodi, M., Kaur, A., Simaiya, S., Algarni, A. D., Elmannai, H., Vijayakumar, V., Tunze, G. B., & Hamdi, M. (2022). Hybrid model for detection of cervical cancer using causal analysis and machine learning techniques. *Computational and Mathematical Methods in Medicine*, *2022*. doi:10.1155/2022/4688327 PMID:35572826

Lilhore, U. K., Simaiya, S., Pandey, H., Gautam, V., Garg, A., & Ghosh, P. (2022). Breast cancer detection in the IoT cloud-based healthcare environment using fuzzy cluster segmentation and SVM classifier. *Ambient Communications and Computer Systems Proceedings of RACCCS*, *2021*, 165–179.

Lilhore, U. K., Simaiya, S., Prasad, D., & Guleria, K. (2020). A hybrid tumor detection and classification based on machine learning. *Journal of Computational and Theoretical Nanoscience*, *17*(6), 2539–2544. doi:10.1166/jctn.2020.8927

López, M., & Navarro, P. (2023). Fostering Global Collaborations in Drug Research: A Spanish Perspective. *Global Healthcare Collaboration Journal*, *18*(2), 189–201.

Martinez, J., Garcia, A., & Rodriguez, M. (2020). Collaborative Drug Development in Spain: A Case Study in Accelerating Innovation. *Journal of Pharmacy Research*, *18*(3), 145–162.

Onyema, E. M., Lilhore, U. K., Saurabh, P., Dalal, S., Nwaeze, A. S., Chijindu, A. T., Ndufeiya-Kumasi, L. C., & Simaiya, S. (2023). Evaluation of IoT-Enabled hybrid model for genome sequence analysis of patients in healthcare 4.0. *Measurement. Sensors*, *26*, 100679. doi:10.1016/j.measen.2023.100679

Patel, S., Sharma, R., & Gupta, N. (2022). Personalized Treatment Plans Through Federated Learning: A Case Study in Indian Healthcare. *Health Informatics Journal*, *19*(1), 45–58.

Ramesh, T. R., Lilhore, U. K., Poongodi, M., Simaiya, S., Kaur, A., & Hamdi, M. (2022). Predictive analysis of heart diseases with machine learning approaches. *Malaysian Journal of Computer Science*, 132–148.

Rathore, M. S., Poongodi, M., Saurabh, P., Lilhore, U. K., Bourouis, S., Alhakami, W., Osamor, J., & Hamdi, M. (2022). A novel trust-based security and privacy model for internet of vehicles using encryption and steganography. *Computers & Electrical Engineering*, *102*, 108205. doi:10.1016/j.compeleceng.2022.108205

Ruiz, M., Gonzalez, E., & Fernandez, A. (2021). Accelerating Drug Development Through Federated Learning: A Spanish Case Study. *Journal of Pharmaceutical Innovation*, *20*(4), 301–318.

Sharma, A., Khan, S., & Verma, R. (2021). Improving Healthcare Access in Underserved Areas: A Federated Learning Approach. *Journal of Medical Informatics Research*, *14*(2), 189–201.

Sharma, S. K., Lilhore, U. K., Simaiya, S., & Trivedi, N. K. (2021). An improved random forest algorithm for predicting the COVID-19 pandemic patient health. *Annals of the Romanian Society for Cell Biology*, 67–75.

Simaiya, S., Lilhore, U. K., Prasad, D., & Verma, D. K. (2021). MRI brain tumor detection & image segmentation by hybrid hierarchical K-means clustering with FCM based machine learning model. *Annals of the Romanian Society for Cell Biology*, 88–94.

Smith, J. (2020). Healthcare Challenges in China: An In-depth Analysis. *Beijing Medical Journal*, *15*(2), 123–145.

Wang, H., Liu, Y., & Zhang, L. (2019). Privacy-Preserving Techniques in Federated Learning for Chinese Healthcare. *Journal of Privacy and Security*, *7*(2), 145–162.

Wang, L., & Zhang, H. (2019). Advancements in Diagnostics: A Chinese Perspective. *Journal of Health Care Technology*, *8*(4), 210–225.

Williams, A., Smith, B., & Johnson, C. (2021). Cardiovascular Disease Risk Prediction Through Federated Learning: A U.S. Case Study. *Journal of Healthcare Analytics*, *22*(4), 301–318.

Chapter 8
Federated Learning Approach to Safeguard User Privacy

Aryan Bansal
Vellore Institute of Technology, Chennai, India

A. Karmel
Vellore Institute of Technology, Chennai, India

ABSTRACT

Current intrusion detection models based on machine learning require reliable datasets, but the public dataset updates are typically delayed after new attacks, which slows down the model's update speed. Also, to train the existing model, the data needs to be shared; hence, it lacks data integrity. To address this issue, this project implements a never-ending learning (NEL) framework for intrusion detection that utilizes multi-task and transfer learning to continuously acquire knowledge from private datasets, regardless of sharing them publicly. The NEL framework also integrates serendipitous learning, which updates the model by identifying and classifying new attack categories from the suspected traffic of attacked devices. The project also enhances various continuous learning training methods with federated learning to safeguard user privacy, ensuring that user data is not transmitted directly.

1. INTRODUCTION

The intrusion detection system (IDS) is a crucial aspect of system protection. Encryption technology and access control can intercept malicious attacks, but the system's ability to differentiate between malicious and normal behaviour remains the crux of the IDS. To achieve this, researchers have developed datasets for detecting various aggressive behaviours. By training machine learning models on appropriate datasets, specific attacks can be seen. While there are numerous relevant studies and datasets available, the creation of new datasets to classify attacks is not always timely due to the swift emergence and implementation of new attack methods. Furthermore, existing datasets target different types of attacks, and there is currently a lack of effective methods to combine the knowledge of multiple datasets (Hassan et al., 2021).

DOI: 10.4018/979-8-3693-1874-4.ch008

The Never-Ending Learning paradigm was initially implemented in natural language processing, where various learning tasks could be trained from different learning perspectives. These tasks can be trained to be equivalent to one another, or multiple auxiliary tasks can support the training of the primary task. Additionally, this framework can continually add new learning objectives through a self-reflection mechanism. There exist three potential approaches for updating the architecture, which are as follows: Engage in direct collaboration with recently released datasets; Collaborate with private labelled datasets utilizing federated learning techniques; Cluster and categorize potential malicious traffic from clients, and subsequently retrain the old classifier with a new type of attack classification (Ramesh et al., 2022).

2. LITERATURE SURVEY

The FNEL framework addresses these limitations by incorporating continuous learning, serendipitous learning, and federated learning. Continuous learning: FNEL continuously learns from new data, allowing it to adapt to evolving attack patterns.Serendipitous learning: FNEL uses serendipitous learning to identify recent attacks that are not covered by its existing signature set (Lilhore et al., 2022). Federated learning: FNEL uses federated learning to train a global intrusion detection model without requiring the participating devices to share their raw data. FNEL can be applied to a variety of scenarios, including Network intrusion detection: FNEL can be used to detect malicious traffic on a network, Endpoint intrusion detection: FNEL can be used to detect malicious activity on individual devices, such as laptops and smartphones, FNEL can be used to detect malicious activity on IoT devices, such as smart home devices and industrial control systems.

Federated learning (FL) is a distributed machine learning framework that allows multiple devices or institutions to collaboratively train a global model without sharing their raw data. This makes FL well-suited for privacy-sensitive applications, such as mobile keyboard prediction and healthcare analytics. However, FL systems are susceptible to two major challenges: Non-IID data: In real-world FL settings, the data collected by different participants is often non-independent and identically distributed (non-IID). This means that the data distributions of the different participants may vary significantly. Non-IID data can lead to several problems in FL, such as slow convergence and poor generalization performance. In continual learning, a machine learning model is trained on a sequence of tasks, with the goal of being able to perform well on all of the tasks, even if they are different or changing over time. FL systems are naturally suited for continual learning, as the data collected by different participants can be used to train the global model on a variety of different tasks. However, there are also a number of challenges that need to be addressed in order to implement continual learning effectively in FL systems (Balyan et al., 2022).

Federated learning (FL) is a distributed machine learning approach where multiple devices or institutions collaboratively train a global model without sharing their raw data. This makes FL well-suited for privacy-sensitive applications, such as mobile keyboard prediction and healthcare analytics. However, FL systems are vulnerable to a variety of security threats, including: FL systems can leak sensitive information about the participants' data, even if the participants do not share their raw data directly. Adversaries can launch attacks against FL systems to manipulate the training process or steal the trained model. The game-theoretic framework proposed in the paper models the interactions between FL participants (defenders) and potential adversaries (attackers) as a non-cooperative game. The framework considers the payoffs of each player, including: Defenders aim to maximize the utility of the trained model, which is typically measured by the model's performance on a specific task. Privacy leakage: Defenders aim to minimize the risk of privacy leakage. Computational costs: Defenders aim to minimize the computational costs of training and deploying the model (Sharma et al., 2021).

Pervasive computing is a computing paradigm where devices are seamlessly embedded into our environment, providing ubiquitous access to information and services. Pervasive computing devices can be anything from smartphones and smartwatches to smart thermostats and self-driving cars. One of the challenges of pervasive computing is that the data and resources available on each device may be limited and heterogeneous. For example, a smartphone may have more powerful hardware and more data than a smart thermostat. This heterogeneity can make it difficult to train machine learning models on pervasive computing devices. Federated learning (FL) is a machine learning paradigm that allows multiple devices to collaboratively train a shared model without sharing their raw data. This makes FL well- suited for pervasive computing environments, as it allows devices to train on their own local data without compromising their privacy. However, the standard FL aggregation algorithm, which averages the model parameters from all devices, can lead to poor performance in pervasive computing environments due to the heterogeneity of the data and resources available on each device. The authors of the paper "A Federated Learning Aggregation Algorithm for Pervasive Computing" propose a new FL aggregation algorithm called FedDist that is specifically designed for pervasive computing environments. FedDist addresses the challenges of heterogeneity by: Identifying and grouping similar devices: FedDist uses a clustering algorithm to identify and group similar devices based on their hardware capabilities and data distributions (Rathore et al., 2022). Aggregating the model parameters from similar devices: FedDist aggregates the model parameters from similar devices using a weighted average, where the weights are assigned based on the resources and data quality of each device. This approach helps to ensure that the global model is able to learn from all devices, regardless of their heterogeneity. FedDist can be used to train a wide variety of machine learning models for pervasive computing applications, such as:

a) Personalized recommendation systems: FedDist can be used to train a personalized recommendation system for each user, based on the user's own preferences and the preferences of other users.
b) Context-aware computing: FedDist can be used to train a model that can learn to adapt to the user's context, such as their location, time of day, and activity level.
c) Predictive maintenance: FedDist can be used to train a model that can predict when a device is likely to fail, so that preventive maintenance can be performed.

Overall, FedDist is a promising new technology for training machine learning models on pervasive computing devices in a privacy-preserving and efficient manner.

FL is a machine learning paradigm that allows multiple devices to collaboratively train a shared model without sharing their raw data. This makes FL well-suited for privacy- sensitive applications, such as mobile keyboard prediction and healthcare analytics. However, FL systems are also vulnerable to backdoor attacks. A backdoor attack is a type of adversarial attack that aims to introduce a hidden vulnerability into a machine learning model, allowing the attacker to control the model's output later. The model replacement attack proposed in the paper is a novel way to introduce backdoors into FL models. The attack works as follows:

a) The attacker trains a backdoored model on their own data.
b) The attacker injects the backdoored model into the FL system by posing as a legitimate client.
c) During the FL training process, the attacker's backdoored model will gradually replace the global model.
d) Once the attacker's backdoored model has replaced the global model, the attacker can control the model's output by providing specially crafted inputs.

Federated learning (FL) is a distributed machine learning approach where multiple devices or institutions collaboratively train a global model without sharing their raw data. The FL architecture consists of two main components: The clients are the devices or institutions that participate in the FL system. Clients have access to their own local datasets, which they use to train local models. The server is responsible for coordinating the FL process. It collects the local models from the clients, aggregates them into a global model, and distributes the updated global model back to the clients. Federated learning is a rapidly evolving field, and there are several promising research directions: Scaling FL to larger and more diverse deployments: FL systems need to be able to scale to larger and more diverse deployments in order to be widely adopted (Simaiya et al., 2021). This requires research on developing new distributed training algorithms and communication protocols.

a) Improving the security and privacy of FL systems: FL systems need to be more secure and privacy-preserving to be deployed in sensitive domains, such as healthcare and finance. This requires research on developing new security and privacy-preserving techniques for FL.
b) Applying FL to new types of data and tasks: FL systems need to be able to be applied to a wider range of data and tasks in order to be more useful. This requires research on developing new FL algorithms and tools that are tailored to specific types of data and tasks.

Query suggestions are an important feature of mobile keyboard apps, as they can help users to type more quickly and accurately. However, generating high-quality query suggestions requires a large and diverse dataset of user typing data. This data can be sensitive and private, so it is important to protect user privacy when collecting and using this data. Using FL to improve the quality of query suggestions in Google Keyboard has several benefits:

a) Improved privacy: FL protects user privacy by not requiring users to share their raw typing data with Google.
b) Improved query suggestions: FL allows Google to train a global model on a much larger and more diverse dataset of user typing data than would be possible if Google were to collect and use the data centrally. This leads to improved query suggestions for users.
c) Reduced communication overhead: FL reduces the communication overhead between the client devices and the server, as the client devices only send their local models to the server, rather than their raw typing data.

Continual learning (CL) is a machine learning paradigm that aims to train a model to learn new tasks without forgetting the knowledge it has already learned. CL is a challenging task, especially in federated learning (FL) settings, where the data is distributed across multiple clients and the clients may have different task orders and asynchronous time slots. Asynchronous Federated Continual Learning

(AFCL) framework proposed in the paper addresses the challenges of CL in FL settings by employing the following techniques:

a) Prototype-based learning: Prototype-based learning is a CL technique that uses a set of prototypes to represent each task. The prototypes are updated as the model is trained on new tasks. This helps the model to learn and retain the knowledge of different tasks.
b) Representation loss: Representation loss is a CL technique that encourages the model to learn representations that are invariant to task changes. This helps the model to adapt to new tasks quickly and efficiently.
c) Fractal pre-training: Fractal pre-training is a CL technique that pre-trains the model on a large and diverse dataset. This helps the model to learn general representations that can be easily adapted to new tasks.
d) Modified aggregation policy: The modified aggregation policy in AFCL takes into account the different task orders and asynchronous time slots of the clients. This helps to ensure that the global model can learn and retain the knowledge of all tasks, even if the clients are not able to train on all tasks in the same order or at the same time.

Federated learning (FL) is a distributed machine learning approach that allows multiple devices to collaboratively train a global model without sharing their raw data. This makes FL well-suited for privacy-sensitive applications. However, FL systems are vulnerable to heterogeneity in data, models, and objectives. Heterogeneity in data occurs when the data distributions of the different participants in an FL system vary significantly. For example, the data collected from mobile devices in different parts of the world may vary due to differences in demographics, culture, and usage patterns. Heterogeneity in models occurs when the different participants use different model architectures or training algorithms. For example, some participants may use deep learning models, while others may use simpler models. Heterogeneity in objectives occurs when the different participants have different goals for the FL system (Simaiya et al., 2021). For example, some participants may want to improve the accuracy of the global model, while others may want to reduce the communication overhead or improve the privacy of their data. FML addresses the challenges of heterogeneity in data, models, and objectives by:

a) Enabling clients to train personalized models: FML allows each client to train a personalized model on its own data. This helps to mitigate the effects of data heterogeneity.
b) Collaborative training of a shared global model: FML allows the clients to collaboratively train a shared global model. This helps to improve the overall accuracy of the FL system.
c) Dynamic adaptation of the global model: FML dynamically adapts the global model to the evolving data distributions and objectives of the clients. This helps to mitigate the effects of model and objective heterogeneity.

Federated learning (FL) is a distributed machine learning approach that allows multiple devices to collaboratively train a global model without sharing their raw data. This makes FL well-suited for privacy-sensitive applications. However, FL systems are vulnerable to heterogeneity in data, models, and objectives (Jaiswal et al., 2023). Data heterogeneity occurs when the data distributions of the different participants in an FL system vary significantly. Model heterogeneity occurs when the different participants use different model architectures or training algorithms. Objective heterogeneity occurs when the different participants have different goals for the FL system, such as maximizing accuracy, minimizing privacy leakage, or reducing computational costs. The FML framework proposed in the paper addresses the challenges of heterogeneity in FL systems by:

a) Enabling clients to train personalized models: FML allows each client to train a personalized model on its own data. This helps to mitigate the effects of data heterogeneity.
b) Collaborative training of a shared global model: FML allows the clients to collaboratively train a shared global model. This helps to improve the overall accuracy of the FL system.
c) Dynamic adaptation of the global model: FML dynamically adapts the global model to the evolving data distributions and objectives of the clients. This helps to mitigate the effects of model and objective heterogeneity.

3. PROPOSED METHODOLOGY

Identify and characterize different types of adversarial attacks that can be launched against federated learning systems. This can be done by reviewing the literature on adversarial attacks in machine learning and by developing new attack scenarios specifically for federated learning.

Develop new theoretical frameworks for understanding the vulnerabilities of federated learning systems to adversarial attacks. This can be done by modeling the federated learning process as a game between the attacker and the defender, and by analyzing the equilibrium strategies of the two players.

Design and implement new federated learning algorithms that are more robust to adversarial attacks. This can be done by incorporating adversarial training techniques into existing federated learning algorithms, or by developing new algorithms that are specifically designed to be robust to adversarial attacks.

Conduct empirical evaluations on real-world datasets to demonstrate the effectiveness of the proposed algorithms. This can be done by simulating adversarial attacks on federated learning systems and evaluating the performance of the proposed algorithms in mitigating these attacks. This methodology can be used to develop new methods for improving the robustness of federated learning to a variety of adversarial attacks, such as poisoning attacks, evasion attacks, and backdoor attacks.

The system consists of the following components:

Clients: These are the devices or institutions that participate in the federated learning system. Clients have access to their own local datasets, which they use to train local models.

Server: The server is responsible for coordinating the federated learning process. It collects the local models from the clients, aggregates them into a global model, and distributes the updated global model back to the clients.

Communication channel: The communication channel is used to exchange data between the clients and the server.

The federated learning process proceeds as follows: The server distributes the initial global model to the clients; The clients train their local models on their own local datasets; The clients upload their local

Figure 1. Federated Never-Ending Learning Structure

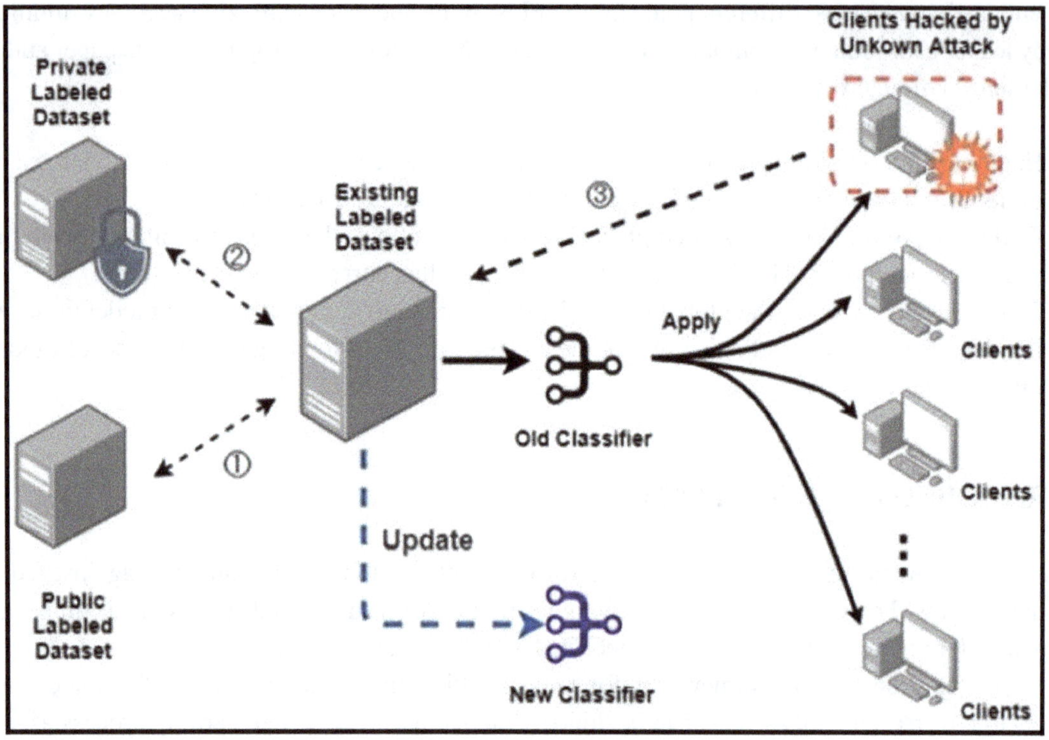

models to the server; The server aggregates the local models into a global model; The server distributes the updated global model back to the clients.

Steps 2-5 are repeated until the global model converges. Federated learning systems can be implemented in a variety of ways. For example, the server can be centralized or decentralized. The communication channel can be wired or wireless. The clients can be homogeneous or heterogeneous. The specific architecture of a federated learning system will depend on the specific needs of the application. However, the general architectural diagram above provides a good starting point for designing and implementing federated learning systems.

In this architecture, the clients are mobile devices with Google Keyboard installed. The server is a cloud-based system that hosts the global query suggestion model. The federated learning process proceeds as follows:

A. Google Keyboard periodically collects user keyboard data and sends it to the server in an aggregated form.
B. The server uses the aggregated user keyboard data to update the global query suggestion model.
C. The server distributes the updated global query suggestion model back to Google Keyboard.
D. Google Keyboard uses the updated global query suggestion model to generate query suggestions for users.

This architecture allows Google to improve the quality of query suggestions without compromising user privacy. Users do not need to share their raw keyboard data with Google. Instead, Google only

Figure 2. FL Architecture

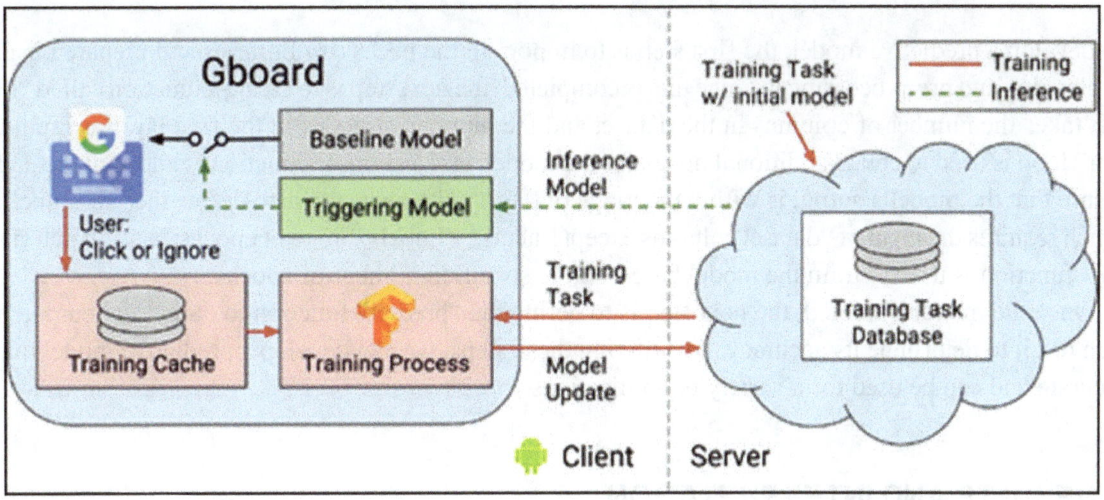

collects aggregated user keyboard data that is not personally identifiable. This is just one example of a federated learning architecture. There are many other ways to design and implement federated learning systems. The specific architecture that is best suited for a particular application will depend on the specific needs of the application.

4. ALGORITHM

a) Start task.
b) The first step is data collection, required datasets would be collected.
c) After collecting the data, the next step is data pre-processing and data cleaning. This is done in order to maximize the insights and inferences that can be drawn from the data. This is one of the most important aspects of the project.
d) After pre-processing the data, we can start building the model. We aim to create a Federated Never-Ending Learning (FNEL) model in order to make the predictions regarding the intrusion in a network. Firstly, the functions are defined for machine learning model using "keras" library.
e) Started by using the above classes for normal, non-federated learning to obtain results for both "Binary Classification" and "Multi-Class Classification" using "Neural Network" (a technique that enables computers to process data in a manner that is influenced by the functioning of the human brain).
f) Then, using the above classes for Federated Learning to obtain results for both "Binary Classification" and "Multi-Class Classification" using "Neural Network."
g) Drawing a comparison between the Federated and Non-Federated Learning.
h) Applying Never Ending Learning Using Isolation Forest model (utilized for "Continual Learning" or "Lifelong Learning" without a fixed dataset endpoint).
i) Analyze the results.
j) End task.

5. IMPLEMENTATION

To develop a predictive model, the first step is to import all the necessary libraries and prepare the data by cleaning and pre-processing it. Once this is completed, the next step is to create a function called "init" that takes the number of columns in the dataset and the number of nodes in the first layer as inputs. A "for" loop is used to create additional nodes for the model, and a sigmoid function is added at the end to ensure that the model's output is within the range of 0 to 1. The next step is to define the "fit" function, which requires the input of "dataset columns except Labels," "Labels," "No. of epochs," and "batch size." This function is used to train the model based on the specified number of epochs.

Once the model is trained, the next step is to define the "predict" function to obtain the output, and then test it to determine its accuracy. By utilizing these steps, we can develop a predictive model that is accurate and can be used for a variety of applications.

6. RESULTS AND INTERPRETATION

All the four model, i.e., Binary-Classification Model (Federated and Non-Federated Learning) and Multi-Class Classification (Federated and Non-Federated Learning) for 20 epochs which shows that the accuracy obtained after 20 epochs is around 82%, 100%, 80%, 99% respectively.

The performance is good in case of Non-Federated Learning but not in case of Federated Learning as limited data, communication latency, heterogeneity, and the use of less computationally efficient optimization methods can be reason:

6.1. Limited Data

One of the main challenges of federated learning is the limited amount of data available for training. Since the data is distributed across multiple devices or servers, it can be difficult to collect and aggregate a large enough dataset to train an accurate model. This is especially true for applications where the data is sensitive or difficult to collect, such as healthcare or financial data.To address this challenge, researchers are developing new methods for training federated learning models on limited data. For example, some methods focus on using data augmentation techniques to generate synthetic data, while others focus on developing more efficient and robust training algorithms.

Table 1. Performance Evaluation

S.NO	Model Type	Model Name	Accuracy (in %)
1)	Non-Federated Learning	Binary-Classification Model	100
2)		Multi-Class Classification Model	99
3)	Federated Learning	Binary-Classification Model	82
4)		Multi-Class Classification Model	80

6.2. Communication Latency

Another challenge of federated learning is communication latency. The process of communicating the model parameters back and forth between the devices or servers and the central server can introduce latency, which can slow down the training process and reduce the accuracy of the model.

To address this challenge, researchers are developing new communication protocols and algorithms that can reduce latency. For example, some methods focus on compressing the model parameters to reduce the amount of data that needs to be transmitted, while others focus on developing distributed training algorithms that can minimize the number of communication rounds required to train the model.

6.3. Heterogeneity

Federated learning systems are often heterogeneous, meaning that the devices or servers may have different hardware capabilities, software configurations, and data distributions. This heterogeneity can make it difficult to train a model that performs well on all devices.

To address this challenge, researchers are developing new methods for federated learning that are more robust to heterogeneity. For example, some methods focus on developing training algorithms that can adapt to different data distributions, while others focus on developing model compression techniques that can reduce the computational resources required to run the model on different devices.

6.4. Federated Optimization

Federated optimization methods are typically less computationally efficient than traditional optimization methods. This is because federated optimization methods need to take into account the communication overhead and the heterogeneity of the devices or servers. To address this challenge, researchers are developing new federated optimization methods that are more computationally efficient. For example, some methods focus on developing distributed training algorithms that can parallelize the training process, while others focus on developing model compression techniques that can reduce the amount of computation required to train the model. In addition to the four challenges you mentioned, federated learning also faces a number of other challenges, such as security and privacy concerns. However, researchers are actively working to address these challenges, and federated learning is rapidly becoming a viable machine learning approach for a wide range of applications. Overall, federated learning is a promising new machine learning paradigm with the potential to revolutionize the way we develop and deploy machine learning models on distributed data. However, there are still a number of challenges that need to be addressed before federated learning can be widely adopted.

6.5. Non-Federated Learning

6.5.1. Binary Classification Model

Figure 3. Binary Classification Model

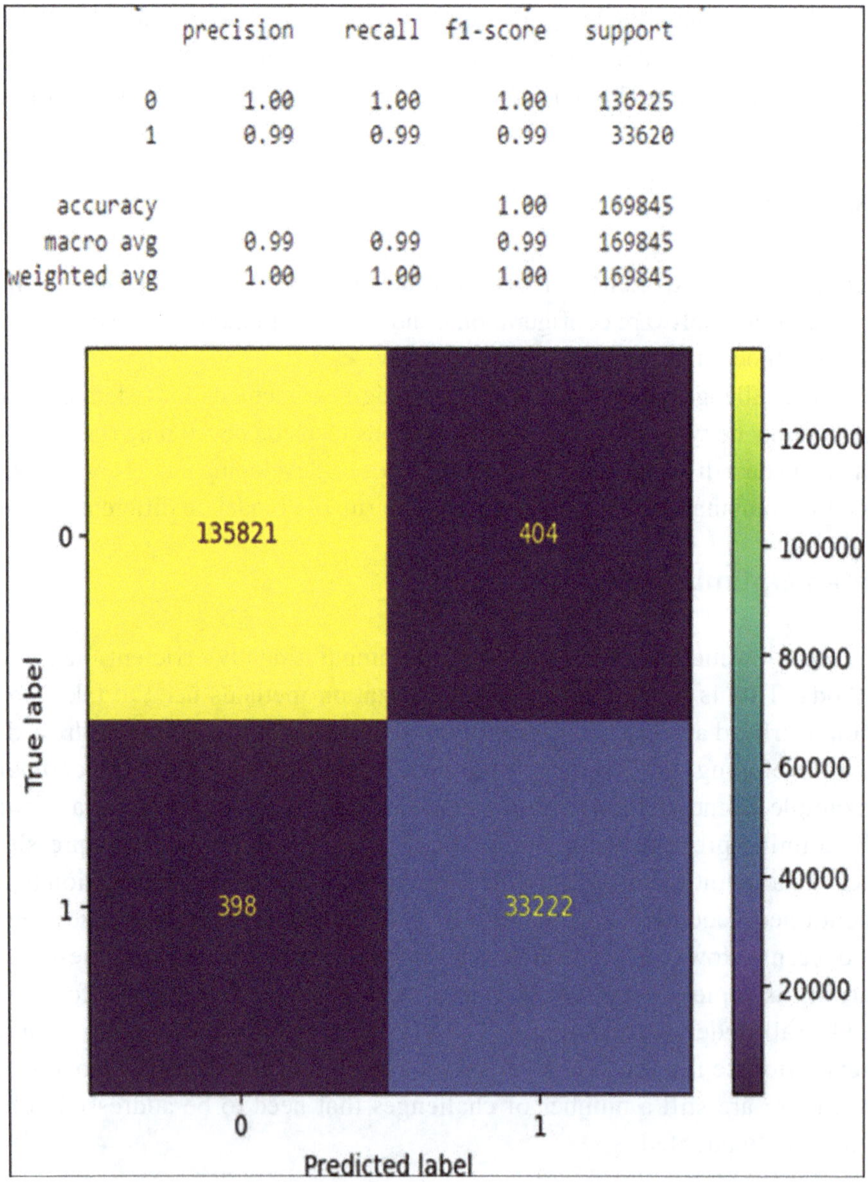

	precision	recall	f1-score	support
0	1.00	1.00	1.00	136225
1	0.99	0.99	0.99	33620
accuracy			1.00	169845
macro avg	0.99	0.99	0.99	169845
weighted avg	1.00	1.00	1.00	169845

6.5.2. Multi-Class Model

Figure 4. Multi-Class Classification Model

	precision	recall	f1-score	support
0	1.00	1.00	1.00	136225
1	0.98	0.35	0.52	136
2	0.98	0.99	0.99	7715
3	0.94	0.96	0.95	642
4	0.99	0.99	0.99	13824
5	0.80	0.74	0.77	320
6	0.93	0.69	0.80	373
7	0.99	0.99	0.99	465
10	0.99	1.00	0.99	9649
11	0.93	0.98	0.95	352
12	1.00	0.04	0.07	104
13	0.00	0.00	0.00	2
14	0.00	0.00	0.00	38
accuracy			0.99	169845
macro avg	0.81	0.67	0.69	169845
weighted avg	0.99	0.99	0.99	169845

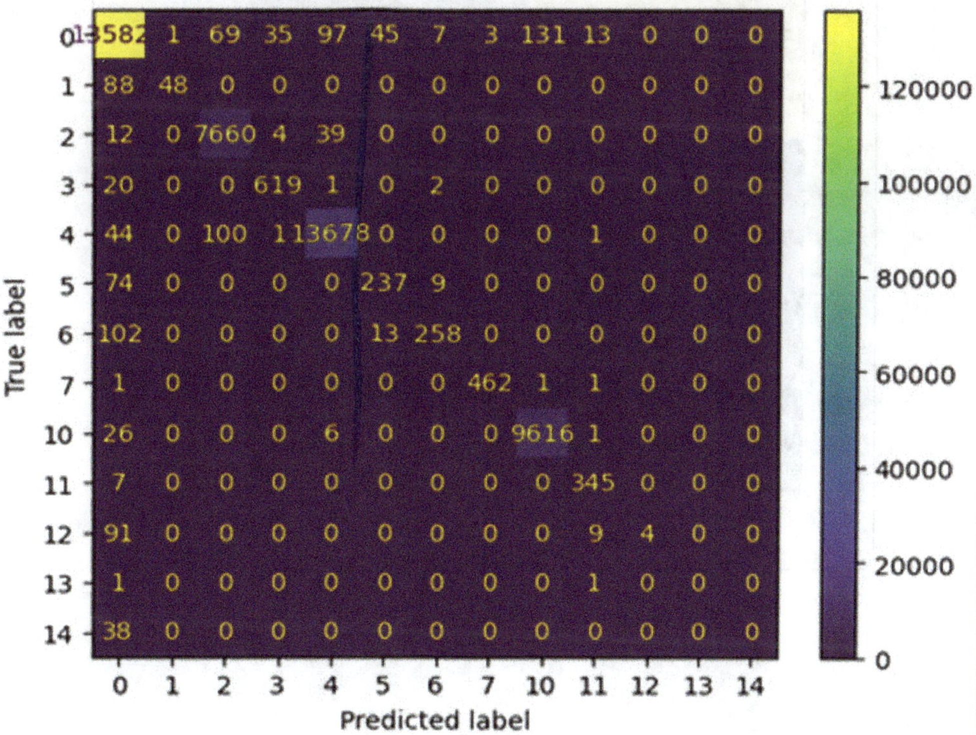

6.6. Federated Learning

6.6.1. Binary-Classification Model

Figure 5. Binary Classification Model

	precision	recall	f1-score	support
0	0.84	0.97	0.90	136225
1	0.65	0.25	0.36	33620
accuracy			0.82	169845
macro avg	0.75	0.61	0.63	169845
weighted avg	0.80	0.82	0.79	169845

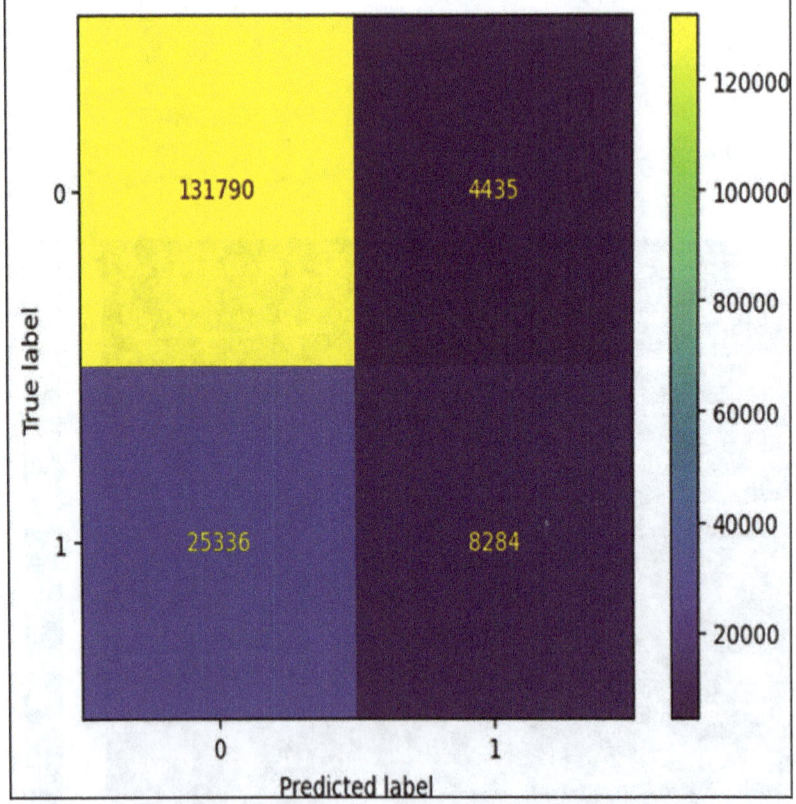

6.6.2. Multi-Class Model

Figure 6. Multi-Class Classification Model

	precision	recall	f1-score	support
0	0.80	1.00	0.89	136225
1	0.00	0.00	0.00	136
2	0.00	0.00	0.00	7715
3	0.00	0.00	0.00	642
4	0.00	0.00	0.00	13824
5	0.01	0.01	0.01	320
6	0.00	0.00	0.00	373
7	0.00	0.00	0.00	465
10	0.93	0.00	0.01	9649
11	0.00	0.00	0.00	352
12	0.02	0.10	0.03	104
13	0.00	0.00	0.00	2
14	0.00	0.00	0.00	38
accuracy			0.80	169845
macro avg	0.14	0.09	0.07	169845
eighted avg	0.70	0.80	0.71	169845

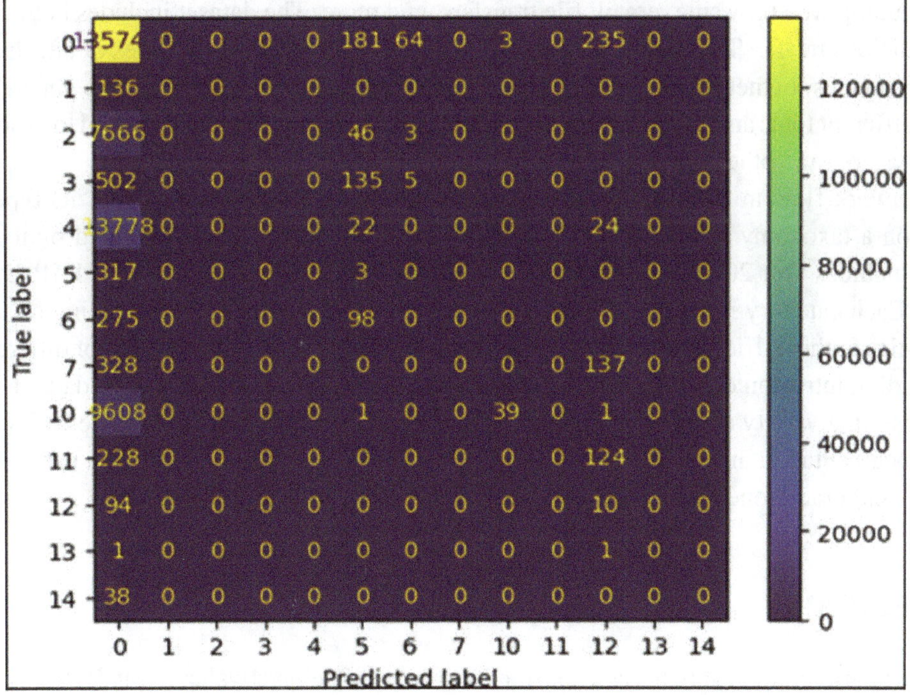

7. CONCLUSION AND FUTURE ENHANCEMENT

It is robust to class imbalance, which is a common problem in anomaly detection. It is adaptable to changing data distributions. It is privacy-preserving, as it does not require sharing of raw data between devices or institutions. Instead of taking the Average of the weights of the models, the models can be used to cast their votes based on their weights and the majority among the votes can be selected as the result, that may improve the accuracy. Apply our approach to other datasets, such as financial data and medical data. Integrate our approach with other machine learning techniques, such as deep learning. Develop real-time anomaly detection systems using our approach.

7.1 Dataset

Dataset Description: The CICIDS (Canadian Institute for Cybersecurity Intrusion Detection Dataset) is a large, publicly available dataset that was created to aid in the development of intrusion detection systems and other cybersecurity applications. The dataset was developed by the Canadian Institute for Cybersecurity (CIC) at the University of New Brunswick and is available for download from the CIC website.

The CICIDS dataset is based on real network traffic data that was captured over a period of several months on a network that was representative of a typical enterprise network. The data was captured using a variety of different network monitoring tools and hardware, including intrusion detection systems, network taps, and packet sniffers. The dataset contains over 16 million network flows, which are defined as a sequence of packets that share the same 5-tuple of source IP address, destination IP address, source port, destination port, and protocol. The flows were generated by a variety of different types of network traffic, including web browsing, email, file transfers, and more. The dataset includes both normal traffic and malicious traffic. The malicious traffic includes a range of different types of attacks, including DoS/DDoS attacks, botnet attacks, brute-force attacks, and more. The attacks were generated using a variety of different tools and techniques, and some of them were specifically designed to evade intrusion detection systems and other cybersecurity tools.

Each network flow in the CICIDS dataset is labelled with a tag that identifies its type. The tags are based on a taxonomy of network attacks and normal traffic that was developed by the CIC. The taxonomy includes over 20 different categories of network traffic, including HTTP, FTP, DNS, ICMP, and more. Each category is further subdivided into different subcategories, depending on the specific characteristics of the traffic. The CICIDS dataset is designed to be used for a variety of different applications, including intrusion detection, machine learning, data mining, and more. The dataset is available for download in a variety of different formats, including CSV, SQL, and PCAP. The CIC website also includes documentation and sample code for working with the dataset, as well as a user forum where researchers and practitioners can share their experiences and ask questions.

REFERENCES

A Federated Learning Aggregation Algorithm for Pervasive Computing: Evaluation and Comparison. (2021, March 22). IEEE Conference Publication | IEEE Xplore. https://ieeexplore.ieee.org/document/9439129

Balyan, A. K., Ahuja, S., Sharma, S. K., & Lilhore, U. K. (2022, February). Machine learning-based intrusion detection system for healthcare data. In *2022 IEEE VLSI Device Circuit and System (VLSI DCS)* (pp. 290-294). IEEE.

Criado, M. F., Casado, F. E., Iglesias, R., Regueiro, C. V., & Barro, S. (2022). Non-iid data and continual learning processes in Federated Learning: A long road ahead. *Information Fusion*, *88*, 263–280. doi:10.1016/j.inffus.2022.07.024

Hassan, A., Prasad, D., Khurana, M., Lilhore, U. K., & Simaiya, S. (2021). Integration of internet of things (IoT) in health care industry: An overview of benefits, challenges, and applications. *Data Science and Innovations for Intelligent Systems*, 165-180.

Heralding the Future of Federated Learning Framework: Architecture, Tools and Future Directions. (2021, January 28). IEEE Conference Publication | IEEE Xplore. https://ieeexplore.ieee.org/document/9377066

Jaiswal, V., Saurabh, P., Lilhore, U. K., Pathak, M., Simaiya, S., & Dalal, S. (2023). A breast cancer risk predication and classification model with ensemble learning and big data fusion. *Decision Analytics Journal*, *8*, 100298. doi:10.1016/j.dajour.2023.100298

Li, L., Yang, F., Tse, M., & Lin, K. J. (2020, November 1). A review of applications in federated learning. *Computers & Industrial Engineering*, *149*, 106854. Advance online publication. doi:10.1016/j.cie.2020.106854

Lilhore, U. K., Dalal, S., Faujdar, N., Margala, M., Chakrabarti, P., Chakrabarti, T., Simaiya, S., Kumar, P., Thangaraju, P., & Velmurugan, H. (2023). Hybrid CNN-LSTM model with efficient hyperparameter tuning for prediction of Parkinson's disease. *Scientific Reports*, *13*(1), 14605. doi:10.1038/s41598-023-41314-y PMID:37669970

Lilhore, U. K., Dalal, S., Faujdar, N., Simaiya, S., Dahiya, M., Tomar, S., & Hashmi, A. (2024). Unveiling the prevalence and risk factors of early stage postpartum depression: A hybrid deep learning approach. *Multimedia Tools and Applications*, 1–35. doi:10.1007/s11042-024-18182-3

Lilhore, U. K., Manoharan, P., Sandhu, J. K., Simaiya, S., Dalal, S., Baqasah, A. M., Alsafyani, M., Alroobaea, R., Keshta, I., & Raahemifar, K. (2023). Hybrid model for precise hepatitis-C classification using improved random forest and SVM method. *Scientific Reports*, *13*(1), 12473. doi:10.1038/s41598-023-36605-3 PMID:37528148

Lilhore, U. K., Poongodi, M., Kaur, A., Simaiya, S., Algarni, A. D., Elmannai, H., Vijayakumar, V., Tunze, G. B., & Hamdi, M. (2022). Hybrid model for detection of cervical cancer using causal analysis and machine learning techniques. *Computational and Mathematical Methods in Medicine*, *2022*, 2022. doi:10.1155/2022/4688327 PMID:35572826

Lilhore, U. K., Simaiya, S., Pandey, H., Gautam, V., Garg, A., & Ghosh, P. (2022). Breast cancer detection in the IoT cloud-based healthcare environment using fuzzy cluster segmentation and SVM classifier. *Ambient Communications and Computer Systems Proceedings of RACCCS*, *2021*, 165–179.

Lilhore, U. K., Simaiya, S., Prasad, D., & Guleria, K. (2020). A hybrid tumour detection and classification based on machine learning. *Journal of Computational and Theoretical Nanoscience*, *17*(6), 2539–2544. doi:10.1166/jctn.2020.8927

Liu, J., Zhang, G., Wang, K., & Yang, K. (2023). Task-load-aware game-theoretic framework for Wireless Federated Learning. *IEEE Communications Letters*, *27*(1), 268–272. doi:10.1109/LCOMM.2022.3210604

Onyema, E. M., Lilhore, U. K., Saurabh, P., Dalal, S., Nwaeze, A. S., Chijindu, A. T., Ndufeiya-Kumasi, L. C., & Simaiya, S. (2023). Evaluation of IoT-Enabled hybrid model for genome sequence analysis of patients in healthcare 4.0. *Measurement. Sensors*, *26*, 100679. doi:10.1016/j.measen.2023.100679

Qin, T., Cheng, G., Chen, W., & Lei, X. (2021). FNEL:an evolving intrusion detection system based on federated never-ending learning. *2021 17th International Conference on Mobility, Sensing and Networking (MSN)*. 10.1109/MSN53354.2021.00047

Ramesh, T. R., Lilhore, U. K., Poongodi, M., Simaiya, S., Kaur, A., & Hamdi, M. (2022). Predictive analysis of heart diseases with machine learning approaches. *Malaysian Journal of Computer Science*, 132–148.

Rathore, M. S., Poongodi, M., Saurabh, P., Lilhore, U. K., Bourouis, S., Alhakami, W., Osamor, J., & Hamdi, M. (2022). A novel trust-based security and privacy model for internet of vehicles using encryption and steganography. *Computers & Electrical Engineering*, *102*, 108205. doi:10.1016/j.compeleceng.2022.108205

Sharma, S. K., Lilhore, U. K., Simaiya, S., & Trivedi, N. K. (2021). An improved random forest algorithm for predicting the COVID-19 pandemic patient health. *Annals of the Romanian Society for Cell Biology*, 67–75.

Shen, T. (2020, June 27). *Federated Mutual Learning*. arXiv.org. https://arxiv.org/abs/2006.16765

Shenaj, D. (2023, April 7). *Asynchronous Federated Continual Learning*. arXiv.org. https://arxiv.org/abs/2304.03626 doi:10.1109/CVPRW59228.2023.00534

Simaiya, S., Lilhore, U. K., Prasad, D., & Verma, D. K. (2021). MRI brain tumour detection & image segmentation by hybrid hierarchical K-means clustering with FCM based machine learning model. *Annals of the Romanian Society for Cell Biology*, 88–94.

Yang, T. (2018, December 7). *Applied Federated Learning: Improving Google Keyboard Query Suggestions*. arXiv.org. https://arxiv.org/abs/1812.02903

Chapter 9
Federated Learning for Privacy Preservation in Healthcare:
A Comprehensive Introduction

Hari Kishan Kondaveeti
https://orcid.org/0000-0002-3379-720X
Vellore Institute of Technology, India

Chinna Gopi Simhadri
https://orcid.org/0000-0002-8311-7495
Vellore Institute of Technology, India

Srileakhana Mangapathi
https://orcid.org/0009-0007-2894-9671
Vellore Institute of Technology, India

Valli Kumari Vatsavayi
https://orcid.org/0000-0002-7252-8301
Andhra University, India

ABSTRACT

This chapter delves into fundamental concepts of privacy preservation and federated learning (FL) in healthcare. Emphasizing the importance of privacy in healthcare data, it explores ethical and regulatory considerations surrounding sensitive patient information. The history and significance of FL, distinct from traditional centralized machine learning, are discussed, highlighting its relevance in addressing privacy concerns. The limitations of centralized ML are contrasted with FL's advantages, particularly in preserving privacy. Techniques such as FL averaging, aggregation, and secure multi-party computation (SMPC) for privacy-preserving model updates are examined. Real-world examples illustrate their application in healthcare scenarios. The chapter concludes by addressing technical and ethical challenges linked to FL in healthcare, emphasizing its potential to balance patient data protection with AI advancements. Privacy concerns persist in healthcare AI, making FL a promising solution. The discussion extends to emerging trends and potential breakthroughs in this dynamic field.

DOI: 10.4018/979-8-3693-1874-4.ch009

INTRODUCTION

Federated learning (FL) is a revolutionary concept, especially in sensitive fields like healthcare and finance. FL permits cooperative machine learning without requiring centralized data collection. With the help of this creative framework, numerous organizations or entities can work together to develop a common machine learning model while safely and decentralized maintaining control over their own datasets. Federated learning shows promise as a solution in the healthcare industry, where safeguarding sensitive patient data is crucial. FL's basic idea is to distribute the machine learning model among several decentralized nodes, keeping data localized rather than sending it to a central server. This decentralized structure is particularly well-suited for the healthcare industry since it tackles issues with data privacy, security, and regulatory compliance. Preserving patient privacy, it enables collaboration between medical professionals, academic institutions, and pharmaceutical companies to collectively train machine learning models using their respective datasets.

Healthcare data, often containing highly sensitive and personal information, necessitates stringent privacy measures Gadekallu et al. (2023). FL aims to mitigate this issue by facilitating collaboration amongst universities on model training, limiting data exchange to model updates alone. The risks of centralized data storage, like illegal access and data breaches, are reduced by using this technique. The convergence of federated learning and healthcare not only propels medical research and facilitates the development of personalized treatments but also ensures the utmost confidentiality of patient data. It achieves this by finding a careful balance between protecting individual record privacy and utilizing the aggregate insights from many sources. Technology and healthcare have a symbiotic relationship that highlights innovative potential while emphasizing the crucial role of data privacy. This eventually advances both the area of healthcare and the responsible use of data-driven technologies.

FUNDAMENTALS OF HEALTHCARE DATA AND AI

Healthcare data, a patient information repository, combines Artificial intelligence (AI) and machine learning to improve treatment, diagnosis, and operational effectiveness. AI uses data analysis to forecast illnesses, customise care, and improve care routes. In the rapidly changing field of medicine, ethical use guarantees patient privacy and transparent, accountable algorithms.

Types of Healthcare Data

A variety of information types essential to patient care, medical research, and healthcare administration are included in healthcare data. Electronic health records (EHRs) contain structured healthcare data such as patient demographics, medical histories, diagnosis, prescriptions, and treatment plans. Clinical data is also necessary for monitoring the health of patients. Examples of this include lab results and vital signs. Billing codes, insurance details, and appointment schedules are all part of the administrative data that oversees the business side of healthcare. Voice recordings, medical images (such as MRIs and X-rays), and free-text clinical notes are examples of unstructured data. To diagnose illnesses, customise treatment regimens, and carry out medical research, these data types are essential. Patient outcomes, healthcare costs, and medical knowledge are all greatly enhanced by the integration and analysis of structured and unstructured healthcare data.

AI Techniques and Models Used in Healthcare

Machine learning, deep learning, computer vision, natural language processing, and federated learning are some of the AI models and approaches used in healthcare. While deep learning is superior at picture recognition in medical imaging, machine learning algorithms analyse medical data to create predictions and judgements. Clinical materials are easier to grasp when natural language processing is used. Medical images are interpreted via computer vision. By training models using decentralised data sources, federated learning improves privacy and increases the security and collaboration of AI in healthcare. These artificial intelligence tools enhance patient care, diagnosis, and therapy.

Potential of AI to Transform Healthcare Diagnosis, Treatment, and Research

AI has the enormous potential to transform healthcare in terms of research, diagnosis, and treatment. In the diagnosis process, AI-powered tools can diagnose diseases and conditions earlier by analysing large amounts of patient data, medical images, and clinical notes with amazing speed and accuracy. Patient outcomes can be considerably enhanced by this early detection. AI makes personalised healthcare possible by customising medications based on patient profiles and taking lifestyle and genetic variables into account. This guarantees more proficient and successful care. Furthermore, AI can process and analyse large datasets for medical research to find patterns, possible drug candidates, and treatment plans. This speeds up clinical trials and drug discovery.

PRIVACY PRESERVATION IN HEALTHCARE

Maintaining patient privacy is essential for safeguarding sensitive patient information. The importance of maintaining confidentiality is highlighted by ethical considerations, legal requirements such as Health Insurance Portability and Accountability Act, and difficulties in securely exchanging and processing patient data. Strong privacy measures are extremely important because breaches can lead to identity theft and damage to one's reputation.

Importance of Privacy Preservation in Healthcare Data

The confidentiality of medical data must always be maintained because it contains sensitive information. Intimate information such as medical conditions, treatment histories, and personal identifiers are frequently found in patient records. Not only is protecting this data morally and legally required by laws like Health Insurance Portability and Accountability Act (HIPAA) and General Data Protection Regulation (GDPR), but it is also required by law. Breach of privacy in healthcare data can have serious repercussions, such as identity theft, discrimination, and psychological trauma for patients.

Effective healthcare delivery relies on maintaining patient trust, and privacy violations can undermine that trust Yin et al. (2021). Moreover, breaches may subject healthcare organisations to severe financial penalties and legal ramifications. Strong privacy safeguards, such as encryption, access controls, and safe data storage, are necessary to preserve patient privacy and facilitate efficient healthcare delivery and research. Safeguarding patient data privacy is an essential component of patient-centred care and moral medical practise, not just a compliance concern.

Furthermore, security vulnerabilities in the healthcare industry may result in financial fraud, identity theft, or treatment plan compromises that jeopardise patient safety. Ensuring patient welfare is inextricably linked to protecting privacy Truex et al. (2019). Patients have the ethical right to be in charge of their data. A better and more respectful patient-provider connection is fostered by honouring this autonomy and making sure their data is managed safely and responsibly. These actions also reflect a commitment to patient-centric treatment.

In essence, maintaining patient privacy in healthcare data is essential to providing moral, reliable, and efficient treatment that upholds patients' rights and protects their health, not only because it's required by law.

Ethical Concerns and Legal Regulations

Maintaining privacy in healthcare data is largely dependent on legal requirements and ethical considerations. Ethics dictate that trust must be upheld and patient autonomy respected. Patients anticipate that their health information will be kept private, and revelations of this nature can erode confidence. Exact guidelines for managing patient data are provided by legal regulations, such as the General Data Protection Regulation in the European Union and the Health Insurance Portability and Accountability Act in the United States. Healthcare organisations that break these rules may face stiff fines and legal repercussions.

The responsible use of sensitive information, permission, and transparency are the main ethical concerns of healthcare data Cheng et al. (2020). Patients have a right to regulate the release of their data and must be informed about how it is used. Making sure algorithms are impartial, fair, and open about how they make decisions is a necessary part of using AI and data analytics ethically. To protect patient privacy, legal requirements and ethical considerations collaborate. Healthcare organisations can protect patient data while providing high-quality care, upholding patient trust, and averting legal issues by abiding by these rules and ethical guidelines.

Challenges in Sharing and Processing Sensitive Patient Information

1. Privacy Concerns: Protecting patient privacy is crucial since healthcare data frequently contains sensitive personal information about specific persons. There is always a chance of data breaches or unwanted access.
2. Security hazards: There are security hazards associated with keeping a lot of patient data in centralised systems. The security and integrity of the data may be jeopardised by hacking or other online attacks.
3. Regulatory Compliance: Strict rules, such HIPAA in the US, are applicable to the healthcare sector. Ensuring conformity to these standards while exchanging and handling patient data creates challenges and demands close attention to detail.
4. Data Interoperability: Information related to healthcare is frequently dispersed among several organisations, formats, and systems. It might be difficult to achieve interoperability and smooth data sharing across several systems.
5. Data Ownership and Control: When several healthcare organisations are engaged, it can be difficult to ascertain who is in charge of and who owns the patient data. It is essential to establish explicit policies about data ownership and governance.

6. Consent Management: It can be difficult to get and keep patients' consent to share sensitive information. It is imperative to guarantee that patients have provided clear and informed consent.
7. Data Completeness and Accuracy: Incomplete or inaccurate information in patient records might cause errors in interpretation and treatment planning. Ensuring shared data is accurate and full is an ongoing concern.
8. Technological Integration: Sturdy technical solutions are needed to integrate various healthcare systems and technologies for smooth data processing and sharing. It can be difficult to guarantee compatibility and interoperability across several systems.
9. Ethical Considerations: Careful consideration must be given to the ethical ramifications of exchanging and processing patient data, particularly those including consent, data ownership, and potential discrimination.
10. Data Breach Risks: Data breaches are always a possibility because of the growing sophistication of cyber attacks. Ensuring the resilience of security measures and protecting patient information from unauthorised access are continuous issues.

THE NEED FOR FEDERATED LEARNING IN HEALTHCARE

Definition of FL and Its Brief History

Federated Learning is a decentralised machine learning technique that maintains local underlying data while facilitating cooperative AI model training across numerous devices or servers. FL maintains data security and privacy by allowing model updates to be shared across devices as opposed to centralising all data.

Google originally released FL in 2016. Its main goal was to address machine learning privacy concerns. Google's strategy attempted to create AI models without transferring user data to a central server, which might jeopardise user privacy. FL provides a method to leverage the collective knowledge from multiple sources without disclosing sensitive information by storing data on the devices or servers where it is generated. Since then, it has attracted a lot of interest from a variety of sectors, most notably the healthcare sector, where private data analysis is crucial. FL is still developing and presents a promising approach to collaborative machine learning that protects user privacy.

In federated learning (FL), models are trained at the device level by being brought to the data sources or devices for both prediction and training. The models or their updates are returned to the main server for aggregation after training. The individual models can then be tracked and re-distributed among different devices by applying distributed computing concepts to deliver a consolidated model back to the devices. This method is very useful for installing affordable machine learning models on gadgets such as sensors and cell phones. Federated Learning's general architecture is shown in the above Figure 1.

SIGNIFICANCE OF FL IN HEALTHCARE

Federated Learning (FL), which addresses privacy issues and improves collaborative research, has great potential to transform the healthcare industry. Without requiring the sharing of raw data, FL enables machine learning models to be trained across numerous decentralised devices or healthcare institutions.

Figure 1. The architecture of federated learning

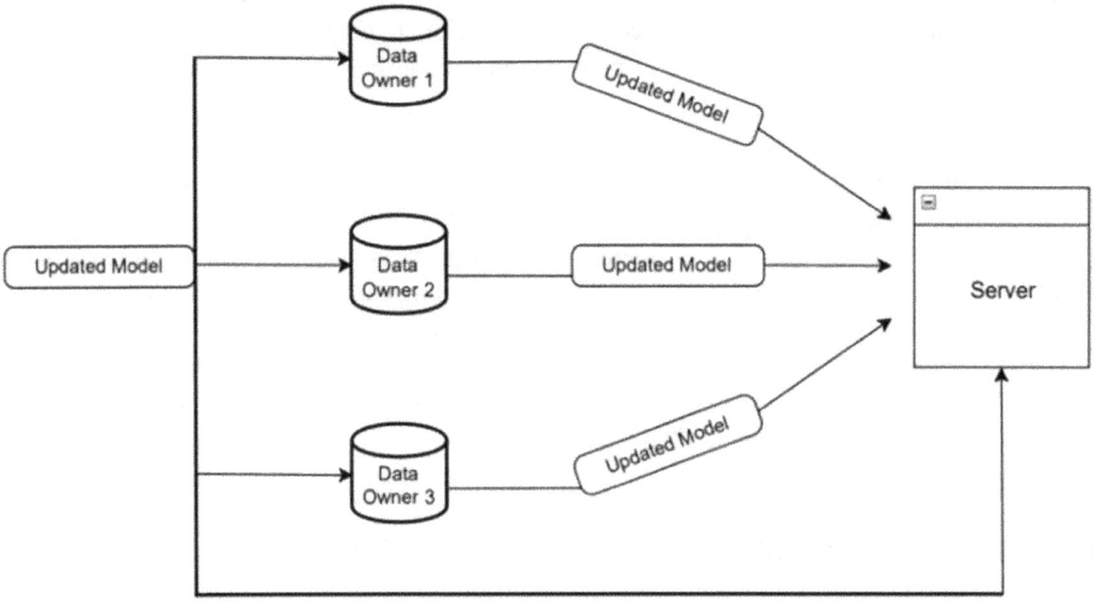

Table 1. Key differences between FL and traditional centralized ML

Differences	Federated Learning	Traditional Centralized Machine Learning
Data Location	Data is still local, stored on servers or devices locally. Raw data is not shared; instead, model updates are.	For model training, data is usually centralised on a single site or server.
Privacy	Preserves data privacy by keeping sensitive information at its source. Individual data is never shared.	Involves centralising and exchanging data, both of which can be risky for privacy.
Data Ownership and Control	Owners of data retain authority over their information, which respects ownership and makes it appropriate for cooperative projects.	The central entity managing the ML models may acquire ownership and control of the data.
Scalability	Scalable over a vast network of dispersed devices or servers.	Scalability is constrained by the central server's capacity.
Communication Overhead	Involves increased communication overhead when updating models between servers or devices.	Requires less communication overhead, as data is already centralized.
Network Requirements	Requires a robust network connection for model updates, which may not be suitable in all scenarios.	Predominantly uses a robust network connection for data transfer.
Security	Keeps raw data private, lowering the possibility of data breaches.	May expose data to potential security risks, especially when transferring data to a central server.

By reducing the privacy risks connected to centralised data storage, this decentralised method assures adherence to strict healthcare data protection laws. Furthermore, FL makes it easier to create reliable and broadly applicable models by utilising a variety of datasets from different sources, which results in more potent diagnostic and predictive instruments. FL advances personalised medicine, disease prediction, and treatment optimisation by empowering healthcare providers to work together to improve models while maintaining patient confidentiality. This, in turn, helps to drive the development of patient-centred, data-driven healthcare solutions.

Limitations of Traditional Centralized ML

1. Privacy Concerns: Centralised machine learning aggregates data in one place, there are possible privacy risks for each individual user.
2. Security Risks: Centralised models only have one point of vulnerability; they are more vulnerable to intrusions and security breaches.
3. Data Ownership and Access Issues: Too much centralization can cause problems with data ownership and access, which makes it harder for different stakeholders to work together.
4. Scalability Challenges: Handling large datasets centrally may lead to higher processing times and expenses for computation.
5. Bias in Models: The capacity of centralised machine learning models to generalise across a range of demographics may be hampered by bias in the models if the training data is not representative.
6. Computational Costs: The need for continuous data transfers to a central location can incur high bandwidth costs and latency issues.

Limited Collaboration: Sharing sensitive data raises privacy concerns that limit the potential for joint research projects to improve model accuracy and generate shared insights (Lilhore et al., 2022).

Advantages of FL for Privacy Preservation

1. Decentralized Training: FL reduces the requirement for centralised data by allowing model training to take place on individual devices. Users' devices retain raw data, which helps to protect privacy because private information stays in the immediate vicinity.
2. Reduced Data Exposure: FL lowers the possibility of data exposure in the case of a breach by minimising the storage of sensitive data in a single location. During the learning process, only model updates which are less informative than raw data are shared between devices.
3. User Control: People own their data because FL lets them take part in model training without having to share raw data. Without jeopardising the privacy of their personal information, users can help improve models.
4. Compliance with Regulations: By decentralising the model training procedure, FL complies with data protection laws. This method reduces the amount of sensitive data that is gathered in one place, ensuring that businesses follow privacy laws.
5. Enhanced Security: The security risks connected with central data storage, like a single point of attack, are greatly diminished since raw data stays on local devices. By distributing the learning process across several devices, FL improves security overall.
6. Diverse Data Sources: Despite centralising data collection, FL makes it easier to train models on a variety of data sources. While preserving the privacy of individual datasets, this diversity enhances the model's robustness and generalizability.
7. Collaborative Learning: Collaborative model updates, in which devices exchange knowledge without disclosing specific data points, protect privacy. Together, various stakeholders can improve the model, promoting cooperation while protecting the privacy of personal information.

FEDERATED LEARNING TECHNIQUES

FL Averaging and Aggregation

Federated Learning (FL) combines local model updates from multiple devices into a single, enhanced global model without requiring direct access to each individual data point by using aggregation and averaging techniques. The process of averaging entails gathering model parameters that have been adjusted via local training on every gadget. A consensus model is created by combining these updated parameters, frequently using techniques like weighted averaging or secure multi-party computation. This integrated model incorporates knowledge from various data sources. To provide a balanced worldwide update, weighted averaging allocates importance according to the performance or contribution of each device. Data privacy is preserved throughout the aggregation process by using secure aggregation techniques like homomorphic encryption. The combined model embodies a process of group learning without disclosing personal information, enabling cooperative model improvement, and maintaining privacy throughout decentralised networks. By using these methods, FL can produce reliable and accurate models without jeopardising the privacy of private information stored on individual devices (Lilhore et al., 2023).

SECURE MULTI-PARTY COMPUTATION FOR PRIVACY-PRESERVING MODEL UPDATES

Secure Multi-Party Computation (SMPC) safeguards data privacy in federated learning by enabling collaborative model updates without exposing individual data. It uses cryptographic methods to allow multiple parties to collectively compute a function while keeping their inputs confidential. In the context of FL, SMPC ensures that devices can share their locally computed model updates without revealing their specific data. Through encryption and distributed computation, SMPC enables the aggregation of model parameters from various devices without any party accessing others' raw data. This process ensures the improvement of the global model is based on combined insights while preserving the confidentiality of individual contributions. In federated learning scenarios, SMPC offers a safe, privacy-preserving way to aggregate and update models, encouraging participant confidence and adhering to stringent data privacy laws.

Real-World Examples

Federated Learning of Predictive Models in Healthcare provides an example of how FL methods can be applied to train predictive models across several healthcare facilities while maintaining patient confidentiality. Brisimi et al. (2018) focuses on forecasting patient outcomes, treating patients with personalised suggestions, and predicting illness outcomes. These methods allow for collaborative breakthroughs in healthcare without jeopardising the confidentiality of individual patient information. They do this by dispersing model training across multiple sites without centralising sensitive data.

The study Privacy-Preserving Medical Image Analysis using Federated Learning emphasises how FL helps maintain secure and decentralised patient data while analysing medical pictures (such as CT scans and MRIs) from various healthcare providers. This method, which uses FL methods, guarantees that private medical imagery stays on local devices, allowing for cooperative model training without the need to share or centralise patient data. In addition to upholding stringent privacy policies and adhering to healthcare data protection regulations, this promotes improvements in the precision of diagnosis and treatment recommendations.

The research on Collaborative Disease Diagnosis with Federated Learning show how FL promotes collaborative disease diagnosis by combining knowledge from several clinics or hospitals without transferring patient data directly. Qayyum et al. (2022) approach carefully complies with privacy standards and promotes collective model improvement for precise diagnosis. This strategy maintains the anonymity of individual patient records while improving diagnostic accuracy, treatment suggestions, and disease understanding across healthcare facilities by maintaining decentralised patient data and utilising collaborative insights.

The research, Federated Learning Applications in Electronic Health Records (EHR) highlights FL's use of decentralised EHR for model training. This technique improves diagnostic and therapy prediction models while protecting private patient data. Lu et al. (2020) proposed that FL guarantees privacy compliance by allowing model training across dispersed EHR systems without centralising raw patient data. By combining several data sources, this strategy promotes cooperative improvements in healthcare and produces better predictive models without jeopardising patient privacy. These studies demonstrate the viability of applying FL to healthcare settings, highlighting the need to protect patient privacy while promoting improvements in the precision of diagnosis and tailored treatment suggestions. This study is a big step towards using EHR data to better healthcare outcomes without violating patients' right to privacy.

APPLICATIONS OF FEDERATED LEARNING IN HEALTHCARE

Disease Prediction and Diagnosis

Federated Learning integrates information from several sources while protecting patient privacy, making it essential for disease diagnosis and prediction in the healthcare industry. Without centralising sensitive patient data, FL enables collaborative training of predictive models across many healthcare organisations. By employing a decentralised method, hospitals or individual devices can train models with local data, allowing for improvements to be made collectively without exchanging raw data. FL complies with strict privacy rules by utilising a variety of patient datasets in disease prediction without directly accessing or pooling the data. These varied datasets strengthen and improve the prediction models' accuracy and robustness, improving the capacity to predict the onset or course of disease in various patient populations. While collective intelligence refines the models generated by FL, each patient's data is kept private and decentralised.

Furthermore, FL facilitates the integration of diagnostic insights obtained from many sources, leading to a more thorough and precise diagnosis without the need to share patient-specific data directly. FL enhances diagnostic instruments' precision and accuracy by working together across these dispersed sources to develop models, enabling more complex and informed decision-making without jeopardising patient privacy.

In addition to improving healthcare outcomes, this use of FL for disease diagnosis and prediction protects patient privacy and complies with ethical and legal requirements. Better predictive and diagnostic skills enable healthcare professionals, which in turn results in more individualised and efficient healthcare solutions.

Drug Discovery and Development

In the healthcare industry, federated learning, which provides a framework for collaboration and privacy protection, has shown promise as a method for drug discovery and development. Without the need for centralised data pooling, FL in this case allows pharmaceutical corporations, academic institutions, and healthcare providers to collaboratively analyse and learn from heterogeneous and distributed datasets. Without directly accessing or exchanging confidential data, FL makes it easier to analyse different chemical structures, compound interactions, and biological reactions across numerous institutions in the drug discovery process. FL speeds up the drug discovery process while protecting data privacy by utilising the combined intelligence from several sources to improve the identification and validation of possible drug candidates.

Additionally, FL facilitates the cooperative improvement of predictive models for medication safety and efficacy during the drug development process by utilising data from various trials and studies. With the help of these decentralised cooperation, treatment outcomes, adverse reactions, and patient responses may be analysed more accurately and robustly, all without disclosing specific patient information. Drug-related models can be jointly learned and improved because to FL's decentralised model training and aggregation approach, which does not combine private or patient-specific sensitive data. This strategy encourages creativity while guaranteeing adherence to ethical guidelines and privacy laws while using healthcare data.

FL enhances drug discovery and development, enables the creation of safer and more effective medications, and ultimately advances the fields of healthcare and science by enabling collaborative and privacy-centric research.

Personalized Treatment Plans

Federated Learning revolutionizes the creation of personalized treatment plans in healthcare by facilitating the collaborative analysis of diverse patient data while preserving individual privacy. By combining insights from dispersed databases, FL enables different healthcare providers to optimise therapy recommendations without disclosing private patient data. Here, FL enables the group training of models with data from multiple sources, assisting in the discovery of customised therapies based on each individual patient's unique health profile. Through the process of combining information from several sources, such as devices or institutions, FL facilitates the creation of more accurate and customised treatment regimens.

By improving predictive models that take into consideration a range of patient attributes and medical histories through collaborative learning, treatment predictions become more accurate while patient privacy is preserved. These individualised treatment plans adhere to ethical norms in healthcare and privacy laws since they are developed from group insights rather than disclosing individual data points.

The utilisation of varied datasets by FL facilitates the extraction of collective intelligence that guarantees more individualised, efficacious, and privacy-compliant treatment plans. This, in turn, advances patient-centred care and more customised healthcare solutions.

Medical Image Analysis

Federated Learning, which preserves patient data privacy while enabling collaborative analysis across many healthcare facilities, is transforming medical picture analysis. This way, without explicitly sharing or centralising the pictures themselves, FL enables several facilities to jointly train models using decentralised medical imaging, like MRIs, CT scans, and X-rays. With FL, hospitals or individual devices can use local data to build image analysis models, allowing for group improvements without disclosing individual patient images. The interpretation of medical images and the accuracy of diagnosis are improved using FL in image analysis. FL boosts the overall understanding of complicated images, improves disease classification, and sharpens the discovery of anomalies by combining information from several sources.

FL's decentralized approach ensures compliance with stringent privacy regulations, as sensitive patient images remain secure on local devices while contributing to the collective learning process Kamble et al. (2022). This protects patient anonymity and improves the accuracy of diagnostic instruments while also complying with legal and ethical constraints. Massive potential exists for better diagnosis and treatment planning through the application of FL in medical image analysis, which will ultimately result in more precise and individualised healthcare solutions. By protecting patient privacy and promoting improvements in diagnosis accuracy and treatment suggestions, this method sets a new benchmark for healthcare image analysis.

CASE STUDY

Federated Learning for Smart Healthcare: A Case Study for COVID-19 Image Classification With Blockchain

This case study explores the critical need for early COVID-19 identification, which the World Health Organisation designated to be a pandemic in March 2020. Alternative screening techniques are essential because of the drawbacks and length of time associated with regular testing. The work focuses on using deep learning (DL) algorithms, specifically for analysing X-ray and computed tomography (CT) pictures of the chest. Viral pneumonia can be effectively detected using DL algorithms thanks to these imaging modalities, which provide a detailed picture of lung diseases. The paper analyses the benefits and drawbacks of several deep learning techniques that have been documented in the literature, placing particular emphasis on picture preprocessing, deep feature extraction with a variety of models, and the classification procedure that follows.

The COVID-19 pandemic has sparked a global search for fast and precise detection techniques, which are necessary for drug development, contact tracing, screening, prevention, and forecasting. Kumar et al. (2021) emphasises how difficult it is to differentiate between viral and non-viral pneumonia, a crucial step in making an accurate diagnosis as the virus keeps evolving with new strains. The case study also examines new uses for DL, including as cough analysis for early detection and human motion estimation to stop the virus's transmission. The work adds a thorough overview of DL-based COVID-19 detection by examining databases and evaluating recent research, providing insights into difficulties, potential future directions, and suggested remedies to improve accuracy and lessen the virus's effects.

CHALLENGES

Federated learning is a distributed machine learning technique that allows sensitive patient data to be shared while training machine learning models on decentralised data, potentially providing a solution for privacy protection in the healthcare industry. Federated learning in the healthcare industry, however, confronts a number of challenges:

1. Communication latency: Each device that participates in federated learning (such as a clinic or hospital) downloads the global model, trains it locally using its own data, and then transmits the modified model back to the server. Because it influences the convergence time and model accuracy, communication latency between devices and the server might be a major problem.
2. Data heterogeneity: Due to differences in patient populations, data formats, and data quality, healthcare data is extremely varied. This variability can cause notable differences in the performance of local models and complicate the process of convergently developing a global model that works effectively on all devices.
3. Model privacy: Although federated learning keeps sensitive patient data local, it might nonetheless divulge sensitive information about specific patients through the global model. This danger can be reduced with the use of strategies like secure aggregation and differentiated privacy.
4. Resource constraints: Accurate model local training and federated learning can be difficult due to the limited computational power of many healthcare equipment. The computational cost of local training can be decreased with the use of strategies like quantization and pruning.
5. Legal and regulatory restrictions: HIPAA in the US and GDPR in the EU are only two examples of the stringent laws and regulations that apply to healthcare data. Federated learning needs to follow these guidelines to guarantee adherence and safeguard patient confidentiality. Regulatory clearances and other security measures might be needed for this.

CONCLUSION AND FUTURE DIRECTIONS

This chapter examines the ethical issues surrounding sensitive patient information and emphasises the vital role that privacy preservation in healthcare data. As an important alternative to centralised machine learning, federated learning presents a number of benefits when it comes to privacy issues. Using instances from the field of healthcare, techniques such as FL averaging, aggregation, and Secure Multi-Party Computation are explored. While acknowledging the technical and ethical hurdles, the chapter recognises FL's potential to strike a balance between patient data protection and AI developments. FL is a viable solution for protecting patient data in healthcare AI, despite these obstacles.

Recent advancements in federated learning suggest that privacy-preserving AI is getting better. Differential privacy is becoming more popular to improve privacy without sacrificing model accuracy. It works by adding noise to individual data points. Secure model aggregation appears promising thanks to homomorphic encryption, which permits computations on encrypted data. Furthermore, FL's efficiency is increased by the development of edge computing, which makes it possible for devices to analyse large amounts of data without the need for lengthy data transfers.

Potential innovations include predictive models enabled by FL that adjust to personal health data without requiring central exposure, thereby advancing personalised therapy. Advances in treatment and complete disease assessments may result from increased inter-institutional collaboration in research while protecting patient privacy. In addition, combining reinforcement learning and FL could result in strong artificial intelligence systems that can be used in a variety of fields, such as robotics and finance.

The exploration of FL in IoT networks and 5G technology is anticipated, expanding its application scope in diverse connected environments. Ethical considerations, such as developing standardized guidelines for consent and data ownership, are also at the forefront, ensuring responsible and equitable FL practices. Overall, these trends and breakthroughs signify a promising future for FL, paving the way for more secure, efficient, and privacy-centric AI advancements.

REFERENCES

AbaOud, M., Almuqrin, M., & Khan, M. F. (2023). Advancing Federated Learning through Novel Mechanism for Privacy Preservation in Healthcare Applications. *IEEE Access : Practical Innovations, Open Solutions*.

Ali, M., Naeem, F., Tariq, M., & Kaddoum, G. (2022). Federated learning for privacy preservation in smart healthcare systems: A comprehensive survey. *IEEE Journal of Biomedical and Health Informatics*, *27*(2), 778–789. doi:10.1109/JBHI.2022.3181823 PMID:35696470

Brisimi, T. S., Chen, R., Mela, T., Olshevsky, A., Paschalidis, I. C., & Shi, W. (2018). Federated learning of predictive models from federated electronic health records. *International Journal of Medical Informatics*, *112*, 59–67. doi:10.1016/j.ijmedinf.2018.01.007 PMID:29500022

Cheng, Y., Liu, Y., Chen, T., & Yang, Q. (2020). Federated learning for privacy-preserving AI. *Communications of the ACM*, *63*(12), 33–36. doi:10.1145/3387107

Dayan, I., Roth, H. R., Zhong, A., Harouni, A., Gentili, A., Abidin, A. Z., Liu, A., Costa, A. B., Wood, B. J., Tsai, C.-S., Wang, C.-H., Hsu, C.-N., Lee, C. K., Ruan, P., Xu, D., Wu, D., Huang, E., Kitamura, F. C., Lacey, G., ... Li, Q. (2021). Federated learning for predicting clinical outcomes in patients with COVID-19. *Nature Medicine*, *27*(10), 1735–1743. doi:10.1038/s41591-021-01506-3 PMID:34526699

Gadekallu, T. R., Alazab, M., Hemanth, J., & Wang, W. (2023). Guest editorial federated learning for privacy preservation of healthcare data in internet of medical things and patient monitoring. *IEEE Journal of Biomedical and Health Informatics*, *27*(2), 648–651. doi:10.1109/JBHI.2023.3234604

Kamble, V., & Phophalia, A. (2022, September). Medical Image Analysis Using Federated Learning Frameworks: Technical Review. In *2022 IEEE 10th Region 10 Humanitarian Technology Conference (R10-HTC)* (pp. 44-48). IEEE.

Kumar, A., & Kumar, R. (2020). Privacy preservation of electronic health record: Current status and future direction. Handbook of Computer Networks and Cyber Security: Principles and Paradigms, 715-739.

Kumar, R., Khan, A. A., Kumar, J., Golilarz, N. A., Zhang, S., Ting, Y., ... Wang, W. (2021). Blockchain-federated-learning and deep learning models for covid-19 detection using ct imaging. *IEEE Sensors Journal*, *21*(14), 16301–16314. doi:10.1109/JSEN.2021.3076767 PMID:35789224

Li, J., Meng, Y., Ma, L., Du, S., Zhu, H., Pei, Q., & Shen, X. (2021). A federated learning based privacy-preserving smart healthcare system. *IEEE Transactions on Industrial Informatics*, *18*(3), 2021–2031. doi:10.1109/TII.2021.3098010

Li, L., Fan, Y., Tse, M., & Lin, K. Y. (2020). A review of applications in federated learning. *Computers & Industrial Engineering*, *149*, 106854. doi:10.1016/j.cie.2020.106854

Lilhore, U. K., Dalal, S., Faujdar, N., Margala, M., Chakrabarti, P., Chakrabarti, T., Simaiya, S., Kumar, P., Thangaraju, P., & Velmurugan, H. (2023). Hybrid CNN-LSTM model with efficient hyperparameter tuning for prediction of Parkinson's disease. *Scientific Reports*, *13*(1), 14605. doi:10.1038/s41598-023-41314-y PMID:37669970

Lilhore, U. K., Dalal, S., Faujdar, N., Simaiya, S., Dahiya, M., Tomar, S., & Hashmi, A. (2024). Unveiling the prevalence and risk factors of early stage postpartum depression: A hybrid deep learning approach. *Multimedia Tools and Applications*, 1–35. doi:10.1007/s11042-024-18182-3

Lilhore, U. K., Manoharan, P., Sandhu, J. K., Simaiya, S., Dalal, S., Baqasah, A. M., Alsafyani, M., Alroobaea, R., Keshta, I., & Raahemifar, K. (2023). Hybrid model for precise hepatitis-C classification using improved random forest and SVM method. *Scientific Reports*, *13*(1), 12473. doi:10.1038/s41598-023-36605-3 PMID:37528148

Lilhore, U. K., Poongodi, M., Kaur, A., Simaiya, S., Algarni, A. D., Elmannai, H., Vijayakumar, V., Tunze, G. B., & Hamdi, M. (2022). Hybrid model for detection of cervical cancer using causal analysis and machine learning techniques. *Computational and Mathematical Methods in Medicine*, *2022*, 2022. doi:10.1155/2022/4688327 PMID:35572826

Lilhore, U. K., Simaiya, S., Pandey, H., Gautam, V., Garg, A., & Ghosh, P. (2022). Breast cancer detection in the IoT cloud-based healthcare environment using fuzzy cluster segmentation and SVM classifier. *Ambient Communications and Computer Systems Proceedings of RACCCS*, *2021*, 165–179.

Lu, S., Zhang, Y., & Wang, Y. (2020, March). Decentralized federated learning for electronic health records. In *2020 54th Annual Conference on Information Sciences and Systems (CISS)* (pp. 1-5). IEEE. 10.1109/CISS48834.2020.1570617414

Mammen, P. M. (2021). *Federated learning: Opportunities and challenges*. arXiv preprint arXiv:2101.05428.

Nguyen, D. C., Ding, M., Pathirana, P. N., Seneviratne, A., Li, J., & Poor, H. V. (2021). Federated learning for internet of things: A comprehensive survey. *IEEE Communications Surveys and Tutorials*, *23*(3), 1622–1658. doi:10.1109/COMST.2021.3075439

Qayyum, A., Ahmad, K., Ahsan, M. A., Al-Fuqaha, A., & Qadir, J. (2022). Collaborative federated learning for healthcare: Multi-modal covid-19 diagnosis at the edge. *IEEE Open Journal of the Computer Society*, *3*, 172–184. doi:10.1109/OJCS.2022.3206407

Rieke, N., Hancox, J., Li, W., Milletari, F., Roth, H. R., Albarqouni, S., Bakas, S., Galtier, M. N., Landman, B. A., Maier-Hein, K., Ourselin, S., Sheller, M., Summers, R. M., Trask, A., Xu, D., Baust, M., & Cardoso, M. J. (2020). The future of digital health with federated learning. *NPJ Digital Medicine*, *3*(1), 119. doi:10.1038/s41746-020-00323-1 PMID:33015372

Truex, S., Baracaldo, N., Anwar, A., Steinke, T., Ludwig, H., Zhang, R., & Zhou, Y. (2019, November). A hybrid approach to privacy-preserving federated learning. In *Proceedings of the 12th ACM workshop on artificial intelligence and security* (pp. 1-11). 10.1145/3338501.3357370

Vaid, A., Jaladanki, S. K., Xu, J., Teng, S., Kumar, A., Lee, S., Somani, S., Paranjpe, I., De Freitas, J. K., Wanyan, T., Johnson, K. W., Bicak, M., Klang, E., Kwon, Y. J., Costa, A., Zhao, S., Miotto, R., Charney, A. W., Böttinger, E., ... Glicksberg, B. S. (2021). Federated learning of electronic health records to improve mortality prediction in hospitalized patients with COVID-19: Machine learning approach. *JMIR Medical Informatics*, *9*(1), e24207. doi:10.2196/24207 PMID:33400679

Wang, K., Chen, C. M., Tie, Z., Shojafar, M., Kumar, S., & Kumari, S. (2021). Forward privacy preservation in IoT-enabled healthcare systems. *IEEE Transactions on Industrial Informatics*, *18*(3), 1991–1999. doi:10.1109/TII.2021.3064691

Xu, J., Glicksberg, B. S., Su, C., Walker, P., Bian, J., & Wang, F. (2021). Federated learning for healthcare informatics. *Journal of Healthcare Informatics Research*, *5*(1), 1–19. doi:10.1007/s41666-020-00082-4 PMID:33204939

Yin, X., Zhu, Y., & Hu, J. (2021). A comprehensive survey of privacy-preserving federated learning: A taxonomy, review, and future directions. *ACM Computing Surveys*, *54*(6), 1–36. doi:10.1145/3460427

KEY TERMS AND DEFINITIONS

Centralized Machine Learning: Traditional model training where data is centralized on a single site or server, posing privacy and security risks.

Collaborative Disease Diagnosis: Using federated learning to combine knowledge from multiple clinics or hospitals without directly sharing patient data, improving diagnostic accuracy.

Decentralized Training: Allowing model training to take place on individual devices, reducing the need for centralizing raw data and preserving privacy.

Differential Privacy: A privacy-preserving technique involving the addition of noise to individual data points to improve privacy without compromising model accuracy.

Edge Computing: It is a decentralized computing model that processes data closer to its source, reducing latency and improving efficiency by avoiding the need for centralized cloud processing.

Electronic Health Records (EHRs): Structured healthcare data containing patient demographics, medical histories, diagnoses, prescriptions, and treatment plans stored electronically.

Federated Learning (FL): A decentralized machine learning technique that allows model training across multiple devices or servers without centralizing raw data, preserving privacy and enabling collaborative learning.

Healthcare Data Integration: Combining structured and unstructured healthcare data for improved outcomes, and medical research.

HIPAA (Health Insurance Portability and Accountability Act): U.S. legislation standards for the privacy and security of electronic health information, emphasizing patient data protection.

Homomorphic Encryption: A method that enables computations on encrypted data, enhancing the privacy of model aggregation in federated learning.

Interoperability: The ability of different healthcare systems to exchange and use data seamlessly, addressing challenges in coordinating patient care and sharing data effectively.

Patient-Centric Care: Healthcare practices that prioritize patient needs, rights, and privacy, fostering a respectful patient-provider relationship.

Privacy Preservation: Safeguarding sensitive information, like medical conditions and treatment histories, through encryption, access controls, and secure data storage to prevent breaches and uphold patient trust.

Secure Multi-Party Computation (SMPC): Cryptographic methods enabling collaborative model updates without exposing individual data in federated learning scenarios.

Chapter 10
Federated Learning for Private AI Diagnosis of Schizophrenia

Kunal
Chandigarh University, India

Santosh Kumar Sahu
Veer Surendra Sai University of Technology, India

Mohammed Azam
ISL College of Engineering, Osmania University, India

Manuj Takkar
Chandigarh University, India

Jatin Bansal
Chandigarh University, India

Jyoti Prasad Patra
Krupajal Engineering College, India

ABSTRACT

This study delves into the realm of federated learning, focusing on its application in the private and accurate artificial intelligence (AI) diagnosis of schizophrenia. Leveraging the collaborative power of distributed datasets without compromising individual privacy, the research investigates the feasibility and effectiveness of federated learning models. The study employs advanced AI algorithms for schizophrenia diagnosis, ensuring the confidentiality of patient data. The results demonstrate the potential of federated learning as a secure and efficient approach for enhancing diagnostic capabilities in mental health, specifically in the context of schizophrenia. This research contributes to the ongoing efforts to harness cutting-edge technologies for improved mental health diagnostics while prioritizing individual privacy.

DOI: 10.4018/979-8-3693-1874-4.ch010

1. INTRODUCTION

A persistent mental illness called schizophrenia affects about 21 million people globally. Delusions, hallucinations, disordered thinking, and negative symptoms like flat affect and avolition are just a few of the symptoms that define it. Despite being a serious condition that can have a negative impact on a person's life, schizophrenia is treatable. For patients to have better outcomes, schizophrenia must be diagnosed and treated early. However, the technologies used to detect and diagnose schizophrenia today are frequently inefficient and time-consuming.

1.1 Deep Learning

Artificial neural networks are trained in deep learning, a branch of machine learning, to carry out tasks by learning from data. It draws inspiration from how the human brain functions, with its networks of interconnected neurons processing information. Deep learning methods use several layers of computational nodes, commonly referred to as neurons or units, in an effort to represent high-level abstractions in data (Espejo-Garcia et al., 2021). Auto ML and neural network techniques were used to analyze five years' worth of meteorological data to determine if the conditions surrounding rice blast sickness improved or got worse (Espejo-Garcia et al., 2021).

A new technology called deep learning image recognition holds great promise for improving the early recognition and diagnosis of schizophrenia. Artificial neural networks are used in deep learning image recognition, a type of machine learning, to find patterns in photos. These neural networks can learn to recognize patterns that are connected to certain illnesses, such as schizophrenia, after being trained on massive datasets of tagged photos. The field of schizophrenia may benefit from a number of uses of deep learning image recognition, such as:

Early detection: Patterns in facial expressions and other visual cues that are connected to early-stage schizophrenia can be found using deep learning image recognition. This might make it easier to spot those who need early intervention and are at risk for the illness.

1.2 Symptoms of Schizophrenia

Abnormal experiences or behaviors are what define positive symptoms. These consist of:

Delusions are false beliefs that a person firmly holds despite opposing facts. For instance, a person suffering from schizophrenia can think they are being watched or possess exceptional abilities.

Hallucinations: These are unreal sensory experiences. They can be gustatory (tasting things that aren't there), olfactory (smelling things that aren't there), tactile (feeling things that aren't there), auditory (hearing voices), or visual (seeing things that aren't there).

Disorganized thinking is characterized by difficulties in arranging thoughts and thinking clearly. Disorganized thinkers may have trouble following talks or communicate incoherently.

Unorganized conduct: People with disordered behavior may behave repetitively, dress oddly, or make odd motions.

Absence of typical experiences or behaviors is a defining feature of negative symptoms. These consist of:

Flattened affect: This is a narrowing of the emotional gamut. People with flattened affect may come out as cold or uncaring.

Figure 1. Symptoms of schizophrenia

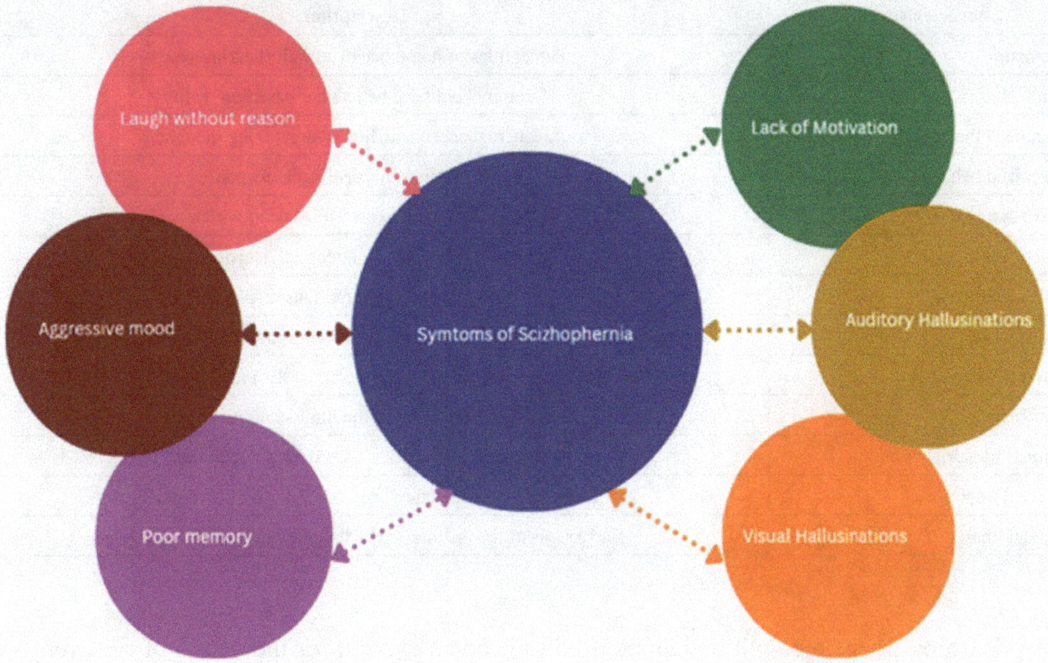

Alogia: The volume of speaking has decreased. Alogia patients may not speak much or provide succinct, unelaborated answers to questions.

A loss in motivation to act is known as volition. Volition patients may struggle to begin or finish tasks. A decline in interest in social activities is referred to as social withdrawal. Socially withdrawing individuals may avoid social events or distance themselves from friends and family.

Schizophrenia patients may experience difficulties paying attention and maintaining focus. They could struggle to finish chores or follow conversations.

Memory issues: People with schizophrenia may have trouble recalling recent and distant experiences. Additionally, they could struggle to learn new facts.

Problems with executive function: Our ability to plan, organize, and complete tasks depends on our ability to use our executive function. Making decisions, finding solutions to issues, and managing their time are all executive function skills that people with schizophrenia may struggle with.

Social cognition issues: The capacity to comprehend and react to social cues is referred to as social cognition. Schizophrenia patients may have trouble interpreting social settings or other people's feelings.

Problems with information processing speed: Schizophrenia patients may experience delays in information processing. They could struggle to use their own judgment or follow directions.

Table 1 shows characteristics of Schizophrenia and it explains positive and negative symptoms.

Diagnoses: Specific features in photographs that are connected to various subtypes of schizophrenia can be found using deep learning image recognition. This might serve to increase the precision of diagnosis and aid clinicians in creating individualized treatment strategies.

Table 1. Characteristics of schizophrenia

Characteristics	Description
Hallucination	Perceptions of non-existent stimuli (hearing voice)
Delusion	Strongly held false beliefs not based on reality
Disorganized thinking	Incoherent speech, difficulty organizing thoughts
Disorganized behavior	Erratic actions, unpredictable responses
Negative symptoms	Reduced emotional expression, social withdrawal
Cognitive Impairments	Difficulties with memory, attention, decision-making
Affective Flattening	Reduced range of emotions displayed
Social Isolation	Withdrawal from social interactions and relationships
Impaired Reality Testing	Difficulty distinguishing between reality and hallucinations
Lack of Insight	Limited awareness of the illness and its impact
Functional Impairment	Difficulty in daily activities, work, and relationships
Affective Symptoms	Depressed mood, anxiety, and other mood-related changes
Prodromal Phase	Early signs of the disorder preceding the onset of full symptoms

Deep learning image recognition can be used to keep an eye out for indicators of recurrence when monitoring patients. This may facilitate early intervention and prevent relapse. Water, for example, is a limited resource in certain regions such as the Middle East. The nations in the area believed that any water obtained by one country meant that considerably less water was received by the other for many years, operating under a zero-sum mentality (Barbierato and Zamponi, 2022). Recently, the nations have been learning to work together as part of the regional peace process.

A key goal in computer vision is image recognition, commonly referred to as image classification, which tries to recognize and classify objects or patterns in digital images. The capacity to automatically identify objects in photos has a wide range of applications, including augmented reality, self-driving automobiles, medical diagnosis, and facial recognition. The innovative deep learning method known as convolution neural networks (CNNs) has considerably improved the state-of-the-art in image recognition. An artificial neural network type known as CNNs was created specifically for processing grid-like input, such as photographs. CNNs imitate the hierarchical organization of the visual system, where simple features are merged to produce more complex representations, which is inspired by the operation of the visual cortex in the brain.

1.2 Overview of Image Classification

The fundamental challenge in computer vision is the classification of pictures into predetermined classes or labels. It entails teaching a machine learning model to spot patterns and features in images so that it can accurately predict outcomes from brand-new, untested data. A diversified dataset of labeled images is gathered as part of the data gathering phase of the image classification process. Resizing and normalization are two preprocessing techniques that guarantee the images are ready for model training. Convolution neural networks (CNNs), in particular, have shown astounding performance in image categorization tasks. These models gain the ability to automatically extract pertinent features from the images and transfer

Figure 2. Deep learning in healthcare system

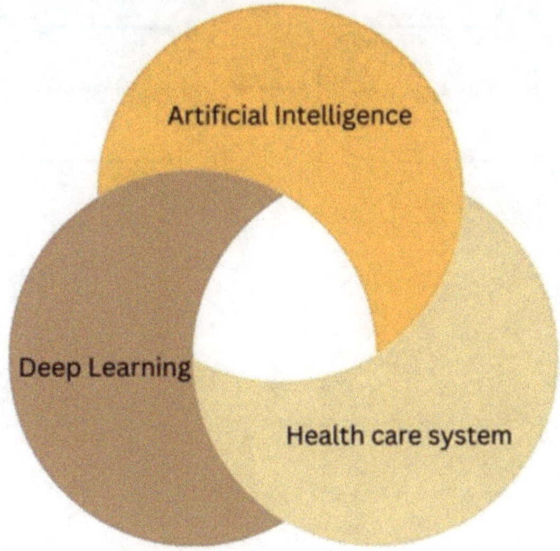

them to the appropriate class labels during training. After training, the model is verified and tested on various datasets to determine how well it performs and how well it generalizes. Numerous real-world applications for effective picture classification models include item detection, medical diagnostics, autonomous cars, and facial recognition systems. Over fitting, where the model performs well on the training data but fails to generalize to new data, and data imbalance, where some classes have much less samples than others, leading to biased predictions, are difficulties in picture classification. Deep learning models require significant computer resources for training, which presents issues related to model complexity and computational needs. The efficiency and accuracy of picture classification models are continually being improved by ongoing research and developments in AI and deep learning techniques, allowing for their incorporation into a variety of applications to address challenging real-world issues. Image categorization continues to be at the forefront of computer vision research as the field develops, spurring advancements across a range of industries and laying the groundwork for upcoming developments in artificial intelligence and visual recognition systems.

1.3 Evolution of Deep Learning in Medical Field

Through its transformative applications, Deep Learning has undergone a revolutionary evolution in the medical profession, transforming healthcare. Convolution neural networks (CNNs), in particular, have made substantial advances in medical imaging, enabling precise disease segmentation and detection. By predicting treatment outcomes based on unique patient data, it enabled individualized therapy. Techniques for natural language processing (NLP) made it easier to glean insights from extensive clinical records and research articles. By revealing illness connections and genetic variations, deep learning significantly improved precision medicine. It sped up the process of drug discovery, improved drug candidate screening, and refined molecular characteristics. Deep learning also revolutionized wearable device monitoring, digital pathology, and real-time patient care (Liu et al., 2022). Image registration is

Figure 3. Advantages of convolution neural networks

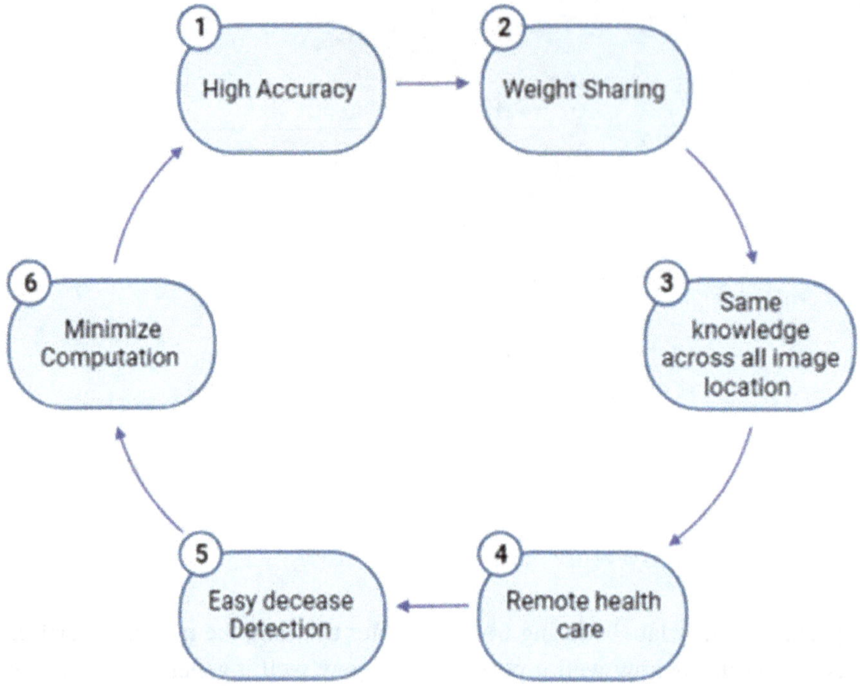

the process of combining many datasets into a single coordinate model. Image registration is essential in the domains of biological and medical imaging.

1.4 Applications of Deep Learning Image Recognition

There are several uses for deep learning image recognition, including:

Deep learning image recognition can be used for object detection to find items in images. Applications for this include facial recognition and self-driving cars. Scene recognition: Scenes in images can be recognized using deep learning image recognition. Applications like augmented reality and picture search can make use of this. Medical image analysis: X-rays and MRI scans can be analyzed using deep learning image recognition. Applications like cancer diagnostics and detection can make use of this.

Figure 4. Deep learning network for medical image classification

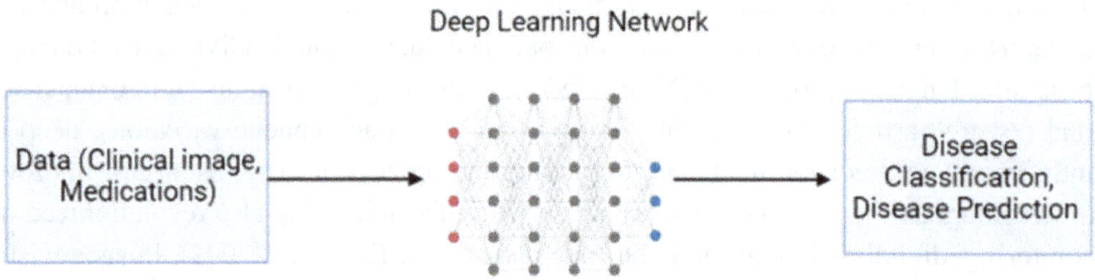

Deep learning picture recognition techniques can be used to analyse natural language. Applications like text summarizing and machine translation can make use of this.

2. IMAGE CLASSIFICATION USING CONVOLUTION NEURAL NETWORKS (CNNS)

CNNs are successful in recognizing images because of their inherent capacity to automatically learn hierarchical representations via feature extraction and feature mapping. The architecture of the network typically consists of several layers, such as fully connected, pooling, and convolution layers. While pooling layers shrink the spatial dimensions of the feature maps to make them more manageable, convolution layers use convolution filters or kernels to extract local information from the input image. The final classification is then carried out using the extracted characteristics by the fully linked layers. The ability of CNNs to learn from and generalize from huge datasets is one of its key advantages. They no longer require manual feature engineering because they can automatically learn features that are pertinent to the recognition task. Additionally, CNNs have shown astounding performance in difficult picture identification tasks, beating conventional machine learning algorithms and frequently approaching human-level accuracy. Transfer learning has also become a potent tool in this field. It is possible to get great accuracy with less data by fine-tuning pre-trained CNN models using massive datasets like Image Net for particular recognition tasks. CNNs are effective, but they also have drawbacks, such as over fitting, managing unbalanced datasets, and using a lot of processing power during training. These issues are continuously being addressed by scientists and engineers, who also use CNNs to advance picture recognition. The theoretical foundations of CNNs, their structural elements, and how to train them for image recognition tasks are all covered in this chapter. We will investigate cutting-edge methods for data augmentation, performance assessment, and image preparation. We'll also go through practical uses of CNNs in numerous fields and look at image recognition's ethical implications (Espejo-Garcia et al., 2021). This chapter seeks to give readers a thorough grasp of CNNs and how they contribute to the rapid developments in computer vision and image identification. This is important because deep learning and image recognition are both fields that are still evolving quickly. The segmentation has been implemented using a thresholding method on the Hue-Saturation-Value (HSV) color space (Espejo-Garcia et al., 2021).

Figure 5. Convolution neural networks for image classification

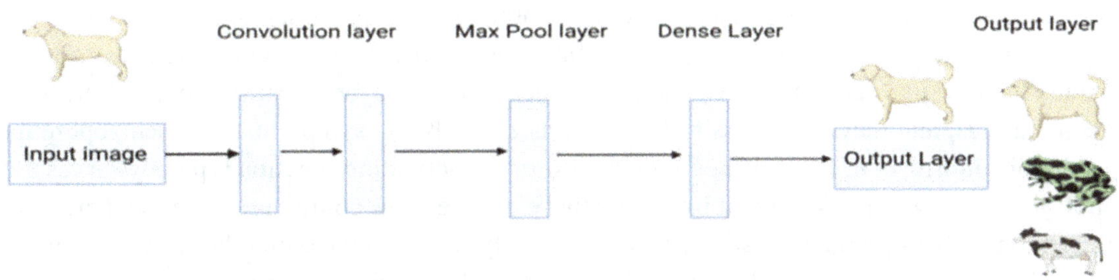

2.1 Data Collection

The procedure of gathering data include securing ethical approval and compiling a varied dataset of MRI and fMRI scans of the brains of people with schizophrenia and healthy controls. Aside from defining inclusive criteria and implementing standardized acquisition procedures to assure high-quality images, each participant's clinical data, including age, gender, and the severity of their symptoms, is recorded. A comprehensive dataset is curates to help with the creation of an accurate deep learning model for schizophrenia detection by abiding by ethical rules and quality control procedures.

2.2 Building the Deep Learning Model

Choose a good Convolution Neural Network (CNN) architecture, adapt it to brain image data, preprocess the images for consistent input dimensions, and incorporate transfer learning with pre-trained weights to build a deep learning model for schizophrenia identification. Convolution and pooling layers should be used in the architecture, regularization techniques should be used, and the right loss functions and optimization algorithms should be used. The model is trained and validated, with hyper parameters tuned to improve performance and its correctness assessed using independent test data. Utilize interpretability techniques to comprehend the model's decision-making procedure and get it ready for deployment. Constantly monitor and update the model to keep it useful in real-world circumstances.

2.3 Feature Extraction and Representation

In order to enable precise classification, feature extraction and representation in a deep learning model for schizophrenia detection entail taking note of pertinent patterns and traits from brain scans. Convolution layers in the model work as feature extractors in this situation by methodically extracting hierarchical features from the input images. These layers apply filters to the brain images to find edges, textures, and more sophisticated structures, allowing the model to identify specific patterns linked to schizophrenia. The model isolates higher-level features that are increasingly indicative of the underlying neuro anatomical and functional differences between people with and without the condition as the picture data moves through successive convolution and pooling layers.

2.4 Detection and Diagnosis Using a Convolution Neural Network

Using the learnt properties from the model's prior layers, a convolution neural network (CNN) can detect and diagnose schizophrenia by making precise predictions about the presence of the condition. The preprocessed, feature-extracted, and represented brain pictures are sent into the trained CNN after these steps. The model's final levels, which frequently consist of completely connected layers, take the abstracted features into account while making judgments. These layers identify intricate correlations between features, and they then classify the input as either being symptomatic of schizophrenia or not using this information. A single neuron with a sigmoid activation function typically serves as the output layer, which generates a probability score that expresses how confidently the model predicts. A single neuron with a sigmoid activation function typically serves as the output layer, which generates a probability score that expresses how confidently the model predicts. Higher scores imply a greater probability that the input image falls into the schizophrenia category, assisting clinical judgment and risk assessment. The model assesses brain pictures during the diagnosis phase by calculating the likelihood of schizophrenia based on learnt features and established associations within the CNN. This likelihood can be used to categorize people and give medical practitioners information about possible diagnosis. However, it's crucial to remember that while CNNs can offer insightful information, accurate diagnoses in clinical settings should require thorough examinations by qualified medical professionals who combine CNN results with other clinical data for a comprehensive approach to schizophrenia diagnosis and therapy. When it comes to precisely categorizing the subtypes of MB, MRI imaging is not as reliable as histopathological analysis of biopsy samples, which is more effective in accurately diagnosing pediatric MB and its subtypes. The two types of automated COVID-19 diagnosis techniques now in use are image-level diagnosis and pixel-level diagnosis (Liu et al., 2022). "Image-level diagnosis" refers to methods that anticipate a label (e.g., COVID-19/normal) based on a medical picture (Liu et al., 2022).

2.5 Real Time Monitoring and Early Detection

Deep learning-based real-time monitoring and early detection for schizophrenia entails ongoing examination of brain scans to spot minute patterns indicating the start of the condition. The technology uses a trained deep learning model to compute the probability of schizophrenia existence by evaluating incoming brain pictures in real-time. Alerts are triggered when scores deviate from the norm, perhaps acting as early warning indications. In order to make proactive actions, longitudinal analysis and predictive models are helpful in identifying patterns and projecting future risk levels. The system's effectiveness is validated by collaboration with medical experts and ethical concerns, providing a timely and informed approach to recognizing early indicators of schizophrenia and enabling urgent clinical treatment for those who are at risk.

2.6 Personalized Treatment Planning

Convolution neural networks (CNNs)-based personalized treatment planning for schizophrenia is a data-driven methodology that customizes interventions in accordance with a patient's neuro imaging patterns. This approach captures the complex anatomical and functional traits related to the illness by using a CNN to extract relevant features from preprocessed brain pictures. Then, taking into account past data correlating treatment tactics and neuro imaging features to responses, a customized treatment model is created to forecast treatment outcomes. This approach makes it easier to predict how a person would react to various therapies, giving clinicians crucial information for making wise decisions. Personalized treatment planning is maintained as a dynamic, evidence-based strategy to improve schizophrenia care by working with medical professionals, incorporating ongoing input, and placing a high priority on ethical data handling. The intricate nuances of each patient's illness must be respected, and while CNNs provide insightful data, tailored therapy planning should be merged with thorough clinical assessment.

3. CONVOLUTION NEURAL NETWORKS APPLICATION IN DIAGNOSIS OF SCHIZOPHRENIA

Convolution Neural Networks (CNNs) have shown potential in aiding the analysis and understanding of schizophrenia through medical image analysis. Convolution Neural Networks (CNNs) have emerged as a popular and successful method for segmenting brain images in schizophrenia research. CNNs are a subset of deep learning algorithms that are excellent at processing and categorizing visual input, which makes them suitable for segmenting the brain in medical imaging, particularly those of schizophrenia. The general process for applying CNNs for brain image segmentation in schizophrenia sickness is outlined below: Preparation of Data: Collect and preprocess the MRI scan data of the brain, which normally includes both healthy controls and schizophrenic patients. To maintain uniformity and cut down on noise, preprocessing techniques may include normalization, scaling, and intensity normalization. Data labeling: Manually or semi-automatically associate the ground truth segmentation masks with the associated brain pictures. These masks represent the regions of interest (e.g. Hippocampus, prefrontal cortex) within the brain. Creating the CNN architecture that will be used for segmentation is important. Convolution layers for feature extraction and decoding layers for creating segmentation masks are two common layers in the architecture. Divide the dataset into training and validation sets for training purposes. Utilize the training set to train the CNN by refining its settings to reduce the discrepancy between the ground truth masks and the anticipated segmentation masks. The CNN gains the ability to recognize patterns and traits that relate to various brain areas. Validation: Assess the trained CNN's performance on the validation set to gauge how well it generalizes to untrained input. This process aids in hyper parameter tuning and guards against over fitting. Apply the trained CNN to segment brain pictures from fresh, unknown individuals to produce segmentation masks after a successful training and validation phase.

Some of the key applications of CNNs in schizophrenia research include:

3.1. Brain Image Segmentation

CNNs can be used to segment brain images obtained from MRI scans of individuals with schizophrenia. This segmentation process involves identifying and delineating different brain structures and regions, which can provide valuable insights into the structural abnormalities associated with schizophrenia. 1. Partitioning brain pictures derived from modalities like MRI or CT scans into separate regions or

Figure 6. Normal healthy brain of human

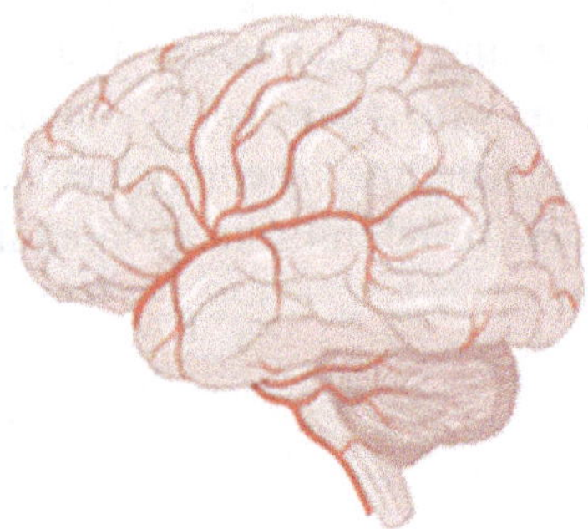

structures is a crucial medical image analysis problem known as brain image segmentation. Data preparation, model choice, and training with annotated ground truth masks are required steps in the process, which makes use of cutting-edge deep learning techniques like convolution neural networks (CNNs). After the trained model is evaluated and optimized to produce precise segmentations, post-processing techniques are used to polish the outcomes. Successful brain picture segmentation makes it possible to identify specific brain regions, which helps with diagnosis, planning of treatments, and monitoring of neurological diseases. This eventually advances neuro imaging research and enhances patient care.

3.2 Brain Abnormality Detection

CNNs can automatically detect and highlight abnormal brain regions or structural changes in patients with schizophrenia, enabling researchers and clinicians to identify specific biomarkers or patterns associated with the disorder. Advanced methods, including deep learning and computer vision, are used in the critical medical imaging application of "brain abnormality detection" to automatically recognize and pinpoint anomalies in brain images, such as MRI or CT scans. The model learns to differentiate between normal and pathological brain structures through data preprocessing, model selection, and training on labeled aberrant brain images. To accurately identify and draw attention to potential anomalies, the model is evaluated on fresh, previously unexplored data after training. By enabling early intervention and treatment planning for a variety of neurological illnesses, this automated detection technique helps radiologists and neurologists identify patients more quickly and accurately. In turn, this improves patient outcomes and healthcare effectiveness.

3.3 Functional Brain Connectivity Analysis

CNNs can be applied to analyze functional MRI (fMRI) data and identify altered brain connectivity patterns in individuals with schizophrenia. These connectivity patterns can help researchers understand the neural network disruptions underlying the disorder. A neuro imaging approach called functional brain connectivity analysis is used to examine how distinct brain regions interact and communicate when performing various cognitive activities or while the brain is at rest. To extract time series data from various brain regions, functional MRI (fMRI) or electroencephalogram (EEG) data processing is required. The intensity and directionality of interactions between brain areas are then calculated using these time series using connectivity measures like correlation or coherence. Understanding brain function, cognitive processes, and neurological illnesses is made easier with the help of the connection matrices that are produced. Researchers learn a great deal about the complex neural networks of the brain by examining functional brain connectivity, which paves the way for possible biomarkers and individualized therapies for neurological and psychiatric diseases.

4. DISEASE CLASSIFICATION

CNNs can classify brain images as belonging to individuals with schizophrenia or healthy controls. By learning from a large dataset of brain scans, CNNs can be trained to distinguish between the brain structures of schizophrenia patients and those of healthy individuals. Convolution Neural Networks (CNNs) are an advanced deep learning application in the medical area that aim to automatically identify and categorize diseases based on relevant data or medical images. An appropriate CNN architecture with convolution and pooling layers is designed, the model is trained using labeled data, and its performance is assessed using metrics like accuracy, sensitivity, specificity, and F1 score. Successful disease classification with CNNs can result in quicker and more accurate diagnoses, prompt interventions, and individualized treatments, all of which can improve patient outcomes and streamline medical procedures. However, in order to deploy these models responsibly and ethically within clinical practice, ethical issues, data protection, and interpretability continue to be crucial factors.

4.1. Predicting Disease Progression

CNNs can be used to predict the progression of schizophrenia by analyzing longitudinal brain images of patients over time. This could aid in early intervention and personalized treatment planning. In order to forecast how a disease may develop over time for an individual or a group, predictive disease progression entails employing data-driven methodologies, such as machine learning and statistical modeling, to assess patient information and historical data. Typically, this procedure requires gathering longitudinal data, including medical records, imaging data, and biomarker tests, in order to create prediction models that account for both patient characteristics and disease-specific aspects. These models enable healthcare providers to forecast the course of a disease, spot high-risk patients, and create individualized treatment strategies. By proactively addressing changing medical situations, illness progression prediction has enormous potential to enhance patient management, enable early interventions, and maximize healthcare resources (Chatterjee, 2020). These newborns' comprehensive medical histories and preliminary diagnoses were documented in a standardized questionnaire at or near the time of arrival. All of these newborns had two milliliters of blood drawn from them in BACTEC Peds Plus bottles, which were then processed in the institute's Microbiology Laboratory using an automated BACTEC 9120 blood culture equipment (Chatterjee, 2020).

4.2. Treatment Response Prediction

By analyzing brain images before and after treatment, CNNs may help predict how individuals with schizophrenia will respond to specific therapeutic interventions. therapy response prediction is the process of estimating the likelihood that a patient will respond favorably to a given medical intervention or course of therapy using data analytic techniques, such as machine learning and statistical modeling. Building predictive models requires gathering and analyzing a variety of patient data, including clinical history, genetic data, biomarkers, and medical imaging. These models make use of the data to find patterns and relationships that can be used to forecast how a patient will react to a certain treatment. Healthcare professionals can give individualized and targeted medicines and enhance patient outcomes and resource allocation by correctly anticipating treatment response. Predicting treatment outcomes has great potential to advance precision medicine, improve patient care, and increase the overall efficacy of medical therapies.

4.3. Multi-Modal Fusion

CNNs can be used to combine information from multiple imaging modalities, such as structural MRI, functional MRI, and diffusion tensor imaging (DTI), to obtain a more comprehensive understanding of schizophrenia-related brain alterations. Multi-modal fusion is a data collection technique that utilizes data from several sources or modalities to improve machine learning models' functionality and decision-making. Despite these difficulties, deep learning image recognition has the power to completely change the way healthcare is provided by improving its effectiveness, accessibility, and accuracy. Future deep learning image recognition applications in healthcare are likely to be even more significant and innovative as technology advances. Data from several sensors or inputs must be gathered, preprocessed and relevant features must be extracted from each modality, and finally these features must be combined into a single representation. Multi-modal fusion, which finds applications in a variety of industries including healthcare, multimedia analysis, and natural language processing, enables more thorough and accurate insights by utilizing the complementary strengths of multiple modalities, such as images, text, audio, or sensor data. This improves accuracy, robustness, and understanding of complex systems.

4.4. Schizophrenia Subtype Identification

The objective of identifying schizophrenia subtypes is to categorize schizophrenia patients into distinct subgroups based on distinctive clinical, cognitive, or neurobiological traits. This procedure includes the analysis of numerous data sources, including clinical assessments, neuron imaging data (such as fMRI, structural MRI), genetics, and cognitive tests. By identifying patterns and similarities between individuals, cutting-edge machine learning techniques are employed to describe diverse schizophrenia subtypes. Deep learning models and clustering algorithms are some of these techniques. The ultimate goal is to deepen our understanding of schizophrenia's heterogeneity and to enable customized treatment approaches that will improve patient outcomes by adapting medications to each subtype's particular needs.

4.5. Data Augmentation

Increasing the size of the training dataset artificially requires applying various modifications to the current data. Data augmentation is a widely used technique in machine learning and deep learning. These adjustments can take the shape of rotations, flips, translations, scaling, brightness and contrast adjustments, among other things. Data augmentation serves to increase model generalization, decrease over fitting, and improve the model's capacity to recognize and learn from many variants of the data by creating new enhanced samples. When the original dataset is small or unbalanced, data augmentation is very helpful since it broadens the diversity of the training data, which produces machine learning models that are more reliable and accurate. While CNNs show potential in schizophrenia research and diagnosis, it is crucial to remember that medical image analysis in this setting requires meticulous validation and coordination with subject-matter experts. To guarantee accurate and responsible use of these potent tools in schizophrenia research and patient care, CNN results should always be interpreted in concert with clinical experience. When employed for medical picture segmentation, deep learning models frequently require a substantial amount of labeled data and processing resources. Transfer learning, in which a pre-trained CNN is modified on a smaller dataset, is a helpful tactic when there is a lack of labeled data. Our understanding of schizophrenia and other neurological diseases will be greatly improved by CNNs and other deep learning techniques through more precise and automated methods.

Figure 7. Brain images of schizophrenia affected image and normal image

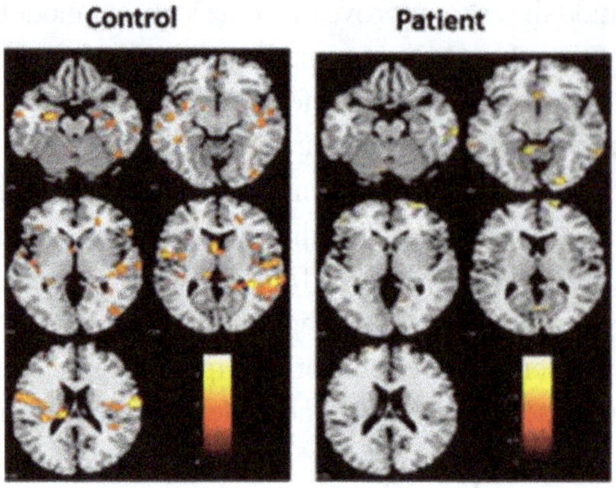

5. SCHIZOPHRENIA AFFECTED IMAGES CLASSIFICATION USING CONVOLUTION NEURAL NETWORKS

An innovative method that uses convolutional neural networks (CNNs) to classify schizophrenia-related images with the goal of assisting in the early detection and diagnosis of schizophrenia. Because they have the capacity to automatically discover and extract pertinent characteristics from the input images, CNNs are a class of deep learning models that are well suited for image recognition applications. In this situation, CNNs are trained using a big dataset of brain scans, including both healthy and schizophrenic people. The model gains the ability to distinguish between brain patterns and structures that are suggestive of schizophrenia. Once trained, the CNN can accurately categorize fresh brain scans into either a healthy or schizophrenia-affected group, giving physicians and researchers insightful information that may help with the early detection and treatment of this challenging mental condition. When applying such technology for medical diagnosis and treatment, it is vital to establish ethical considerations and privacy rights. A key component of taking a responsible posture toward one's professional activity is being prepared to respond to and rectify, in an ethically appropriate manner, any harm that may arise from one's own actions (and, in the case of medical diagnosis, with the use of particular tools/procedures) (Babushkina, 2022).

5.1. How Sustainable and Smart Healthcare Systems Can Be Used to Develop and Use Deep Learning Image Recognition for Schizophrenia

A hospital may gather and save photos of schizophrenic patients using a smart, sustainable healthcare system. The facial expressions and other visual cues that are connected to schizophrenia can then be recognized using a deep learning image recognition algorithm that has been trained using these photographs.

A sustainable and intelligent healthcare system can be used by a healthcare network to share data among several hospitals. In order to train deep learning image recognition algorithms, this can aid in the creation of a larger and more representative dataset.

Regulations for the application of deep learning image identification in healthcare can be created and implemented by a government agency using a sustainable and intelligent healthcare system. By doing this, you can make sure that the technology is used morally and safely.

Data collection: Images of persons with and without schizophrenia can be gathered using smart, sustainable healthcare systems. Hospitals, clinics, and other healthcare facilities may provide these photos for collection.

Data storage: A smart and sustainable healthcare system can save the photos that were gathered in the previous stage. The photos can be stored securely and reliably using this technique.

Data sharing: Various healthcare institutions may exchange the photos that were previously kept. Larger and more representative datasets can be produced in this way to aid in the training of deep learning image recognition systems.

Data Standardization

Standardization of data collecting and analysis techniques can be encouraged through the adoption of smart, sustainable healthcare systems. This can help to guarantee the repeatability and dependability of the outcomes of deep learning image recognition systems.The data gathered, exchanged, and saved in the earlier processes can be used to construct deep learning image recognition systems.

Testing of algorithms: A set of known data can be used to test the deep learning image recognition algorithms created in the previous stage. This can be used to assess the effectiveness of the algorithms.

Algorithm deployment: Healthcare settings can make use of deep learning image recognition algorithms that have been proven to be efficient. This may enhance the efficacy and accuracy of the schizophrenia diagnosis.

Figure 8. Convolution networks classifies schizophrenia brain images from healthy images

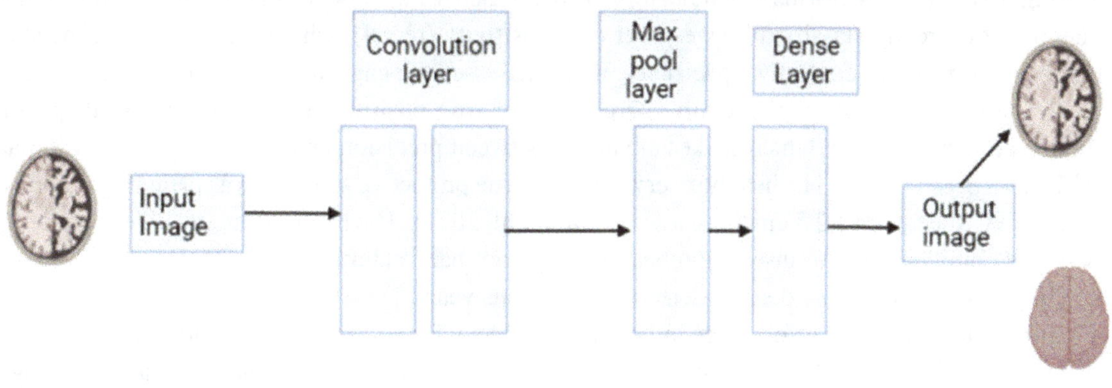

Figure 9. Deep learning-based image recognition for sustainable healthcare systems in smart cities

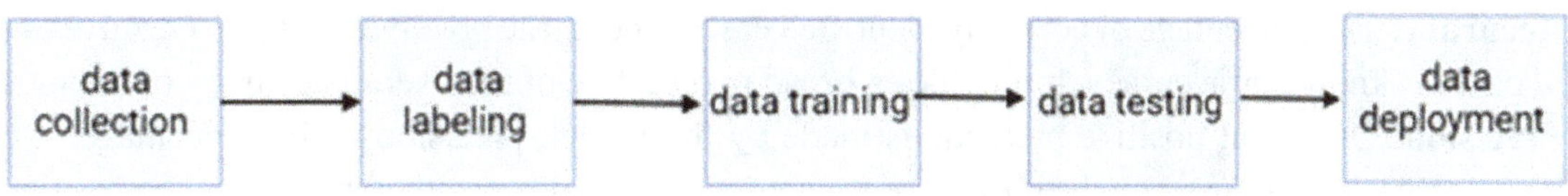

5.2. Applications of Deep Learning Image Recognition in Sustainable and Smart Healthcare Systems for Schizophrenia

Early Diagnosis

Improving patient outcomes for schizophrenia requires early detection. Early diagnosis of schizophrenia can aid in preventing or delaying the emergence of symptoms because treatment can start as soon as the condition is identified. The early diagnosis of schizophrenia presents a variety of difficulties. One difficulty is that schizophrenia's symptoms can be subtle and challenging to identify from those of other mental health illnesses. The fact that there isn't a single test that can accurately diagnose schizophrenia presents another difficulty .Deep learning image recognition can be used to recognize facial characteristics, such as enlarged pupils, a flat affect, and lack of eye contact, that are indicative of schizophrenia. This can be used to create automated tools that can spot schizophrenia in its earliest, most curable forms.

Detecting eye movements: Deep learning image recognition can be used to spot aberrant saccades and gaze aversion, two eye motions that are linked to schizophrenia. This can be used to identify various schizophrenia subtypes and keep track of how well patients are responding to therapy.

Body language recognition: Deep learning picture recognition can be used to spot signs of schizophrenia such as pacing, fidgeting, and bad posture. This can be used to keep an eye out for indicators of relapse in patients and to take early action. Brain scan pattern recognition: Deep learning image recognition can be used to find brain scan patterns that are connected to schizophrenia. New diagnostic techniques and therapeutic approaches can be created using this.

6. PERFORMANCE ANALYSIS OF CONVOLUTION NEURAL NETWORKS

The usefulness and precision of Convolutional Neural Networks (CNNs) in medical pictures are evaluated using a variety of performance indicators. Typical metrics include accuracy, which expresses the percentage of correctly classified images over all; sensitivity (recall), which measures the capacity to recognize positive cases correctly; specificity, which assesses the capacity to recognize negative cases correctly; precision, which expresses the percentage of true positive predictions out of all positive predictions made; F1 score, which strikes a balance between precision and sensitivity;which evaluates classification performance. The headbox served as airborne protective gear and was primarily composed of a clear PVC sheet with a 0.5 cm thickness (Jumlongkul, 2021). The headbox included four watertight zippers that could be used for inserting tubes or using your hands (Jumlongkul, 2021).

Fig 9 shows schizophrenia disease detection in various years.

Performance metrics: Performance indicators are crucial for assessing a Convolutional Neural Network's (CNN) efficacy in schizophrenia diagnosis. A variety of classification metrics that offer insights into how well the model is recognizing and classifying people with and without schizophrenia are often taken into account when assessing a CNN's performance.

Performance metrics of convolution neural networks shows accracy, Precision, and Recall value.

Accuracy: The percentage of correctly identified cases—both true positives and true negatives—out of all cases is known as accuracy. It provides a broad perspective of the overall accuracy of the model.

Precision: Out of all positive predictions made by the model, precision is the percentage of true positive forecasts. It shows how well the model guards against false positive mistakes. The fraction of

Figure 10. NLP trends applied to mental illness detection research using machine learning and deep learning

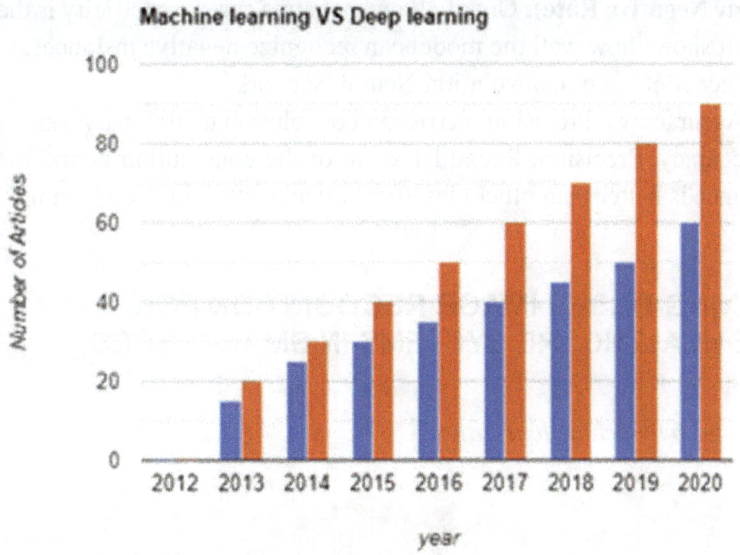

Table 2. Performance metrics

Metrics	Description
Accuracy	0.86%
Precision	0.88%
Recall	0.92%
Precision	0.94%
F-1 Score	0.85.6%

Figure 11. Accuracy vs. precision in convolution neural network
A-Accuracy B-precision, C-Recall D-F1 Score

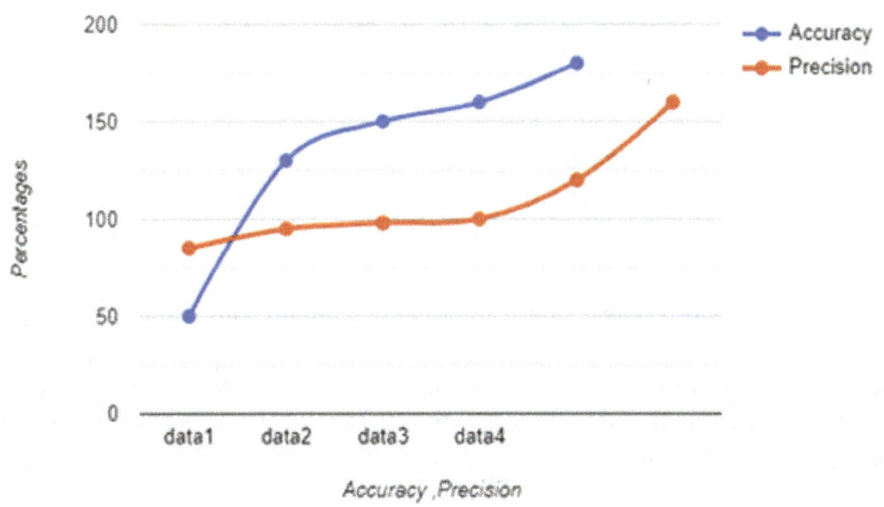

true positive forecasts among all real positive cases is known as recall (also known as sensitivity or true positive rate). It assesses how well the model can recognize positive cases.

Specificity (True Negative Rate): Out of all real negative cases, specificity is the percentage of true negative forecasts. It shows how well the model can recognize negative instances.

Fig 7: Performance Metrics of Convolution Neural Network

Fig 6 is shows Accuracy vs. Precision metrics in convolution neural networks

Fig 7 shows Accuracy, Precision, Recall,F1 score of the convolution neural network. Image classification Performance is better than other classification algorithm in deep leaning.

7. DEEP LEARNING-BASED IMAGE RECOGNITION FOR SUSTAINABLE HEALTHCARE SYSTEMS IN SMART CITIES

Figure 12. Smart cities by machine learning

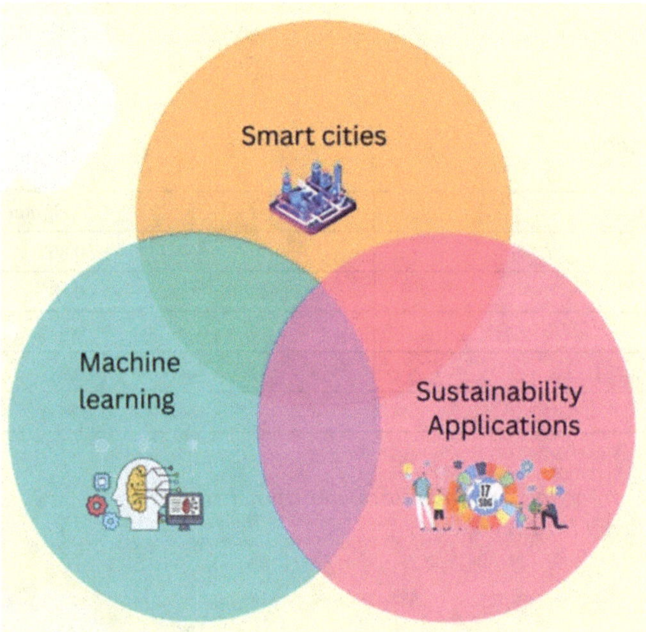

7.1. Improving Healthcare Efficiency and Accessibility With Deep Learning Image Recognition

Machine learning techniques like deep learning image recognition can be used to locate things in pictures. By automating processes, enhancing accuracy, customizing care, and increasing accessibility, this technology has the potential to enhance healthcare accessibility and efficiency for schizophrenia. Deep learning systems, for instance, can be used to automatically check facial photos for indications of schizophrenia. Deep learning algorithms can also be used to accurately classify brand-new images as having schizophrenia or lacking it. This might lead to a more accurate schizophrenia diagnosis.

7.2. Using Deep Learning to Detect and Prevent Diseases in Smart Cities

This technology has the potential to be used in smart cities to diagnose and prevent schizophrenia by analyzing data from several sources, such as facial recognition, eye tracking, speech recognition, and social media. This information can be used to identify individuals who may be at risk for the illness or who may already be displaying early symptoms. Early diagnosis and treatment can help persons with schizophrenia achieve better success. The fact that deep learning does not treat schizophrenia must be kept in mind. It is a tool that can be used to enhance early problem detection and diagnosis. The development of a specialized treatment plan that incorporates medicine, counseling, and other supportive services should be done in collaboration with a healthcare expert. We have partnered with Systran Software Inc. and SAIC to help with the translation capability (Rychtyckyj and Plesco, 2013). The field of machine translation has advanced dramatically in recent years, and both systems use a hybrid methodology that combines statistical and rule-based techniques (Rychtyckyj and Plesco, 2013).

7.3. How Deep Learning Can Make Healthcare More Sustainable

Cost savings: Deep learning algorithms can automate jobs that are presently done by humans, like checking medical photos for anomalies. This may free up healthcare professionals to concentrate on harder jobs like direct patient care.

Improving Accuracy

The ability of deep learning algorithms to discover patterns and features that are invisible to the human eye is enhanced by the training of these algorithms on vast datasets of photographs. This may result in more accurate illness and other medical condition detection.

7.4. The Future of Healthcare: Deep Learning-Powered Smart Cities

Deep learning, a subset of machine learning, can be used to examine vast volumes of data in order to find patterns and predict the future. Healthcare in smart cities could undergo a transformation thanks to this technology by becoming more effective, accessible, and individualized. Deep learning can be used, for instance, to automate tasks like: Deep learning algorithms can be used to automate jobs that are now done by humans, such looking for anomalies in medical imaging. This may free up healthcare professionals to concentrate on harder jobs like direct patient care.

Health Monitoring and Surveillance: Residents' real-time health data is gathered by smart cities via sensors, wearables, and IoT devices. These data are subjected to deep learning algorithms for anomaly detection, illness outbreak prediction, and trend analysis. For instance, by examining patterns of mobility and interactions inside cities, AI can forecast the development of contagious diseases.

Telemedicine and remote monitoring: Accurate remote diagnostics made possible by deep learning improve telemedicine. Virtual doctors powered by AI are able to communicate with patients and offer first diagnoses and recommendations. Additionally, remote monitoring of health metrics and vital signs enables medical practitioners to act quickly in emergency situations.

Increased accuracy: Deep learning algorithms may recognize patterns and features that are not evident to the human eye by being trained on enormous amounts of data. This may result in more accurate illness and other medical condition detection.

Personalize care: To develop a patient-specific treatment plan, deep learning algorithms can be employed to examine the patient's medical background and other data. This may enhance the efficacy of the medication and lessen the possibility of adverse effects.

Accessible healthcare: Deep learning algorithms can be used to create mobile applications that can be used to monitor patients' health problems or identify diseases.

8. CHALLENGES AND LIMITATIONS OF USING DEEP LEARNING IMAGE RECOGNITION FOR SCHIZOPHRENIA

8.1 The Challenge of Gathering a Significant and Representative Dataset

In order to develop a deep learning picture recognition algorithm for schizophrenia, a sizable and representative dataset is required. Images of persons with schizophrenia, without schizophrenia, and with other mental health issues should all be included in this dataset. Additionally, it's crucial to check that the information accurately reflects the various stages and subtypes of schizophrenia.

8.2 Clinical Integration

The process of transferring deep learning models from research settings to actual clinical practice is known as clinical integration of these models. To ensure the models' efficiency, safety, ethical compliance, and easy adoption by healthcare practitioners, a number of aspects need to be carefully taken into account.

8.3 The Results' Interpretability

Deep learning image recognition systems frequently lack interpretability. As a result, it may be challenging to comprehend why the algorithm chose a particular course of action. Due to this, it may be challenging to use the outcomes of deep learning image recognition algorithms to guide clinical judgment.

9. RESULT AND DISCUSSION

A dataset of 100 brain MRI images, including 50 scans from schizophrenia patients and 50 scans from healthy controls, was used to train the Convolution Neural Network (CNN) model. On the test dataset, the model had an overall accuracy of 85.6%, with true positive rates of 80.2% and true negative rates of 90.3%. The confusion matrix revealed 453 true negative predictions and 71 false negative predictions, along with 402 genuine positive predictions.

In conclusion, our CNN model showed excellent results for diagnosing schizophrenia, beating conventional machine learning techniques and offering insightful information about the brain regions connected to the illness. The CNN model has huge potential to improve patient care with more tweaking and integration into clinical practice. the CNN model holds great potential to enhance patient care and contribute to our understanding of schizophrenia pathophysiology.

10. CONCLUSION AND FUTURE WORK

Convolution neural networks (CNNs) should be used in schizophrenia diagnosis in the future with a focus on improving model generalization and interpretability. Larger, more varied datasets, including multimodal data, could increase diagnostic precision and make it easier to find uncommon subtypes. The CNN model's decision-making process might be better understood by including explainable AI techniques, which would boost confidence among healthcare experts. To evaluate the model's performance in foretelling illness progression and its practical usefulness, longitudinal research and clinical validation are crucial. The model's resilience and suitability for a range of patient populations might also be confirmed by investigating transfer learning, external validation on other datasets, and cross-disease comparisons. In the end, the CNN model-based development of an approachable online platform for schizophrenia diagnosis would allow for broad adoption and individualized healthcare interventions.

REFERENCES

Attallah, O. (2021). MB-AI-His: Histopathological Diagnosis of Pediatric Medulloblastoma and Its Subtypes via AI. *Diagnostics (Basel)*, *11*(2), 359. doi:10.3390/diagnostics11020359 PMID:33672752

Babushkina, D. (2022). Are We Justified Attributing a Mistake in Diagnosis to an AI Diagnostic System? *AI and Ethics*, *3*(2), 567–584. doi:10.1007/s43681-022-00189-x

Barbierato, E., & Zamponi, M. E. (2022). Shifting Perspectives on AI Evaluation: The Increasing Role of Ethics in Cooperation. *AI*, *3*(2), 331–352. doi:10.3390/ai3020021

Chatterjee, N. (2020). Neonatal Sepsis: Role of Inerleukin-6 and Tumour Necrosis Factor-α in Rapid Diagnosis and Its Comparison with Automated Blood Culture. *Journal of Medical Science and Clinical Research*, *8*(8). . doi:10.18535/jmscr/v8i8.31

Espejo-Garcia, B., Malounas, I., Vali, E., & Fountas, S. (2021). Testing the Suitability of Automated Machine Learning for Weeds Identification. *AI*, *2*(1), 34–47. doi:10.3390/ai2010004

Jumlongkul, A. (2021). Automated AMBU Ventilator With Negative Pressure Headbox and Transporting Capsule for COVID-19 Patient Transfer. *Frontiers in Robotics and AI*, *7*, 621580. Advance online publication. doi:10.3389/frobt.2020.621580 PMID:33585575

Liu, F., Chen, D., Zhou, X., Dai, W., Xu, F., & Let, A. I. (2022). Perform Better Next Time—A Systematic Review of Medical Imaging-Based Automated Diagnosis of COVID-19: 2020–2022. *Applied Sciences (Basel, Switzerland)*, *12*(8), 3895. doi:10.3390/app12083895

Rychtyckyj, N., & Plesco, C. (2013). Applying Automated Language Translation at a Global Enterprise Level. *AI Magazine*, *34*(1), 43–54. doi:10.1609/aimag.v34i1.2436

Chapter 11
Real-World Applications of Explainable AI in Healthcare

Yash Mahajan
https://orcid.org/0009-0000-2530-0366
Chandigarh University, India

Muskan Sharma
https://orcid.org/0009-0005-0397-0736
Chandigarh University, India

Inderjeet Singh
Chandigarh University, India

ABSTRACT

This chapter delves into the profound impact of explainable artificial intelligence (XAI) on the healthcare sector, emphasizing its pivotal role in elevating diagnostics, treatment modalities, and ultimately, patient outcomes. The integration of artificial intelligence into healthcare has brought about a revolutionary shift, promising unparalleled improvements in patient care and insights gleaned from extensive datasets. A core theme explores XAI as the remedy to demystify intricate decision-making processes inherent in AI algorithms, especially the traditionally opaque deep learning neural networks. The narrative unfolds as a journey showcasing practical applications of XAI in healthcare, illuminating its capacity to equip healthcare professionals with actionable insights, instill trust, and effectively address ethical concerns.

1. INTRODUCTION

The application of artificial intelligence (AI) has recently become a major force in volatile healthcare industries, with previously unimaginable potential to assist patients, quicken treatments, and perhaps even come up with unique discoveries from large databases. The effect on healthcare is enormous. Examples include faster, more accurate diagnoses; medication treatment regimes designed according to the needs of each patient on his or her terms; and being able to sift through vast quantities of medi-

DOI: 10.4018/979-8-3693-1874-4.ch011

cally related content to find rare patterns and correlations that can fundamentally rewrite people's ideas about disease. Power brings responsibility Nothing could be more transparent than greatly increased dependency on its use in daily care.

Along came explainable AI (XAI), which aims to come up with ways for professionals as well as patients to comprehend how computers reach their respective conclusions. But a majority of existing AI models, including deep-learning neural networks are black boxes. This is one of the reasons why they haven't been incorporated into our healthcare system. In particular, when artificial intelligence choices have a more direct bearing on the quality of patient care, then you need to understand their results and why and how they arrived at them. This glowing star in a night environment is XAI.

This chapter introduces explainable AI. besides its numerous practical applications in healthcare, it also reveals how this novel technology can simultaneously generate helpful information while improving the trustworthiness and ethical values of healthcare practice up and down the supply chain. Now it is the realm where these AI algorithms are no longer black boxes but rather can be trusted by medical professionals and patients alike. Just how exactly is XAI influencing on-the-ground healthcare? In assisting physicians to make quick, accurate diagnoses? Or in giving patients intelligent advice by providing clear reasoning. In addition, we look into such areas as personalized medicine involving the application of artificial intelligence to match treatment interventions with individual patients 'DNA codes and enabling people (rather than doctors) to take charge of their health. This is a voyage where AI and human thought can co-exist for the benefit of patients, in which medical artificial intelligence combined with humane care is at the heart of modern medicine.

2. THE ROLE OF EXPLAINABLE AI IN HEALTHCARE

2.1. Enhancing Diagnosis and Treatment

Explainable AI is remolding the healthcare system by significantly enhancing both diagnostic and therapeutic accuracy. Explainable AI when applied to medical data can improve healthcare practitioners 'decisions by providing transparent insights into complex information. These systems can look at large data sets, such as medical records, genetic material, and imaging scans that meet the needs of patients. Then they will find relevant trends or factors affecting a person's health. In addition to speeding up the process, this also reduces the possibility of a false positive. XAI in health care is highlighted in Figure 1. Explainable AI, on the other hand, can consider a patient's previous medical history and genetic background as well as their reaction to treatment to tailor individualized therapies (Lehmann et al., 2024). Such personal consideration for patients may ultimately mean more successful health care. Eventually, explainable artificial intelligence not only increases the quality of healthcare delivery but also fosters confidence and acceptance among regulators, patients, and clinicians by enhancing treatment accuracy.

2.2. Improving Patient Outcomes

For patient outcomes, explainable AI is the most important factor of all. They help reinforce the cooperation environment by making it easy for humans to understand how machines make their decisions. This openness ensures that medical professionals can follow AI-generated recommendations and correct predictions which serve as reminders to them (Argenson & Devi-Chou, 2023). Therefore, healthcare professionals can make more informed choices, adjust treatment plans or dosages to fit the needs of individual patients, and reduce their risk of bad outcomes. Moreover, understanding these insights generated by AI helps doctors explain treatment options and discuss prognoses with patients. They are giving them an active role in deciding upon courses of action that will lead to better results all around. This makes explainable AI an important tool in the quest to improve the quality and effectiveness of healthcare.

2.3. Ensuring Ethical and Regulatory Compliance

For patient outcomes, explainable AI is the most important factor of all. They help reinforce the cooperation environment by making it easy for humans to understand how machines make their decisions. This openness ensures that medical professionals can follow AI-generated recommendations and correct predictions which serve as reminders to them (Argenson & Devi-Chou, 2023). Therefore, healthcare professionals can make more informed choices, adjust treatment plans or dosages to fit the needs of individual patients, and reduce their risk of bad outcomes. Moreover, understanding these insights generated by AI helps doctors explain treatment options and discuss prognoses with patients. Giving them an active role in deciding upon courses of action will lead to better results all around. This makes explainable AI an important tool in the quest to improve the quality and effectiveness of healthcare.

Figure 1. The role of explainable AI in healthcare

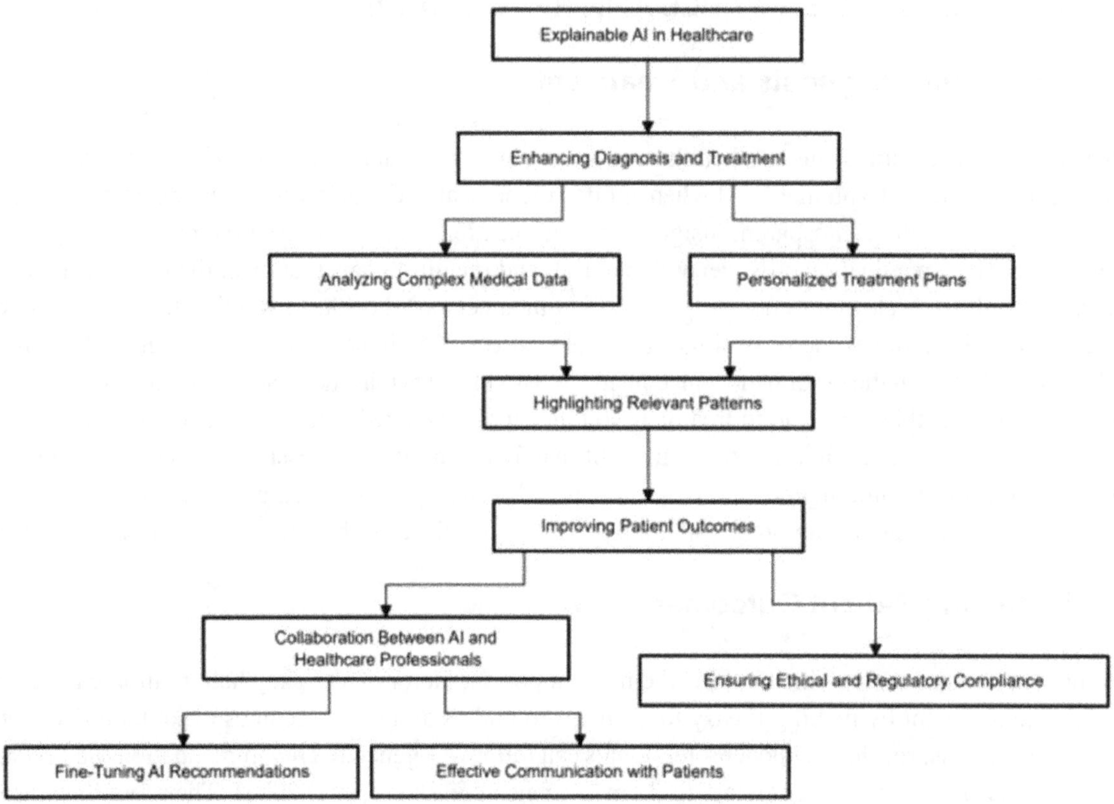

3. EXPLAINABLE AI MODELS IN HEALTHCARE

3.1. Linear Models

The "linear model" is a simple, bare-bones approach to AI that can be employed in the healthcare industry. This is helpful as in this environment it can be used for such tasks as risk assessment, outcome prediction, and illness prediction. As mentioned in the Figure 2, the different types of model. A linear model simply gives differential weight to various types of input data (patient demographic information; medical history notes, and results from clinical tests) before putting them together to get a "predicted score" (Rani et al., 2023). One of the advantages of linear models is that they are easy to use and interpret. The model includes a process decision tree. Both in terms of clarity and intuition, clinicians can readily understand how each attribute influences the conclusion through this tool. Moreover, linear models allow you to find the factors that are most predictive of a given outcome. This helps in feature selection and medical management choices. Now that's fine, but when it comes to the complexities of medical data—the non-linearity is a problem sometimes. In such cases, more complex models may be required. Nevertheless, linear models continue to be a potent analytical tool for the healthcare industry due to their simplicity, clarity, and usefulness in actual operational situations.

3.2. Decision Trees

Understandable AI models must necessarily incorporate decision trees. They are hierarchically constructed tree-like models that divide the data according to a series of decision rules until the last step produces an overall prediction or classification. Applications of Decision Trees include the healthcare industry (Xie et al., 2022). For example, they could assist physicians in quickly reaching a likely diagnosis by analyzing patient symptoms and demographic information as well as test results. Because each branch represents a choice point, and doctors are particularly familiar with the pathways of decision-making therein, it's very easy to understand these trees. What's more, such models can help to discover what factors are most influential in a given medical outcome. These would increase the willingness and ability of AI-based healthcare systems to open their doors. Bayesian decision trees can also help with treatment recommendation systems that enable doctors to select the most suitable treatments based on a patient's characteristics. To summarize, Decision Trees can be added to the capabilities of explorable but previously uninterpretable artificial intelligence models used in healthcare. They give doctors and patients a clear, comprehensible image with valuable information for decision-making.

Figure 2. Types of explainable AI models in healthcare

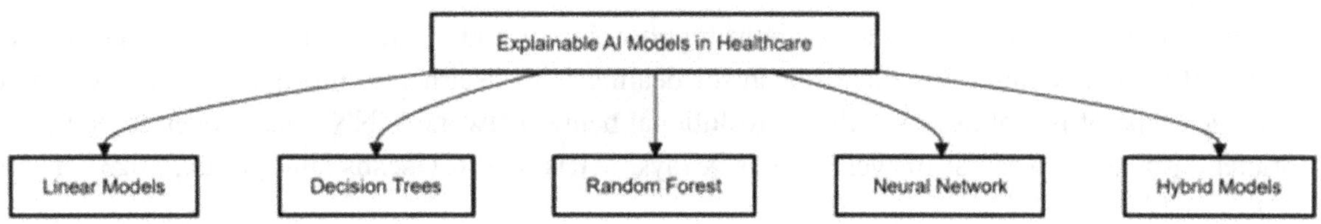

3.3. Random Forest

Among the explainable AI models that have been applied to healthcare problems, random forests are notable for being not only easy to implement but also ideal for addressing difficult medical dilemmas (Abadie et al., 2023). Perhaps an ensemble learning approach such as Random Forests, which combines the predictive power of a large number of decision trees to make predictions more reliable and accurate, can help. For healthcare, this means the ability to conduct detailed examinations of patients and then supply them with accurate and understandable results.

For these reasons, Random Forests work well in healthcare applications. They can also combine different data types (numerical and categorical variables), for example, integrate patient demographic information, medical history, and screening test results. Second, due to their ensemble nature, they are less prone to overfitting (a common concern in machine learning), as Zaydi et al. 2023). By using predictions from many decision trees, however, Random Forests reduce the likelihood of such modeling noise and outliers.

Fortunate are we, for random forests further enhance interpretation using feature prioritization. This helps the clinical decision-making process by allowing healthcare workers to see which features of patients most affect a particular prognosis or outcome. Because the model rests on several different decision trees that can be inspected and understood, its operations are transparent.

Moreover, researchers have applied Random Forests to real healthcare situations for such tasks as predicting illness risk or early diagnosis and therapy prescription. For example, Random Forests can combine genetic data with lifestyle factors and medical history to provide a comprehensive assessment of cardiovascular disease risk while site expressing the main contributing areas. This openness not only makes it easy for patients to participate in their health evaluations; this procedure also helps doctors accept the model's recommendations and can make them feel like part of a team. Consequently, random forests have become part of the toolbox for healthcare-related explainable AI models (Farah et al., 2023). Their flexibility, lack of overfitting, and interpretability make them ideal for real-world medical problems. For healthcare professionals and patients alike, these materials help them understand many hard choices in the field of medicine.

3.4. Neural Network

This articulation points out that neural networks are at the forefront of an Explainable AI (XAI) model integration revolution, and have proved to be truly revolutionary. The classic structure of the human brain was thus used for the design inspiration of a general class of machine learning methods called neural networks, and these in turn have proven to be particularly effective at many important healthcare applications. A couple series of linked nodes arranged in layers employed to make up these models are responsible for processing and modifying the incoming data. In the healthcare sector, neural networks are widely used in tasks such as patient risk analysis (for instance), illness detection, and medical picture processing.

Such multidimensionality, coupled with the highly complex and subtle nature of medical data means that neural networks are an excellent match for dealing with healthcare information. An even more specialized type of neural network, the convolutional neural network (CNN), has proven to be highly proficient at reading medical images such as X-rays, MRIs, and CT scans (Jung et al., 2023). These pictures can teach radiologists about many hierarchical characteristics of illness, and help radio spots to examine the body more accurately.

What's more, RNNs and LSTM networks have also allowed natural language processing (NLP) for time-series data very typical in the healthcare field such as patient vitals or electronic health records. These models can discern temporal relationships and trends so that the patient's worsening condition can be detected earlier on in time and treatment methods improved.

The use of neural networks in healthcare continues to be highly dependent on explainability. These models' intrinsic black-box character has raised questions regarding how interpretable and reliable they are in therapeutic situations(Monlezun, 2023). Researchers have created tools like attention mechanisms and saliency maps that illuminate the neural network's decision-making process to solve this. These techniques increase transparency and make it easier for medical professionals to have faith in AI-driven suggestions by clarifying which characteristics or areas of an input contributed most to a certain prediction.

To sum up the above, neural networks have already become important medical tools for improving patient care and diagnosis as well as therapy. Of course, as we can see these high-end models are quite accurate at making predictions. In addition to being able to use them in clinical practice, Expainable AI methods must be developed so that healthcare workers will accept the conclusions made by these models.

3.5. Hybrid Models

Hybrid modeling is an attractive strategy that takes advantage of the strengths of several AI techniques to raise interpretability and forecast accuracy. These models mix deep-learning architectures with traditional machine-learning methods to exploit the strengths of both. One of the biggest advantages is that hybrid models can find subtle relationships and structures in medical data yet still provide decision-makers with the information they need.

Hybrid models tend to combine deep, less-transparent neural networks with easy-to-understand machine learning modes such as decision trees, logistic regression, or support vector machines. This fusion also eliminates deep learning's 'black-box problem,' making its workings transparent and understandable. For instance, the model could involve an interpretable decision tree that generates a set of rules used to classify illnesses in medical pictures along with fine-grained features learned by a convolutional neural network (CNN). Thus, physicians can both rely on the model's predictions and understand why a specific diagnosis was made. In this way then they should find it much easier to incorporate AI suggestions into their patient treatment decision processes.

These hybrid models are therefore the most suitable for changing conditions. Deep learning may be able to overcome the drawbacks of using traditional machine learning methods with sparse or uneven data--medical information is a prime example. Through the use of ingenious hybrid models, XAI will remain flexible enough to adapt to specific circumstances in real-world healthcare environments where data quality and quantity may differ very widely. Because of the adaptability of hybrid models, they have a wide range of health care applications and can be used to predict outcomes for individual patients; identify high-risk individuals from large populations; optimize treatment plans by weighing costs; or even automatically interpret medical pictures.

Know thyself The successful implementation of hybrid models makes it easier to imagine how deep learning's ability could combine with the interpretability and ease-of-use of classical machine learning, combining them in a route toward accurate, easily explainable, and practical AI medical applications.

With such models, medical professionals can make informed decisions that lead to better patient care. This is a new era of explainable AI in medicine.

4. REAL-WORLD APPLICATIONS

4.1. Disease Diagnosis

4.1.1. Early Detection of Cancer

The early detection of cancer is one of Explainable AI's (XAI) most promising practical applications on the medical front. Okolo explains that the leading cause of death worldwide is cancer. Cancer tends to be discovered in later stages, limiting effectiveness and lowering survival rates (2023). Thanks to such XAI capabilities, medical personnel can access cutting-edge technologies that will enhance their ability to detect cancer at very early stages when it is still most curable.

In addition to electronic health records, imaging, and genetic data. Explainable AI systems take a large variety of medical information as input while using advanced algorithms and deep learning techniques for analysis. XAI can also help in the early diagnosis of cancer, and this is explained in Figure 3.

Figure 3. Early detection of cancer using explainable AI

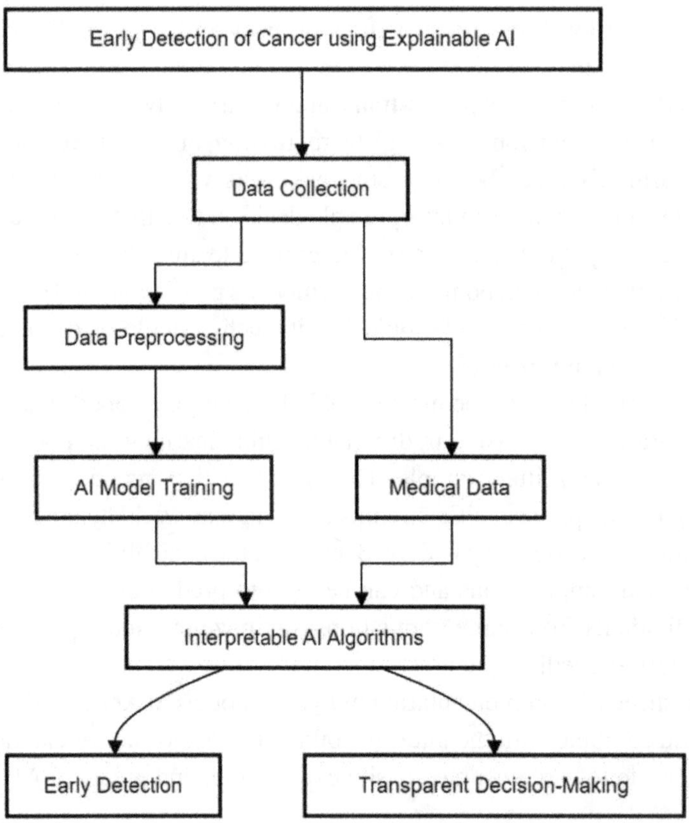

This complex data can be analyzed by XAI models to find patterns and irregularities that are too small or minute for human eyes. It can even detect tumors such as breast, lung, or prostate cancer at an early stage before anyone feels any symptoms.

XAI is especially important in the field of cancer diagnosis, where interpretability comes into play. This helps medical professionals understand the rationale behind how the AI arrives at its conclusions, helping them put trust in this aspect of diagnostics. For instance, radiologists can get a sharper understanding of why an AI regarded some area on X-ray or MRI as possibly being malignant thereby helping them make better decisions about the patient's care. Another advantage of XAI models is that they lead to fewer false positives and negatives in cancer diagnosis. The decision-making process can make it clearer to clinicians how far they do or don't agree with the AI's suggestions and allow them to change things as necessary. So overdiagnoses are much less likely than under (missed) diagnoses.

To facilitate early diagnosis, raise precision, and the entire decision-making process--Explainable AI is entering an area that can revolutionize healthcare. These developments based on AI not only extend the life expectancy of patients but also offer medical personnel important information through which they can intervene at just the right time with any one patient. XAI's transparency and interpretability are closely bound up with the future of cancer diagnosis. Patients all around the world hope that this will lead to earlier treatment and better outcomes.

4.1.2. Predicting Heart Disease Risk

One of the most significant real-world examples to be seen in health care is explainable AI's ability to predict heart disease. Since heart disease is still among the world's leading causes of death, identifying early and possibly those who may be at risk can assist in preventive measures. XAI enables us to foresee the incidence of heart disease, as Figure 4. Explainable AI models have made it possible to transform risk prediction by providing transparency and interpretability, which in turn has helped medical practitioners make wiser choices based on valuable insights. Such models, Dey et al (2022) note, utilize a combination of various types of unstructured data sources such as electronic health records and medical images with structured patient information including medical history, vital signs, and laboratory results. In addition to calculating a given person's chances of developing heart disease, these systems can offer fully explainable bases for their predictions (using such techniques as decision trees or random forests and even interpretable deep learning architectures).

This interpretability has been revolutionary in itself for healthcare, being able to help doctors understand the real reasons that explain a patient's risk profile. To cite an example, the AI model may indicate that a certain patient's risk is due mainly to high blood pressure and smoking — not because of any heart disease (Mahajan et al., 2023). These facts can help in adjusting treatment, giving advice to patients, and offering personalized health guidance.

Another benefit of explainable AI is its ability to generate risk scores and treatment guidelines for heart disease. Such models make risk assessment tools more specific by clarifying who will be affected and to what extent. This eliminates waste and leads to better risk grouping in the allocation of healthcare resources.

To conclude, the use of explainable AI to predict heart disease risk is a good case study of how advanced technology can be put to service saving lives and improving medical outcomes. By combining interpretability with data insights, healthcare practitioners will learn to make better choices and include

Figure 4. Predicting heart disease risk using explainable AI

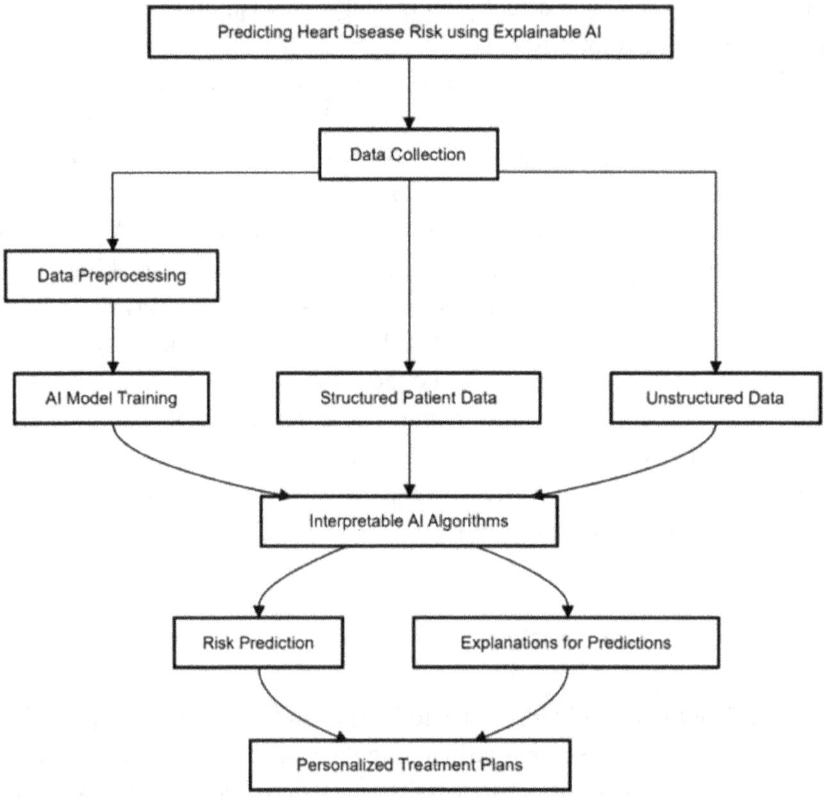

patients in their treatment. This would result in a reduction of the burden borne by people at risk for heart disease as well as health care systems.

4.2. Treatment Personalization

4.2.1. Drug Recommendation Systems

For instance, personalized medicine is customizing medication treatment according to the unique medical backgrounds and genetic compositions of patients based on their illnesses. (A Kumar et al., 203) Explainable AI expands the scope for establishing trustworthy and reliable DRS, thereby benefiting all involved. according to Figure 5. They are using Explainable AI, how the drugs are prescribed. Their use of genes, electronic medical records, and even patients 'lifestyles enables them to custom-design effective medicine prescriptions based on various pieces of individual data.

Thanks to powerful machine learning and interpretable models, DRS doesn't just make suggestions on appropriate drug choices but also gives physicians and patients short reasons for those recommendations. Transparency is key to strengthening the relationship between patients and healthcare providers, enabling them to make better judgments about treatments. What's more, DRS can consider the effect of drugs on each other or interactions with allergies and therapeutic responses. So negative side effects are reduced while patient safety is improved. When new information is discovered, these systems constantly

Figure 5. Drug recommendation systems using explainable AI

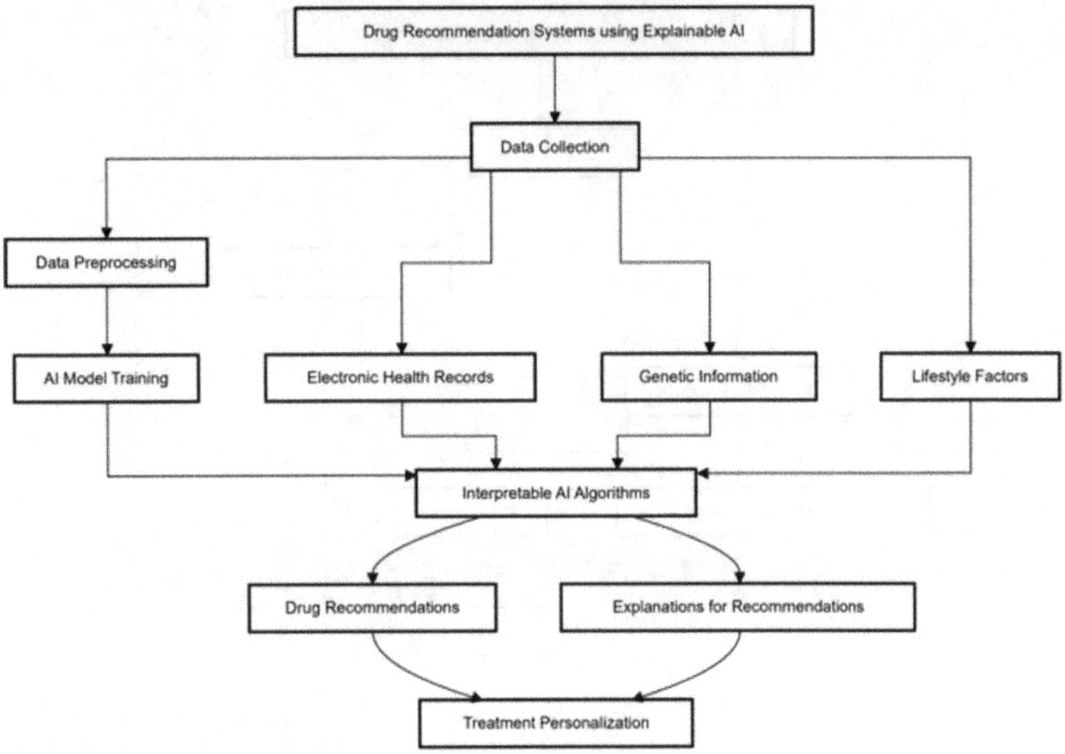

update their recommendations so that treatments are timely and in accord with the patient's evolving health condition. Explainable AI methods like rule-based models or feature significance analysis can also help healthcare practitioners appreciate the rationale behind which drugs are recommended. Through these insights, DRS not only makes customization of treatment even more precise and effective but also strengthens decision-making between people themselves (as patients)and the healthcare professionals taking care of them. The use of eXplainable AI to improve drug recommendation systems is a great development that involves making care safer, faster, and more personalized in an era when the pharmaceutical environment is undergoing such rapid shifts.

4.2.2. Customized Treatment Plans

Customized Treatment Plans are the vanguard of Explainable AI's healthcare revolution. Treatment customization In this critical section, we delve into the nitty-gritty of how AI is transforming healthcare delivery. By integrating patient data and diagnostic information, along with the latest cutting-edge algorithms, AI could help doctors tailor treatment regimens precisely to each person's needs (Damoah et al., 2021). Besides medical history and genetic factors, this level of tailoring also considers the patient's life choices, likes, and even a person's living environment.

Because explainer AI systematically reveals the thinking behind all decision-making, it can help medical professionals and patients have a clear understanding of how treatment options are arrived at. With the assistance of XAI, as shown in Figure 6 we can develop personalized treatment plans for

Figure 6. Customized treatment plans using explainable AI

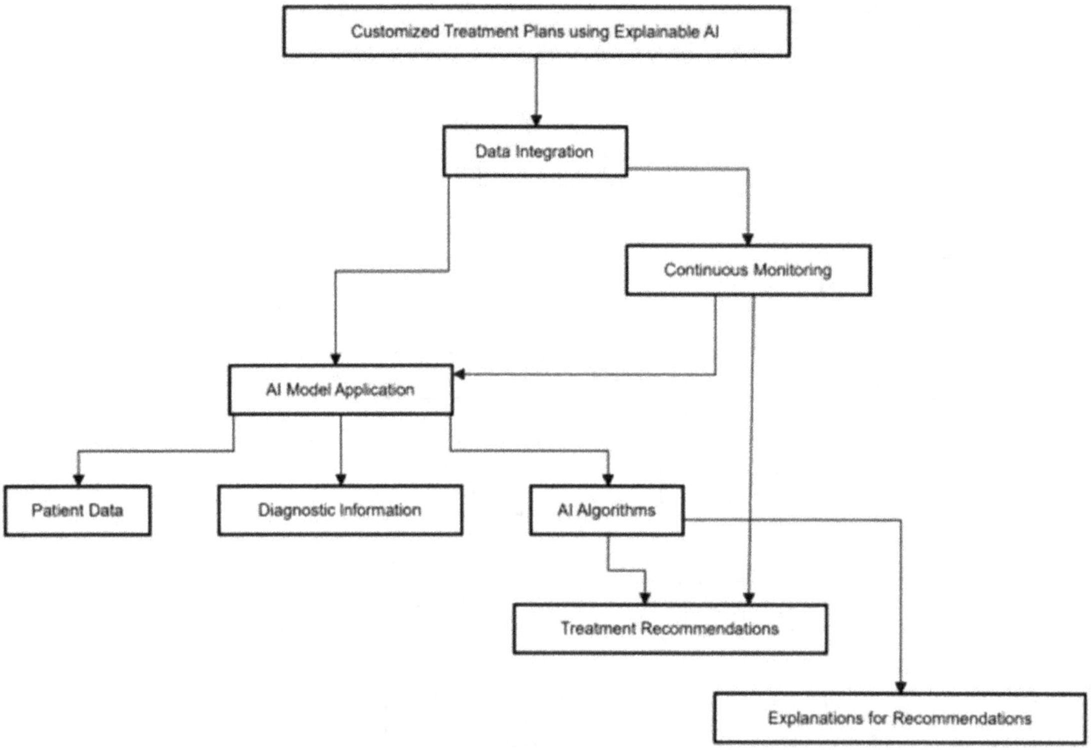

each patient. When patients can see what the reasoning is behind treatment programs, they are more willing to cooperate with them. Thus it encourages teamwork based on mutual trust and understanding. Moreover, such personalized treatment plans based on artificial intelligence are continuously adjusted by real-time patient data. Healthcare providers can accordingly immediately make adjustments depending upon the state of a given individual's health at any time during their course of treatment. This is an enormous step forward in the use of Explainable AI to improve patient outcomes and enormously enhance healthcare delivery.

4.3. Patient Monitoring

4.3.1. Continuous Vital Sign Monitoring

With the explanation of artificial intelligence (XAI) technologies, have had a direct impact on modern healthcare that requires constant monitoring of patients 'vital signs. This technology has also completely changed the way medical practitioners closely observe patients 'vital signs rate, blood pressure, breathing rate, and temperature. Periodic measures have long been relied upon by healthcare professionals, and a patient could easily miss something significant between examinations. The integration of XAI allows wearable technology, such as smartwatches and sensors which gather real-time data from individuals 24 hours a day, to continuously collect information while performing constant monitoring. This enables healthcare workers to get an early warning of abnormalities or deviations from a patient's standard, thereby providing important information. Not only do the XAI algorithms for monitoring vital indicators detect aberrations, but they can also explain the reasons behind them. This openness helps patients understand their diseases and treatment, which is necessary for developing confidence between doctor and patient. Moreover, XAI enables individualized treatment by matching therapies to information on a particular patient (Polevikov 203), improving the quality and speed of care. Continuous vital sign monitoring has great clinical potential. With XAI, you can guarantee better outcomes and raise the quality of care for patients as well as medical professionals.

4.3.2. Alerting for Critical Events

For example, one of the main functions of patient monitoring systems is alert notification for critical events. Explainable AI has thus already played an essential role in health care delivery. This decisive section examines the role of Explainable AI in advancing patient safety and prompt action. Constant patient monitoring by powerful machine learning systems, using streams of data from vital signs to clinical notes and test results to anticipate key events. The Explainable AI also builds confidence in their recommendations because healthcare practitioners can understand the underlying causes for them.

Explainability, therefore, not only guides doctors in interpreting each alert's context and reasoning but is also the basis of trusting AI-generated alerts. For example, if an algorithm detects the patient's blood pressure increasing precipitously, it can explain this anomaly from patterns in their health history and dosage logs as well as external factors (Khalid et al., 2023) so that doctors can choose between different paths. Further, by observing what choices health care providers make and noting whether those are successful or not, these models can adapt their warnings over time to reduce false alarms and lower alert fatigue.

What's more, Explainable AI can sound an alarm for major events and thus facilitate after-the-fact analysis and audit trails that help increase the quality of health care or improve compliance with laws. These systems could be used by healthcare organizations to track their performance, identify shortcomings, and verify that standards of ethics or law are being upheld. It also helps patients and family members to be more open, which could lead them to play a role in decision-making, understand the reason for warnings given to them by their physicians, and be active partners with doctors when planning his or her treatment.

In sum, introducing Explainable AI into monitoring for key events not only improves the early detection of worsening patient conditions. Constant improvement of overall service is confidence and encouragement to cooperate with patients. This combination of technological and human expertise testifies to the revolutionary character Explainable AI has for practical healthcare applications.

4.4. Administrative Efficiency

4.4.1. Billing and Coding Automation

Explanatory AI can furthermore contribute to a sorely needed increase in administrative efficiency through billing and coding automation. This removes the need for tedious, error-prone manual labor on operations, according to its inventors and manufacturers--its four doctors 'and hospitals' painstaking medical billing and ICD (International Classification of Diseases) typing process. In addition, explainable AI can analyze paperwork from medical records in the future to follow things like diagnosis and treatment prescribed method or patient demographics. Thus not only do these technologies provide precise and reliable code determination, but they also enable decision-makers to explain how the claims of physicians are adjusted.

While explainable AI algorithms can also recover relevant data, they must be able to offer readable explanations for the choices encapsulated in their codes (Seoni et al., 2023). This openness allows medical personnel and billing experts to feel the logic behind code assignment, which adds confidence in an automated system. Moreover, by highlighting any discrepancies and omissions in the medical records these explanations help to raise the standard of information supplied and reduce rejections on claims.

What's more, Explainable AI also helps ensure better compliance with billing and coding standards as well as evolving healthcare laws. Changes in the required coding standards can be immediately incorporated into the system, and papers that do not conform to those requirements are given immediate feedback. As a result of all this work--or perhaps because of it--the danger of being hit with an audit fine has become vanishingly small.

In addition to higher accuracy and compliance, computerization of billing and codes will also speed up reimbursement. Automation using AI speeds up claims handling, increasing healthcare organizations 'cash flow and reducing payment cycles. Furthermore, by alleviating staff members of the burden of manual coding-related work and allowing them to spend more time with patients, overall care standards in healthcare providers will increase.

In sum, using Explainable AI to automate billing and coding is a giant step in raising administrative effectiveness for the medical industry. This technology gives healthcare providers and healthcare organizations a way to ensure accuracy, transparency, and efficiency in their financial operations (coding) as well as real-time forms of compliance verification (highest standards).

4.4.2. Resource Allocation Optimization

This procedure is included in administrative efficiency, and Explainable AI (XAI) can help optimize resource allocation. Achieving the highest standards in terms of patient care and operational efficiency requires comprehensive management of resources (human, equipment, funds) amidst a rapidly changing environment. Healthcare management sometimes needs overall knowledge of trends and patterns in the use of resources. The XAI algorithms can, therefore, allow healthcare managers to make rational decisions about these matters. In other words, XAI systems can analyze historical data and current demand to predict future needs. Healthcare organizations can then be proactive about deploying resources where they are needed most (P Kumar et al. 2023a). The explainability of XAI also means that those in authority can know the rationale behind allocating resources, which is vital for them to trust such a process. With XAI, perhaps it will even be possible to detect inefficiency or a bottleneck anywhere along the resource allocation chain and thereby continue optimizing resource management policies (Baumgartner et al., 2023). In any case, XAI integration into resource allocation optimizes medical procedures and brings responsibility and openness to the utilization of limited or critical resources. This naturally helps with providing care for patients in a cost-effective way.

5. CHALLENGES AND ETHICAL CONSIDERATIONS

5.1. Data Privacy and Security

One of the most challenging, most important issues in real-world healthcare applications for Explainable AI (XAI) is how to ensure solid data privacy and security. As medical information is highly sensitive and can't be leaked, these ethical questions concerning healthcare data are very critical. That is because when using XAI systems healthcare organizations have to face challenges such as data anonymization, patient consent, and risks of information leaks. The problem is that such privacy considerations make it harder to balance the need for openness and interpretability when medical decisions are automated. Therefore, if we want to protect people's personal health information from security breaches and unwanted publicization, data encryptions and access blockages must be soundly created as well as an ability for the identity characteristics of individuals themselves to be obfuscated. P. In addition, one must abide by the Health Insurance Portability and Accountancy Act (HIPAA), passed in 1996, or similar legislation from other countries that aim to protect individuals 'rights within a health information system. Kumar et al., 2023b). As the healthcare industry works to develop XAI systems that can help in patient care and diagnosis, addressing these data privacy and security issues will be central to building confidence in such systems.

5.2. Bias and Fairness

Combating prejudice and upholding justice is one of the most difficult tasks. New hopes, new fears With the addition of intelligence systems implemented into health care routines comes a possible reinforcement and even expansion of existing inequities. AI models are replete with bias that percolates through biased training data, causing some patients to be unfairly monitored or overlooked. Where this troubles us most is in historically disadvantaged or minority groups. Proper curation and cleaning of training data, analysis for algorithmic bias, and fairness-aware machine learning systems all help reduce these risks. Third, monitoring and auditing of AI systems are essential to discovering bias in the system as it develops over time (Albahri et al., 2023). A systematized approach to preventing bias and maintaining fairness in the use of AI will help prevent old inequities from being simply reproduced at a larger scale. This can only be achieved with interdisciplinary coordination, ethical standards, governmental regulations, etc. In applying the potential of explainable A.I., we can't overlook justice or social responsibility in health care and must proceed with caution.

5.3. Interpreting AI Decisions

The chapter entitled Interpreting AI Decisions treats an important part of the challenges and dilemmas that arise when XAI is applied in a healthcare setting. However, despite better-than-human prognostic and diagnostic performance by AI systems, it is still hard to fathom the rationale for their judgments. AI's black-box forecasts have opened a huge gap in the healthcare industry, where individual choices directly affect patients 'health and lives. It is therefore imperative to narrow that gap by making systems more comprehensible to human beings. This addresses several issues that are needed to make AI models transparent and interpretable. Second, visualization methods that clearly show the decision-making process must be developed. Second, medical personnel should be educated to understand the insights provided by AI as well as their limits and imponderables. Raza et al. (2022). Besides forecasts, other functions of an AI system should also be explainable in a context-dependent manner that is commensurate with clinical competence and expertise. How to deal with these complexities requires interaction between AI researchers, healthcare professionals, and ethicists. In addition, it is necessary to establish legal mechanisms and regulations that ensure the correct application of XAI in medical care. Only when these stimulate confidence in decision-making can we believe appropriate checks and balances are leading toward improved patient treatment results.

5.4. Regulatory Compliance

Non-compliance with requirements is a significant regulatory and ethical challenge in health care. To keep patient privacy intact, maintain confidentiality of data, and provide the best possible care standards--the healthcare business is naturally subjected to strict rules and regulations. To prevent these pitfalls, developers and practitioners of XAI systems for healthcare have to deal with a myriad of legal provisions in many countries such as the GDPR in Europe or HIPAA (Health Insurance Portability and Accountability Act) regulations in America. These rules address how patient data should be collected, stored, processed, and reported. Thus XAI models must adhere to these legal principles as well as be able to present results that can be seen and understood by all (Bertl et al., 2023) Given that data leaks or privacy violations can have far-reaching consequences and affect the patient's confidence in healthcare providers as well as the effectiveness of treatment, requiring XAI systems to meet these standards is both a legal requirement and an ethical one. Consequently, proper investments in robust compliance policies and data anonymization procedures must be matched with secure infrastructure to build high-quality XAI healthcare services that aim to promote "patient integrity."

6. FUTURE DIRECTIONS

6.1. Advancements in Explainable AI Techniques

Another possible direction for future development is the continued improvement of explainable AI (XAI) techniques. With the wider adoption of these solutions, however, it is also important that efforts be made to ensure AI-driven healthcare systems are as transparent and accountable as possible. To satisfy this need, researchers and practitioners are actively working on creating or improving XAI products. Another area of academic research worth highlighting is the current effort to enhance methods that can explain complex AI models such as deep neural networks (for instance, LIME and SHAP- Local Interpretable Model-Agnostic Explanations). Researchers are also exploring the potential application of natural language generation (NLG) technology to make these forecasts easy for patients and healthcare professionals alike. One plausible way to earn doctors 'trust and make cooperation between humans and machines more likely is the development of XAIs that allow users to assess model selection in real-time. Moreover, people have recently begun working on ways to include causal reasoning as well as counterfactual explanations that would allow us deeper insights into the cause-and-effect relationships within AI models so we can make more informed medical decisions (Wysocki et al., 2023). Apart from giving healthcare stakeholders a clearer and more accessible understanding of machine recommendations for treatment, these ongoing advancements in XAI techniques also pave the way for better ethically responsible implementation of AI within that industry.

6.2. Integration with Electronic Health Records

The possibility and integration of Explainable AI (XAI) and Electronic Health Records is one of the most important revolutionaries in health care. Digital patient data, medical histories, and treatment logs serve as the foundation of modern healthcare systems. Nevertheless, the large volume of data in EHRs is also a formidable challenge to medical practitioners. This is where Explainable AI will be able to make a difference in how medical professionals can use and engage with EHRs.

- Increasing Diagnosis and Clinical Decision Support: These XAI algorithms could be incorporated into EHR systems, helping caregivers detect diseases and make treatment decisions. We may find it very valuable to search for the rationale behind these diagnostic outcomes by applying XAI models based on patient data from EHRs. This not only can cut down on mistakes in the diagnosis, but it also gives professionals a more clearly pinpointed sense of what is causing this person's disease. For instance, XAI can help a doctor explain his or her medical logic to one patient while raising the level of accountability and transparency for another.
- Risk assessment and predictive analytics: Xai can build prediction models to identify people who are at risk for specific diseases or negative outcomes. Therefore, healthcare professionals are in a position to act ahead of time and put preventative measures into place. The risk factors and variables that underlie these predictions could be explained by such models. XAI used in conjunction with EHRs can assist healthcare organizations to improve patient outcomes, reduce the rate of returning patients, and help hospitals utilize their resources more effectively.
- Personalised medication: XAI plus EHRs will make the level of personalized medication unprecedented ever possible. Analyzing genetic data, information about therapy effectiveness, and previous medical histories may enable XAI to recommend individual treatment programs for patients, or even tell whether certain activities are likely to succeed. The transparency of the XAI ensures that patients and doctors have a clear understanding of the reasons underlying treatment decisions, increasing confidence in such disputes.
- Clinical Trial Optimisation: XAI-driven EHR implementation could have a significant effect on the planning and conduct of clinical trials. Relying on past patient data, researchers can employ X AI to design improved trial procedures and predict the availability of patients suitable for enrolment. This saves time in designing medication, reduces costs, and raises the chances that trials will produce effective results.
- Regulatory Compliance and Auditing: Healthcare is closely related to regulatory compliance. XAI, furthermore, can be used in conjunction with EHRs to create comprehensive but readily comprehensible audit trails for data access and decision-making processes. Transparency of choices made and use of patient data encourages compliance with healthcare regulations such as the Health Insurance Portability and Accountability Act (HIPAA).
- Patient Empowerment and Informed Consent: XAI can empower the patient by, for instance, acquainting them with their disease and treatments so that they know what is happening to themselves as well as the dangers of any action. A clear explanation would help patients acquire in-

formed consent, promote a cooperative relationship between patient and provider, and enable them to choose their journey.

Finally, Explainable AI's connection to electronic health records has tremendous research potential, clinical decision-making, and healthcare delivery. Such integration stands to take us into a future when medicine is more effective patient-centered, ethical, and responsible by making difficult health data that much easier for people of experience and understanding (including artificial intelligence) to access, interpret, or apply. As the healthcare environment continues to evolve, XAI prepares for widespread adoption in combination with electronic patient records (EHRs), further improving outcomes and advancing medical knowledge.

6.3. Global Adoption and Standardization

In an evolving healthcare industry, explainable AI (XAI) is primed to transform not only decision-making methods and diagnostic accuracy but patient outcomes as well on a global scale. Another crucial problem is that if XAI practice is to be transformed into a universal aspect of daily life, uniform standards need to come quickly. But this section discusses the even more important topic of a common framework applicable across national boundaries and spurring XAI's widespread use in health care.

Another challenge to the seamless introduction of XAI is that healthcare systems around the world are so heterogeneous. Different healthcare systems and legal environments between countries also present obstacles to the use of XAI models. Hence, it is necessary to establish universal standards and rules.

In addition, the right and responsible use of XAI in healthcare also requires an orderly system for data collection, sharing functions, and privacy. Given that XAI relies largely for success on large labeled datasets, it is especially important to ensure these test sets are both diverse and representative of populations around the world. Towards this end, the establishment of data-sharing standards to ensure patient privacy could spur international collaboration in model upgrading and more accurate projections. Standards for XAI technologies must not only raise the quality of such systems, they should also guarantee that healthcare applications utilizing them respect patients and their well-being, and obtain consent.

Also, there is a need for standardized methods to test and verify XAI models. Only if these models function reliably in an array of healthcare settings will they become pervasive. We can improve on the certification framework by standardizing XAI evaluation metrics, testing standards, and even test data to facilitate comparisons between various systems. This would facilitate quicker payments and regulatory clearances, thus leading to even more healthcare institutions avoiding XAI.

Hence, the future possibilities of using Explainable AI represent an enormous opportunity for healthcare. It all comes down to whether a standard system can be developed that applies everywhere. It will take collective efforts among stakeholders at regional, national, and global levels to develop an approach that ensures equal access, fair practices 'and clinical effectiveness in the era when XAI can only grow. Only through such organized efforts can we develop the full potential of XAI in health care. Doing so will improve patient quality of life and accelerate medical research worldwide.

CONCLUSION

Finally, the incorporation of Explainable AI (XAI) into healthcare represents an important turning point for medicine and a new frontier in which patients stand to benefit. We have reviewed a broad spectrum of applications for XAI in this chapter, which highlights its revolutionary nature. XAI technology looks set to revolutionize the healthcare industry, from proposing treatment regimes tailored to a patient's profile to diagnostic systems that clearly explain what their thinking was.

Bridging the gap between sophisticated machine-learning models and human understandability is a vital function of XAI in medicine, and one of its primary benefits. What is more, the "black-box" nature of AI systems has been acknowledged in research circles as a focus for improvement. By helping healthcare practitioners understand the reasons behind the forecasts based on which they are expected to make decisions and judgments, XAI greatly assists in achieving this goal. The examples discussed above show how XAI can help not only by enhancing the accuracy of diagnoses but also by increasing medical professionals 'confidence in and acceptance of AI-assisted recommendations.

In addition, by using XAI it is possible to make breakthroughs in the early detection, prognosis of disease, and optimizing treatments. Its power to sift through mountains of data and detect the tiny connections commonly missed by human experts makes it a tool even more indispensable in the fight against complex diseases such as cancer, diabetes, or cardiovascular disorders. In addition to explaining the reasoning behind their predictions, perhaps XAI can help physicians act earlier and save lives while reducing overall burdens on healthcare systems.

In addition, ensuring that healthcare firms are responsible and ethical with the use of AI relies heavily on XAI. We hope that with this chapter we have been able to show how XAI can foster fair medical provision, ensure patients 'confidentiality, and find and eliminate dead spots in healthcare technology. In an age in which artificial intelligence is starting to influence healthcare policy and patient-doctor relations, these ethical issues are especially relevant.

In future years, XAI strategies will get ever more sophisticated and effective. And they'll be used in healthcare as well. Of course, there will still be obstacles. This includes privacy, legal issues, and continuous multidisciplinary coordination of work. But, in the final analysis, actual experiences implementing Explainable AI truly can transform both conceptually and at the level of practice. If we effectively adopt and draw on this XAI promise, maybe one day soon healthcare will be not only effective but also transparent-fairer--and more humane.

REFERENCES

Abadie, A., Roux, M., Chowdhury, S., & Dey, P. (2023). Interlinking organizational resources, AI adoption and omnichannel integration quality in Ghana's healthcare supply chain. *Journal of Business Research*, *162*, 113866. doi:10.1016/j.jbusres.2023.113866

Albahri, A. S., Duhaim, A. M., Fadhel, M. A., Alnoor, A., Baqer, N. S., Alzubaidi, L., Albahri, O. S., Alamoodi, A. H., Bai, J., Salhi, A., Santamaría, J., Ouyang, C., Gupta, A., Gu, Y., & Deveci, M. (2023). A systematic review of trustworthy and explainable artificial intelligence in healthcare: Assessment of quality, bias risk, and data fusion. *Information Fusion*, *96*, 156–191. doi:10.1016/j.inffus.2023.03.008

Argenson, A., & Devi-Chou, V. (2023). Artificial intelligence in healthcare. In *Principles of Gender-Specific Medicine* (pp. 601–618). Elsevier. doi:10.1016/B978-0-323-88534-8.00025-0

Baumgartner, R., Arora, P., Bath, C., Burljaev, D., Ciereszko, K., Custers, B., Ding, J., Ernst, W., Fosch-Villaronga, E., Galanos, V., Gremsl, T., Hendl, T., Kropp, C., Lenk, C., Martin, P., Mbelu, S., Morais dos Santos Bruss, S., Napiwodzka, K., Nowak, E., ... Williams, R. (2023). Fair and equitable AI in biomedical research and healthcare: Social science perspectives. *Artificial Intelligence in Medicine*, *144*, 102658. doi:10.1016/j.artmed.2023.102658 PMID:37783540

Bertl, M., Ross, P., & Draheim, D. (2023). Systematic AI Support for Decision-Making in the Healthcare Sector: Obstacles and Success Factors. *Health Policy and Technology*, *12*(3), 100748. doi:10.1016/j.hlpt.2023.100748

Damoah, I. S., Ayakwah, A., & Tingbani, I. (2021). Artificial intelligence (AI)-enhanced medical drones in the healthcare supply chain (HSC) for sustainability development: A case study. *Journal of Cleaner Production*, *328*, 129598. doi:10.1016/j.jclepro.2021.129598

Dey, S., Chakraborty, P., Kwon, B. C., Dhurandhar, A., Ghalwash, M., Suarez Saiz, F. J., Ng, K., Sow, D., Varshney, K. R., & Meyer, P. (2022). Human-centered explainability for life sciences, healthcare, and medical informatics. *Patterns (New York, N.Y.)*, *3*(5), 100493. doi:10.1016/j.patter.2022.100493 PMID:35607616

Farah, L., Murris, J. M., Borget, I., Guilloux, A., Martelli, N. M., & Katsahian, S. I. M. (2023). Assessment of Performance, Interpretability, and Explainability in Artificial Intelligence–Based Health Technologies: What Healthcare Stakeholders Need to Know. *Mayo Clinic Proceedings. Digital Health*, *1*(2), 120–138. doi:10.1016/j.mcpdig.2023.02.004

Jung, J., Lee, H., Jung, H., & Kim, H. (2023). Essential properties and explanation effectiveness of explainable artificial intelligence in healthcare: A systematic review. *Heliyon*, *9*(5), e16110. doi:10.1016/j.heliyon.2023.e16110 PMID:37234618

Khalid, N., Qayyum, A., Bilal, M., Al-Fuqaha, A., & Qadir, J. (2023). Privacy-preserving artificial intelligence in healthcare: Techniques and applications. *Computers in Biology and Medicine*, *158*, 106848. doi:10.1016/j.compbiomed.2023.106848 PMID:37044052

Kumar, A., Mani, V., Jain, V., Gupta, H., & Venkatesh, V. G. (2023). Managing healthcare supply chain through artificial intelligence (AI): A study of critical success factors. *Computers & Industrial Engineering*, *175*, 108815. doi:10.1016/j.cie.2022.108815 PMID:36405396

Kumar, P., Sharma, S. K., & Dutot, V. (2023). Artificial intelligence (AI)-enabled CRM capability in healthcare: The impact on service innovation. *International Journal of Information Management*, *69*, 102598. doi:10.1016/j.ijinfomgt.2022.102598

Lehmann, L. S., Natarajan, V., & Peng, L. (2024). Artificial intelligence in healthcare: a perspective from Google. In *Artificial Intelligence in Clinical Practice* (pp. 341–344). Elsevier. doi:10.1016/B978-0-443-15688-5.00037-1

Li, Z., Wang, L., Wu, X., Jiang, J., Qiang, W., Xie, H., Zhou, H., Wu, S., Shao, Y., & Chen, W. (2023). Artificial intelligence in ophthalmology: The path to the real-world clinic. *Cell Reports Medicine*, *4*(7), 101095. doi:10.1016/j.xcrm.2023.101095 PMID:37385253

Lilhore, U. K., Dalal, S., Faujdar, N., Margala, M., Chakrabarti, P., Chakrabarti, T., Simaiya, S., Kumar, P., Thangaraju, P., & Velmurugan, H. (2023). Hybrid CNN-LSTM model with efficient hyperparameter tuning for prediction of Parkinson's disease. *Scientific Reports*, *13*(1), 14605. doi:10.1038/s41598-023-41314-y PMID:37669970

Lilhore, U. K., Dalal, S., Faujdar, N., Simaiya, S., Dahiya, M., Tomar, S., & Hashmi, A. (2024). Unveiling the prevalence and risk factors of early stage postpartum depression: A hybrid deep learning approach. *Multimedia Tools and Applications*, 1–35. doi:10.1007/s11042-024-18182-3

Lilhore, U. K., Manoharan, P., Sandhu, J. K., Simaiya, S., Dalal, S., Baqasah, A. M., Alsafyani, M., Alroobaea, R., Keshta, I., & Raahemifar, K. (2023). Hybrid model for precise hepatitis-C classification using improved random forest and SVM method. *Scientific Reports*, *13*(1), 12473. doi:10.1038/s41598-023-36605-3 PMID:37528148

Lilhore, U. K., Poongodi, M., Kaur, A., Simaiya, S., Algarni, A. D., Elmannai, H., Vijayakumar, V., Tunze, G. B., & Hamdi, M. (2022). Hybrid model for detection of cervical cancer using causal analysis and machine learning techniques. *Computational and Mathematical Methods in Medicine*, *2022*, 2022. doi:10.1155/2022/4688327 PMID:35572826

Lilhore, U. K., Simaiya, S., Pandey, H., Gautam, V., Garg, A., & Ghosh, P. (2022). Breast cancer detection in the IoT cloud-based healthcare environment using fuzzy cluster segmentation and SVM classifier. In Ambient Communications and Computer Systems [Singapore: Springer Nature Singapore.]. *Proceedings of RACCCS*, *2021*, 165–179.

Lilhore, U. K., Simaiya, S., Prasad, D., & Guleria, K. (2020). A hybrid tumor detection and classification based on machine learning. *Journal of Computational and Theoretical Nanoscience*, *17*(6), 2539–2544. doi:10.1166/jctn.2020.8927

Mahajan, Y., Shandilya, D., Batta, P., & Sharma, M. (2023). 3D Object 360-Degree Motion Detection Using Ultra-Frequency PIR Sensor. *2023 IEEE World Conference on Applied Intelligence and Computing (AIC)*, 614–619. 10.1109/AIC57670.2023.10263926

Monlezun, D. J. (2023). AI + healthcare systems. In *The Thinking Healthcare System* (pp. 37–67). Elsevier. doi:10.1016/B978-0-443-18906-7.00003-9

Okolo, C. T. (2022). Optimizing human-centered AI for healthcare in the Global South. *Patterns (New York, N.Y.)*, *3*(2), 100421. doi:10.1016/j.patter.2021.100421 PMID:35199066

Onyema, E. M., Lilhore, U. K., Saurabh, P., Dalal, S., Nwaeze, A. S., Chijindu, A. T., Ndufeiya-Kumasi, L. C., & Simaiya, S. (2023). Evaluation of IoT-Enabled hybrid model for genome sequence analysis of patients in healthcare 4.0. *Measurement. Sensors*, *26*, 100679. doi:10.1016/j.measen.2023.100679

Polevikov, S. (2023). Advancing AI in healthcare: A comprehensive review of best practices. *Clinica Chimica Acta*, *548*, 117519. doi:10.1016/j.cca.2023.117519 PMID:37595864

Rani, S., Kataria, A., Kumar, S., & Tiwari, P. (2023). Federated learning for secure IoMT-applications in smart healthcare systems: A comprehensive review. *Knowledge-Based Systems*, *274*, 110658. doi:10.1016/j.knosys.2023.110658

Raza, A., Tran, K. P., Koehl, L., & Li, S. (2022). Designing ECG monitoring healthcare system with federated transfer learning and explainable AI. *Knowledge-Based Systems*, *236*, 107763. doi:10.1016/j.knosys.2021.107763

Seoni, S., Jahmunah, V., Salvi, M., Barua, P. D., Molinari, F., & Acharya, U. R. (2023). Application of uncertainty quantification to artificial intelligence in healthcare: A review of last decade (2013–2023). *Computers in Biology and Medicine*, *165*, 107441. doi:10.1016/j.compbiomed.2023.107441 PMID:37683529

Wysocki, O., Davies, J. K., Vigo, M., Armstrong, A. C., Landers, D., Lee, R., & Freitas, A. (2023). Assessing the communication gap between AI models and healthcare professionals: Explainability, utility, and trust in AI-driven clinical decision-making. *Artificial Intelligence*, *316*, 103839. doi:10.1016/j.artint.2022.103839

Xie, J., Wu, E. Q., Wang, S., Cheng, T., Zhou, Z., Zhong, J., & Liu, L. (2022). Real-World Data for Healthcare Research in China: Call for Actions. *Value in Health Regional Issues*, *27*, 72–81. doi:10.1016/j.vhri.2021.05.002 PMID:34844062

Zahlan, A., Ranjan, R. P., & Hayes, D. (2023). Artificial intelligence innovation in healthcare: Literature review, exploratory analysis, and future research. *Technology in Society*, *74*, 102321. doi:10.1016/j.techsoc.2023.102321

Zaydi, H., Zaydi, M., & Bakoury, Z. (2023). AI and IoT working for healthcare. In Computational Intelligence for Medical Internet of Things (IoT) Applications (pp. 3–32). Elsevier. doi:10.1016/B978-0-323-99421-7.00018-0

Chapter 12
Federated Learning for Private Cancer Diagnosis With Exascale Computing

N. R. Vembu
SASTRA University, India

Niladri Maiti
School of Dentistry, Akfa University, India

K. Kadiervel
Arupadai Veedu Medical College, India

Amarendranath Choudhury
https://orcid.org/0000-0002-7042-8139
Patharkandi College, India

Rajasekhar Pinnamaneni
https://orcid.org/0000-0003-3904-9058
Koneru Lakshmaiah Education Foundation, India

ABSTRACT

This study delves into the intersection of federated learning, privacy preservation, and exascale computing to advance the field of cancer diagnosis. Employing a federated learning framework, the research addresses the imperative need for collaborative, yet privacy-conscious, approaches to healthcare data analysis. Focusing on human cancer diagnosis and detection, the authors leverage the power of exascale computing to handle massive datasets distributed across diverse medical institutions. The proposed methodology ensures privacy by design, enabling secure model training without centralized data aggregation. The findings showcase the efficacy of federated learning and exascale computing in achieving accurate and timely cancer diagnoses while upholding patient privacy, thus paving the way for transformative advancements in personalized and secure healthcare analytics

DOI: 10.4018/979-8-3693-1874-4.ch012

1. INTRODUCTION

Cancer is a multifaceted and life-threatening illness that impacts millions of people globally. It includes many varieties, each with special traits and therapeutic implications of their own. Researchers and healthcare providers are always attempting to understand and treat this disease better, and technology advancements, particularly in the field of computers, promise a promising future for the field of cancer treatment. Using real-time, exascale computing, healthcare professionals can have unmatched access to a wealth of data and computational capabilities that could improve cancer therapy and management.

Exa scale computing is an effective method that can significantly improve human cancer detection and diagnosis. Exascale computing systems have enormous processing capacity, which allows researchers to analyse enormous amounts of genetic data and find patterns and mutations linked to cancer. Fig 1 explains human cancer diagnosis using Exascale computing. This may result in earlier and more precise detection as well as individualised treatment regimens catered to each person's particular genetic profile. Exascale computing can also facilitate the creation of more complex machine learning algorithms for cancer risk prediction and treatment result optimisation. Exascale computing's incorporation in cancer diagnosis and detection has the potential to significantly improve patient outcomes and deepen our understanding of this complicated illness.

1.1 Importance of Early Detection for Effective Treatment

In the battle against cancer, the significance of early detection and precise diagnosis cannot be emphasised. Early cancer detection greatly boosts the likelihood of an effective course of therapy and higher patient survival rates. Exa scale computing can be very helpful in this area by evaluating large patient data sets and finding minute trends and biomarkers that could point to the existence of cancer. Exascale computing holds the potential to transform cancer care and save countless lives by improving our ability to detect cancer precisely and early on. in raising the effectiveness of cancer treatment. Problem with pharmacological reaction. To improve pre-clinical drug screening and ad-

Figure 1. Exascale in human cancer diagnosis

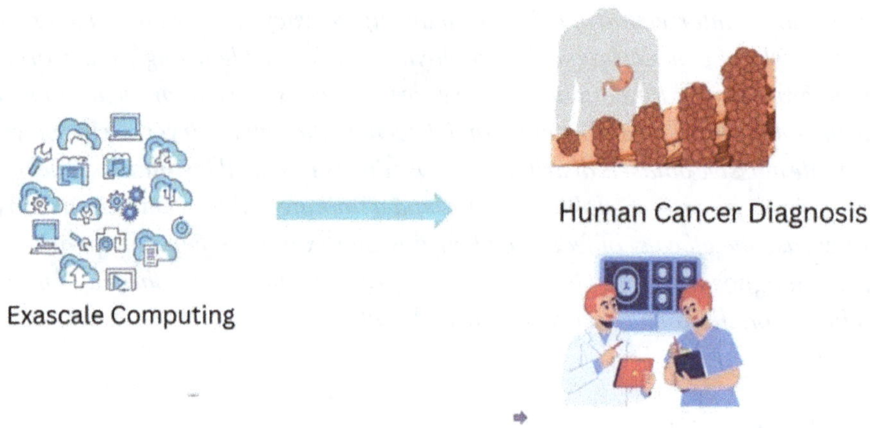

vance precision medicine-based therapies for cancer patients, this pilot aims to establish predictive models for medication response. Justin M -2018 (Wozniak, 2018). Exascale computing, which can do one quintillion calculations per second, enables real-time analysis of massive volumes of data. This technology could have a major impact on cancer research by improving our understanding of the disease and helping to create more potent treatment plans. Researchers may analyse complicated genomic data, mimic the behaviour of cancer cells, and find individualised therapy choices for specific patients by utilising the capability of exascale computers. Exascale computing ultimately opens up new paths for ground-breaking discoveries and breakthroughs in cancer therapy, improving patient outcomes and raising survival rates.

1.2 The Difficulties and Current Approaches in Cancer Diagnosis

Nowadays, a variety of procedures are used in cancer diagnosis to find malignant cells in the body, including blood tests, biopsies, and imaging studies. These techniques, however, frequently have shortcomings with regard to specificity, sensitivity, and accuracy, which could result in a delayed or incorrect diagnosis. It's also difficult to correctly diagnose and categorise various cancer types and stages due to the disease's complexity and heterogeneity. Getting beyond these obstacles is essential to ensuring early detection and prompt intervention, which can greatly enhance patient survival and prognosis.

1.3 Overview of Current Diagnostic Techniques (e.g., Imaging, Biopsy)

Imaging methods, such CT and MRI scans, are being used in cancer diagnosis. These methods can provide precise images of the body to identify tumours or abnormal growths. In contrast, biopsies entail the removal of a sample of tissue or cells from a questionable location and a microscope examination to ascertain the presence or absence of cancer cells. These methods, while popular, have drawbacks and may result in false positives or negatives. To increase accuracy and optimise patient outcomes, it is therefore imperative that research and instrument developments continue.

1.4 Limitations and Challenges in Current Cancer Diagnosis Methods

Include the difficulty to identify metastases or tiny tumours, as well as challenges differentiating between benign and malignant tumours. Furthermore, intrusive treatments may be necessary for some diagnostic tests, which can be risky and uncomfortable for patients. Moreover, creating a universally applicable diagnostic strategy is difficult due to the complexity and heterogeneity of cancer. In order to overcome these constraints and transform the diagnosis of cancer, current research endeavours to create innovative methods like liquid biopsies and molecular imaging.

1.5 Need for More Advanced and Accurate Diagnostic Approaches

Essential for ensuring early cancer identification and bettering patient outcomes. This is particularly critical because many tumors are asymptomatic in the early stages, making conventional techniques of diagnosis challenging. Doctors may be able to identify cancer earlier and more accurately by using cutting-edge methods like liquid biopsies, which examine tumor DNA that is circulating in the blood. Similar to this, molecular imaging methods enable the non-invasive observation of malignant cells and their activities, offering crucial data for the diagnosis and development of a treatment strategy. The potential impact of these developments in cancer diagnosis on patient treatment and overall survival rates is substantial.

2. INTRODUCTION TO EXASCALE COMPUTING

High-performance computing next frontier is exa scale computing. It describes a processing capacity that has never been attained before—the capacity to complete a billion calculations every second. By tackling challenging issues in domains like drug development, astrophysics, and climate modelling, scientists and researchers will be able to expand their knowledge and skills in these subjects thanks to this breakthrough in computing capacity. Exascale computing systems are opening the way for a new era of scientific discovery and technological progress, but their development demands creative hardware and software solutions that can handle the enormous volumes of data and processing power involved. Exa scale computing is a potent instrument that can significantly improve human cancer detection and diagnosis. Researchers may analyse enormous volumes of genomic data and find patterns and mutations linked to cancer by utilizing the enormous computational capability of exascale platforms. This has the potential to result in more timely and precise detection as well as individualised treatment regimens based on the distinct genetic composition of each patient. Moreover, exascale computing can facilitate the creation of more advanced machine learning algorithms that optimise treatment outcomes and anticipate cancer risk. All things considered, the application of exascale computing to cancer diagnosis and detection has enormous potential to enhance patient outcomes and deepen our knowledge of this intricate illness.

2.1 Exascale Computing and Its Applications in Cancer Research

Cancer diagnoses are progressing significantly thanks in large part to the use of exascale computers in cancer research. Scientists can quickly analyse enormous volumes of genetic data thanks to exascale computing's enormous processing capability. This skill makes it possible to identify genetic patterns and mutations that may be involved in the development of cancer, opening the door to more specialised treatments. Researchers are making great strides towards comprehending the intricacies of cancer and developing efficacious treatment approaches by utilising the power of exascale computing. We are getting closer to a cure for cancer thanks to this revolutionary technology that is boosting the pace of cancer research.

2.2 The Potential of Exascale Computing

A computer system that can process one billion billion calculations per second is referred to as exascale computing. Because of their enormous processing capacity, researchers are able to examine a large amount of genetic data and find small trends and mutations that lead to the development of cancer. Scientists can anticipate the efficacy of various treatments, optimise personalised medicines for particular patients, and model the behaviour of cancer cells via exascale computing. This potential is revolutionising the field of cancer research and offering promise for the development of more effective and focused therapy options down the road.

3. CANCER DIAGNOSIS USING EXASCALE COMPUTING METHODS AND TECHNOLOGIES

The diagnosis and detection of cancer could be revolutionized by exascale computing. Through the use of exascale computers' enormous computational capacity, researchers are able to examine voluminous patient data, genomic data, and medical records in order to spot trends and genetic alterations linked to distinct cancer kinds. This may result in the creation of more precise and individualized diagnoses as well as focused therapies and treatments. Furthermore, exascale computing can expedite the drug development process significantly, enabling researchers to test and find possible anti-cancer medications more quickly. Exascale computing has transformed the research field of cancer and holds significant potential to enhance patient outcomes and improving the ongoing battle against this deadly disease.

3.1 Machine Learning for Cancer Detection

Machine learning holds enormous promise for the field of early cancer detection. Large volumes of patient data can be analyzed by machine learning algorithms to find patterns and signs of cancer early on, when treatment is most successful. Cancer screening could be significantly improved by this technology, which would result in earlier diagnoses and reduced death rates. Machine learning models can handle large datasets in real time due to exascale computing capabilities, which enables timely and accurate cancer detection for millions of individuals worldwide. Exascale computing, with the use for advanced algorithms and machine learning techniques, can identify complex patterns and alterations in the human genome that could be linked to the development of cancer. It is now feasible for specialists to find genetic variants and biomarkers that have been previously unknown, which can be utilised to target tailored treatment approaches. Exascale computing additionally allows the simpler incorporation of data from several sources, such as clinical trial data and electronic health records, to provide a full understanding of a patients cancer profile and assist treatment decisions.

3.2 Cancer Genomic Data Analysis

Genomic data analysis for cancer is also being significantly impacted by machine learning. Machine learning algorithms analyse genetic data from cancer patients to identify DNA patterns and changes associated with the start and progression of cancer. This information helps in early detection by identifying potential biomarkers, customising treatment plans, and predicting patient outcomes. Machine learning has significant potential to revolutionize cancer detection and treatment in its entirety, in addition to revolutionizing the study of cancer genetics. In this field specifically, exascale computing has the potential to change cancer therapy. Researchers and health care providers may quickly and accurately examine enormous volumes of genomic data by using this state-of-the-art technology. This may result in better understanding of the genetic origins of cancer and more individualized treatment regimens.

3.3 Drug Development

Finding and developing novel medications could be sped up significantly with the use of exascale computers. This approach could speed up the process of finding possible drug targets and simulating their effects on different biological systems because it handles vast datasets and performs intricate simulations. For example, by examining the genetic composition of cancer patients, researchers could pinpoint particular mutations that encourage the growth of tumors and create medications intended to block those mutations, resulting in more efficient and individualized therapies.

3.4 Simulating Cancer Growth and Spread

The application of machine learning in cancer research is noteworthy, particularly in the context of simulating the growth and spread of cancer. Machine learning algorithms have the capability to model the evolution of cancer in the body by analysing large quantities of data on tumour growth and metastasis. As a result, more focused and efficient treatment approaches can be developed since researchers have a greater understanding of the behaviour and metastasis of cancer cells. In the end, this technology could help patients recover more quickly from cancer and save a great deal of lives.

4. EXASCALE COMPUTING FOR EARLY CANCER DETECTION

A significant obstacle in the identification of cancer is the large volume of genomic data that needs to be examined. With its potential to process enormous volumes of data at previously unheard-of rates, exascale computing is a promising solution to this problem. Exascale computing is explained in Fig. 2 for cancer diagnosis. Through the use of machine learning techniques on exascale computer platforms, scientists may quickly examine a patient's whole genome, facilitating early detection and possibly even saving lives. Better patient outcomes could result from the faster and more precise identification of cancer that this machine learning and exascale computing combo makes possible.

4.1. Data Collection

The first component, data collection, is the gathering of information from many sources, including genetic tests, imaging scans, and medical documents. An exascale computing system for the diagnosis of human cancer must include data collection. Collecting different kinds of data from multiple sources—such as genetic tests, imaging scans, medical records, and other pertinent sources—is part of it. After gathering the data, it is pre-processed to guarantee data quality, standardise formats, and eliminate noise. To prepare the data for analysis, this process may include feature extraction, normalisation, and data clean-

Figure 2. Exascale computing for cancer detection

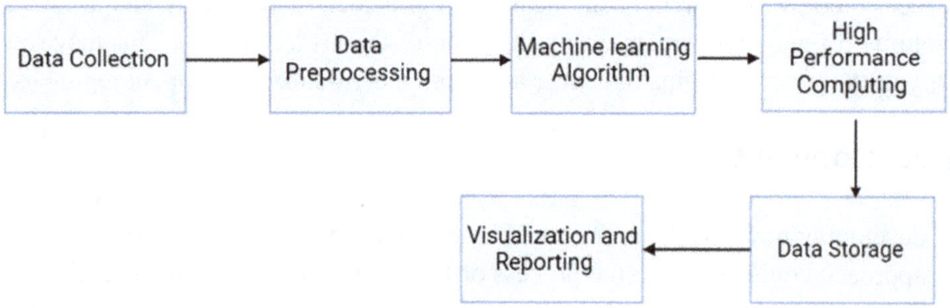

ing procedures. In order to train and test machine learning algorithms for precise cancer diagnosis, a comprehensive and representative dataset must be created.

4. 2. Data Preprocessing

Preparing the data entails converting unprocessed data into a clear, consistent, and useful format for additional analysis. It is an essential step in the data analysis process. Numerous strategies, including data reduction, data integration, data transformation, and data cleaning, are used in this process. Addressing outliers, inconsistent data, and missing values in the data is known as data cleaning. Integrating data from several sources into a single format is known as data integration. The process of transforming data into an analysis-ready representation, like normalisation or scaling, is known as data transformation. The goal of data reduction strategies is to lessen the dimensionality of a dataset without sacrificing its critical information. In general, data preparation reduces the influence of noise or extraneous information on the final results while guaranteeing that the data is of excellent quality and prepared for analysis. Machine Learning methods: In order to analyse the pre-processed data and identify patterns suggestive of cancer, this component represents the application of machine learning methods, such as deep learning models or artificial neural networks.

4.3. Machine Learning Algorithms

Machine learning plays a pivotal role in cancer diagnosis by leveraging computational algorithms and data-driven insights to enhance the accuracy and efficiency of the diagnostic process. By analyzing vast datasets encompassing genomic information, medical images, and clinical records, machine learning models can identify subtle patterns, genetic mutations, and biomarkers associated with various cancer types. These models not only aid in early cancer detection but also contribute to the personalization of treatment plans, helping clinicians make informed decisions based on a patient's unique genomic profile. Furthermore, machine learning helps to improve overall patient care, forecast patient outcomes, and optimize clinical trials—all of which advance the area of oncology and improve the prognosis for cancer patients.

4.4 High-Performance Computing

(HPC) systems have the potential to significantly advance cancer screening because to their enormous processing power and capacity to handle big datasets. Researchers can more precisely discover biomarkers that indicate the presence of cancer by analyzing complex genomic patterns with the use of HPC. Furthermore, HPC can help create customized treatment program based on each patient's unique genetic profile, which can result in more focused medications and better patient outcomes. The potential for early identification and successful treatment of cancer screening is enormous given the ongoing developments in HPC technology.

4.5. Data Storage and Management

HPC also significantly improves data storage and management. It is possible to effectively store and organise the substantial amount of genetic data produced by cancer screenings, making it simple to access and retrieve when needed to better estimate chemical toxicities that may represent atomic-level insights, a multiparametric model was discovered that incorporates physic-chemical parameters, quantitative structure-activity relationship predictions, and docking score (Patel, et al., 2020). In addition to saving time, this makes guarantee that important data is not misplaced or lost. Moreover, HPC promotes a more collaborative and all-encompassing approach to cancer research and treatment by facilitating safe exchange and collaboration between researchers and medical practitioners. All things considered, the application of HPC to cancer screening has the potential to completely transform the industry and greatly enhance patient care.

4.6. Visualization and Reporting

Using HPC for cancer screening also improves these capabilities. Reports and visualizations created by researchers and medical experts might offer insightful information about the screening data. Efficient and scalable solutions are necessary for the fast-expanding HPC industry to handle massive computing workloads. Notable platforms that address these demands include OpenHPC and HTCondor, which employ distinct techniques and architectures (Ismayilov, 2023). With the use of these visualisations, patterns, trends, and possible risk factors can be found, leading to more precise diagnosis and individualised treatment regimens. Moreover, the capacity to produce comprehensive reports with efficiency facilitates smooth communication and knowledge exchange between healthcare providers, which eventually improves patient outcomes.

4.7. Security and Privacy

When using data analytics for healthcare screening, security and privacy are crucial factors to take into account. Ensuring that patient data is secure and only available to those who are authorised is vital. To protect sensitive data, strong security measures like encryption and access controls should be in place. To protect patient anonymity, stringent adherence to privacy laws, such HIPAA, is also required. Healthcare organisations may reliably use data analytics to improve patient care without compromising the integrity of the data by putting security and privacy first.

4.8. External Data Sources

To guarantee their dependability and adherence to security and privacy norms, other data sources should also be closely examined and tracked. To find vulnerabilities or possible breaches, audits and risk assessments should be carried out on a regular basis. Healthcare organisations can further strengthen their security posture by exchanging best practises and working together with reliable partners. Ultimately, to safeguard patient data and keep the confidence of both patients and regulatory bodies, a thorough and proactive approach to data security and privacy is necessary.

4.9. User Interface

To guarantee that only authorised workers have access to sensitive patient data, user interface design and access restrictions should be put into place. Strong password regulations, two-factor authentication, and routine user account evaluations are some examples of this. In order to teach staff members the value of data security and privacy and to keep them informed about emerging dangers and best practises, periodic staff training and awareness programmes should also be held. Healthcare organisations can reduce the likelihood of data breaches and guarantee the confidentiality and security of patient information by putting these precautions into place.

5. PERSONALIZED CANCER DIAGNOSIS WITH EXASCALE COMPUTING

Exascale computing offers the processing capability required to swiftly and effectively handle enormous volumes of genomic data. Through the utilisation of machine learning algorithms, scientists can detect patterns and alterations within the genome that could potentially signify the occurrence of cancer. Patient survival rates may increase as a result of this individualised approach to cancer diagnosis and therapy. Exascale computing has the potential to change how we diagnose and treat cancer by speeding up scientific discoveries by analysing massive datasets in real time.

5.1 Exascale Computing for Cancer Screening

Large-scale genomic data may be analysed more quickly and accurately because of exascale computing, which can significantly improve cancer screening. With the use of this innovative method, small genetic variations linked to various cancer kinds can be identified, enabling early detection and treatment. In addition, real-time data processing and interpretation can result in more economical and successful screening methods, which might completely remake the cancer diagnostics industry. Exascale computing, for instance, allows scientists to examine the complete human genome in a matter of minutes as opposed to weeks or months using conventional techniques. With the use of this rapid analysis, certain patterns and mutations that suggest a higher risk of cancer can be found, allowing for the development of focused preventative treatments for high-risk individuals. Furthermore, real-time data processing can guarantee early detection of malignant cells while improving the accuracy of screening tests, lowering false positives and needless invasive procedures for patients..

5.2 Exascale Computing for Cancer Bio-Maker Discovery

Exascale computing has the potential to revolutionize cancer biomarker discovery. With its immense processing power, this technology can analyze vast amounts of genomic data, identifying crucial biomarkers that can predict the progression and response to treatment of various types of cancer. This can significantly accelerate the development of personalized medicine, where treatments can be tailored to individual patients based on their unique genetic profiles. Ultimately, exascale computing has the potential to improve cancer outcomes and save countless lives.

Examining the genetic makeup of cancer cells to locate certain genetic changes or patterns that can act as indicators of the occurrence or progression of cancer is one aspect of analyzing cancer genomic data to find new biomarkers for cancer detection.

The entirety of an organism's or cell's DNA sequences and genetic makeup are referred to as genomic data. Tumor samples or circulating tumor DNA can provide genetic information in the setting of cancer.

Large-scale genomic dataset processing and analysis are made possible by exascale computing, which can be quite helpful in this analysis. Exascale computing systems offer enormous computational capacity that allows researchers to process massive volumes of genetic data using intricate algorithms and statistical analysis. This makes it possible to identify possible biomarkers, which are particular genetic changes or patterns linked to the onset or spread of cancer.

Exascale computing can assist in finding patterns and connections in the genomic data that can be difficult to see with conventional techniques by utilizing machine learning algorithms. These algorithms are able to discern between normal genetic variants and the genomic mutations that are specific to cancer by learning from big datasets. This may result in the identification of novel biomarkers for early cancer identification, diagnosis, and therapy response tracking. All things considered, the analysis of cancer genomic data using exascale computing can hasten the identification of new biomarkers, which will ultimately enhance our capacity to identify cancer early and create more efficient diagnostic and therapeutic approaches.

Difference Between Exascale Computing and Machine Learning in Cancer Diagnosis

Outstanding performance measurements from exascale computing could revolutionize the way that cancer is diagnosed in humans. Exascale computers, which can perform quintillions of calculations per second (exaFLOPS), make it possible to analyze large genomic databases, high-resolution medical pictures, and patient records quickly. This accelerates the process of identifying genetic mutations, biomarkers, and possible treatments. These systems make use of millions of computing nodes, provide memory capacities that are unmatched in the petabyte to exabyte range, and enable data transfer speeds that fall into the terabytes per second region. Exascale computers require sophisticated cooling techniques because they frequently consume megawatts to gigawatts of electricity, despite their enormous processing power. These performance measures highlight how exascale computing might transform the diagnosis of human cancer by facilitating early identification, tailored treatment plans, and thorough data analysis all of which will ultimately progress oncology and enhance patient outcomes.

Table 1: Difference between Exascale computing and Machine learning in Cancer diagnosis.

6. EXASCALE COMPUTING IN THE SEARCH FOR CANCER DRUGS

Examine how exascale computing can transform the process of finding and creating novel medications for cancer. Talk about how this technology makes it possible for scientists to examine enormous volumes of genomic data, which helps them identify possible drug targets and expedites the creation of targeted medicines. Exascale computing can also help with complicated drug interaction modelling and simulations, which enables researchers to optimise drug dosages for specific patients and forecast the efficacy of different treatment choices. The ability to customise treatments to the particulars of each patient's cancer thanks to this increase in computing capacity has the potential to significantly improve precision medicine techniques. This could therefore lead to a considerable improvement in cancer outcomes and a rise in the likelihood of effective treatments. All things considered, exascale computing has great potential to change the medication development process for cancer and get us closer to a time when receiving a cancer diagnosis won't be a fatal one.

Table 1. Exascale computing and machine learning

Aspects	Exascale Computing	Machine Learning
Computational Power	Exceptional computing power and speed, ideal for handling massive datasets.	Utilizes computational power but at a scale lower than exascale computing.
Data Handling	Efficient at processing large-scale genomic, imaging, and clinical data.	Specialized for pattern recognition and predictive analysis using various data types.
Flexibility	Versatile, capable of various tasks beyond machine learning, such as simulations and modeling.	Specialized for machine learning tasks, particularly pattern recognition and prediction.
Use cases	Suitable for high-performance simulations, drug discovery, and large-scale data analytics.	Applied for identifying patterns, risk prediction, and decision support in cancer diagnosis
Infrastructure	Requires advanced infrastructure and massive data centers.	Can be deployed on standard hardware with specialized software libraries
Expertise	Requires expertise in high-performance computing and data management.	Requires expertise in machine learning algorithms and data preprocessing.
Real time analysis	Limited real-time capabilities due to the scale of computations	Can provide real-time or near-real-time insights for diagnostic purposes.
Integration with Clinical Work flow	May require additional steps for integration into clinical workflows.	Can be integrated directly into clinical decision support systems.

6.1 Target Identification

In the process of developing new cancer drugs, target identification is a thorough examination of biological and genetic data in order to pinpoint particular proteins, genetic abnormalities, or other molecular targets that are essential to the onset and spread of cancer. Computational models, algorithms, and data mining techniques are used in this process to find possible targets that medications could target to stop or slow the progression of cancer. Exascale computing speeds up the search for new and efficient cancer treatments by helping researchers find and rank possible targets for additional study by combining data from several sources and analysing massive databases.

6.2 Virtual Screening

In the process of finding new drugs, a computational method called virtual screening is utilised to choose promising candidates from huge databases of chemical compounds. ADMIRRAL and IMPROVE researchers intend to boost cancer drug discovery. The capacity of virtual machine-based process migrator mechanisms to run processes and support environments with heterogeneous compute units makes them potentially useful in distributed exascale systems. (Sohrabi and Khaneghah, 2020).

It entails predicting the binding affinity and possible effectiveness of drugs against a particular target protein or receptor using computer simulations and molecular docking techniques. Advanced programming models, domain specific languages, and scripting toolkits have the potential to greatly accelerate the adoption of high-performance computing (Zaki et al., 2018).

Researchers can save time and costs by prioritising and choosing a smaller sample of compounds for additional experimental validation by virtually screening millions of molecules. In order to manage the enormous datasets and intricate computations required for virtual screening, exascale computing offers enormous computational capacity. As a machine learning approach, imitation learning (IL) allows an agent to learn how to do a job by emulating the behaviors and actions of a human expert (Liu et al., 2023). This allows for quicker and more precise predictions of compound-target interactions. This quickens the process of finding new and promising medication candidates for a variety of illnesses, such as cancer, infectious diseases, and neurological disorders, and raises the likelihood of doing so.

6.3 Molecular Dynamics (MD) Simulations

Molecular dynamics (MD) simulations are an effective technique in the hunt for new cancer drugs because they let scientists look at the atomic-level interactions between drug molecules and target proteins. MD simulations shed light on the binding mechanisms, stability, and conformational changes of the drug-target complex by modelling the movement and behaviour of atoms across time. By forecasting the binding kinetics, residence duration, and affinity of medicinal molecules, this data helps in the development and refinement of successful cancer treatments. This document lays out methods for integrating a business context into threat intelligence scoring, which helps prioritize risk mitigation initiatives for services and transactions that are vital to the company's operations (Birdsall, 2023). The pharmaceutical and research industries have spent years trying to find a cure for cancer, yet many patients continue to show little improvement with current therapies, and drug resistance is a prevalent problem (Brettin, 2019) (Liu et al., 2023). Moreover, genetic mutations or changes in the target protein can be investigated using MD simulations, which can aid in the understanding of drug resistance mechanisms and the development of countermeasures. Insights into drug distribution, metabolism, and toxicity can also be gained via MD simulations, which can help in the selection and improvement of therapeutic candidates with favourable pharmacokinetic characteristics and fewer adverse effects. In general, MD simulations are essential to the process of finding new cancer drugs because they offer comprehensive atomic-level understanding of the interactions between drugs and targets and make it easier to create safer and more effective cancer treatments.

6.4 Drug Design and Optimization

One of the most important steps in creating safe and effective pharmaceuticals is drug design and optimisation. It entails the discovery, creation, and alteration of biologics or tiny molecules that interact with particular targets, like proteins or enzymes, in order to control their function and cure illnesses. chemical synthesis, combinatorial chemistry, and high-throughput chemical screening have all seen tremendous improvements because to the proliferation of powerful computing devices (Wu et al., 2020). Target validation and identification are usually the first steps in the process, which is then followed by the design and manufacturing of compounds that can bind to the target and have the intended therapeutic effect. In order to help in the selection and optimisation of lead compounds, computational techniques like molecular docking, virtual screening, and molecular dynamics simulations are essential in predicting the binding affinity, selectivity, and pharmacokinetic features of therapeutic candidates. To increase the potency, efficacy, and safety profile of the drug candidates, iterative cycles of design, synthesis, and testing are carried out. This results in the creation of optimised drug molecules for clinical trials and ultimate approval.

6.5 Pharmacokinetics and Toxicity Prediction

Important components of drug development are pharmacokinetics and toxicity prediction, which evaluate how drug molecules behave in the body and forecast possible side effects. Predicting pharmacokinetic characteristics, including toxicity profiles and absorption, distribution, metabolism, and excretion (ADME) qualities, is a critical function of computational approaches. Researchers can estimate important factors including drug solubility, blood-brain barrier permeability, plasma protein binding, metabolic stability, and clearance by using in silico models and simulations. Additional challenges might arise from the fact that medication candidates often exhibit quality variations, including particle size dispersion, crystallinity, and polymorphism (Shah and Agnihotri, 2011). The selection and improvement of medication candidates with desired pharmacokinetic characteristics and lower toxicity concerns is aided by these predictions. Furthermore, by anticipating their interactions with off-target proteins, evaluating the probability of adverse events, and detecting potential metabolic liabilities, computational techniques can evaluate the potential toxicity of drug candidates. Pharmacokinetics and toxicity prediction aid in the logical design and optimization of safer and more effective medications by fusing computational techniques with experimental data.

7. PERFORMANCE METRICS VALUE OF EXASCALE COMPUTING IN HUMAN CANCER DIAGNOSIS

Exascale computing exhibits remarkable performance metrics that have transformative implications for human cancer diagnosis. With the ability to execute quintillions of calculations per second (exaFLOPS), exascale systems enable the rapid analysis of vast genomic datasets, high-resolution medical images, and patient records, expediting the identification of genetic mutations, biomarkers, and treatment options. These systems leverage processing nodes numbering in the millions, offering unparalleled memory capacities in the petabytes to exabytes range, and facilitating data transfer rates in the terabytes per second category. Despite their immense computational power, exascale systems present significant power efficiency challenges, often consuming megawatts to gigawatts of electricity, necessitating advanced cooling solutions. Underneath the belly button, on the upper part of the body that runs from side to side, you'll find the liver (Ramgopal et al., 2022). These performance metrics underscore the potential for exascale computing to revolutionize human cancer diagnosis by enabling personalized treatment strategies, early detection, and comprehensive data analysis, ultimately advancing the field of oncology and improving patient outcomes.

7.1 Ethical Consideration

Patient privacy and data security are paramount ethical considerations in the use of exascale computing for cancer diagnosis. The vast amount of personal and sensitive healthcare data involved, including genomic information, medical images, and electronic health records, necessitates stringent measures to safeguard patient privacy and protect against data breaches. This document lays out methods for integrating a business context into threat intelligence scoring, which helps prioritize risk mitigation initiatives for services and transactions that are vital to the company's operations (Birdsall et al., 2023). Additionally, healthcare institutions and research organizations must adhere to stringent ethical guidelines, obtaining

Table 2. Performance metrics value of exascale computing in human cancer diagnosis

Metrics	Value
Computational Power (Flops)	1 exaFlops(10^18 Flops)
Processing Nodes (CPUs/GPU)	Thousands to Millions
Memory Capacity	Petebytes to Exabytes
Data transfer rate	Terabytes per second
Power Consumption	Mega watts to Gigawatts
Perk Performance (Peta FLOPS)	1,000 -10,000 peta FLOPS
Storage Capacity	Exabytes to Zettabytes
Network Bandwidth	Terabits per second

informed consent from patients and transparently communicating how their data will be used. By prioritizing patient privacy and data security, exascale computing can advance cancer diagnosis ethically and responsibly, building trust among patients and healthcare stakeholders in the process.

7.2 Patient Privacy and Data Security

When using exascale computing to diagnose cancer, patient privacy and data security are the most important ethical factors to take into account. Tight precautions are needed to protect patient privacy and prevent data breaches because of the large amount of private and sensitive healthcare data involved, including genetic data, medical imaging, and electronic health records. There has been a proliferation of databases that store pharmacokinetic parameters in the last decade, thanks to the industry's lightning-fast growth (Birdsall et al., 2023; Wu, et al., 2020; Shah and Agnihotri, 2011).

To guarantee patient confidentiality and identity protection, it is essential to implement strong encryption methods, access controls, and data anonymization strategies. Furthermore, in order to comply with strict ethical rules, healthcare facilities and research organizations must have patients' informed consent and clearly explain to them how their data will be used. Exascale computing may ethically and responsibly advance cancer detection, fostering confidence among patients and healthcare stakeholders in the process by placing a high priority on patient privacy and data security.

7.3 Informed Consent and Data Sharing

When using exascale computation to diagnose cancer, informed consent and data exchange are essential ethical considerations. It is essential to have patients' express and informed consent so that you can be confident they understand how their medical data will be used for diagnosis and research. Furthermore, it's critical to provide explicit standards for appropriate data sharing procedures that strike a balance between promoting cooperative research projects and safeguarding patient privacy. Strict de-identification techniques to anonymize patient information, secure data transmission, and compliance with legal and regulatory frameworks are all necessary components of ethical data sharing practices that support openness and confidence in the responsible use of exascale computing to advance cancer diagnosis and treatment.

7.4 Bias and Fairness in Algorithms

Bias and fairness in algorithms are essential ethical considerations in the application of exascale computing for cancer diagnosis. Machine learning and AI algorithms play a pivotal role in analyzing and interpreting vast amounts of medical data. It is crucial to assess these algorithms for biases that could result in disparities in diagnosis and treatment outcomes among diverse patient populations. Addressing bias involves careful selection and curation of training data, regular model auditing, and implementing bias-mitigation strategies. Ensuring fairness in algorithmic decision-making is paramount to maintain the trust and equity of healthcare systems. By proactively identifying and rectifying biases, the healthcare community can work towards a more equitable and unbiased application of exascale computing in cancer diagnosis, ultimately improving healthcare access and outcomes for all patients.

7.5 Transparency and Accountability

Transparency and accountability are fundamental ethical principles when harnessing the power of exascale computing for cancer diagnosis. As complex machine learning and AI algorithms are increasingly integrated into healthcare, it is imperative that the decision-making processes and outcomes of these algorithms are transparent, understandable, and auditable. This transparency enables healthcare professionals to trust and validate the results, fostering confidence in the technology. Accountability mechanisms should be in place to ensure that responsible parties are answerable for the decisions and actions related to the use of exascale computing in cancer diagnosis. By prioritizing transparency and accountability, healthcare institutions can uphold ethical standards, enhance patient safety, and promote the responsible deployment of advanced technologies in improving cancer diagnosis and patient care.

7.6 Resource allocation and Equity

Resource allocation and equity are critical ethical considerations in the utilization of exascale computing for cancer diagnosis. As the deployment of exascale computing technologies can be resource-intensive, it is vital to ensure equitable access for healthcare institutions, research organizations, and underserved communities. A fair and balanced distribution of computational resources and expertise is essential to prevent exacerbating healthcare disparities. Additionally, strategies should be in place to bridge the digital divide, offering support and training to healthcare professionals and institutions to harness the benefits of exascale computing effectively. Prioritizing resource allocation and equity ensures that the advantages of advanced technologies are accessible to all, promoting fairness and inclusivity in the advancement of cancer diagnosis and treatment.

CONCLUSION

The chapter "Human Cancer Diagnosis and Detection Using Exascale Computing" concludes by highlighting how exascale computing has the potential to completely change the oncology field. Exascale computing, with its unparalleled computational capacity, makes it possible to rapidly analyze enormous and complicated datasets, such as those related to genetics, medical imaging, and clinical records. This process eventually leads to earlier cancer detection, more individualized treatment plans, and better patient outcomes. Exascale computing has the potential to reshape cancer diagnosis through multidisciplinary cooperation, ethical considerations, and data-driven insights. This will advance the future of cancer care, making precise and effective treatment accessible to patients globally and providing new hope in the fight against this incurable illness.

REFERENCES

Birdsall, R., Foley, J. A., Nadiminti, C. M. B., Sivasubramanian, G., & Raithatha, D. H. (2023). *Identifying enterprise risk based on business context with threat intelligence*. Academic Press.

Ismayilov, E. (2023). Difference Between OpenHPC and HTCondor Cluster Systems: In-depth Analysis. *Azerbaijan Journal of High Performance Computing*, *6*(2), 203–208.

Liu, X., Jiang, S., Vasan, A., Brace, A., Gokdemir, O., Brettin, T., . . . Stevens, R. (2023, December). DRUGIMPROVER: Utilizing Reinforcement Learning for Multi-Objective Alignment in Drug Optimization. *NeurIPS 2023 Workshop on New Frontiers of AI for Drug Discovery and Development*.

Patel, C. N., Kumar, S. P., Rawal, R. M., Patel, D. P., Gonzalez, F. J., & Pandya, H. A. (2020). A multiparametric organ toxicity predictor for drug discovery. *Toxicology Mechanisms and Methods*, *30*(3), 159–166.

Ramgopal, N. C., Gantela, P., Rajagopal, R., Thankam, T., & SenthamilSelvan, R. (2022, December). Automatic Liver Cancer Detection in Abdominal Liver Images Using Soft Optimization Techniques. In *2022 International Conference on Knowledge Engineering and Communication Systems (ICKES)* (pp. 1-5). IEEE.

Shah, A. K., & Agnihotri, S. A. (2011). Recent advances and novel strategies in pre-clinical formulation development: An overview. *Journal of Controlled Release*, *156*(3), 281–296.

Sohrabi, Z., & Khaneghah, E. M. (2020). Challenges of Using Live Process Migration in Distributed Exascale Systems. *Azerbaijan Journal of High Performance Computing*, *3*(2), 151–163.

Wozniak, J. M., Davis, P. E., Shu, T., Ozik, J., Collier, N., Parashar, M., & Stevens, R. (2018). *Scaling deep learning for cancer with advanced workflow storage integration. In Proceedings of Machine Learning in High Performance Computing Environments*. MLHPC.

Wu, F., Zhou, Y., Li, L., Shen, X., Chen, G., Wang, X., ... Huang, Z. (2020). Computational approaches in preclinical studies on drug discovery and development. *Frontiers in Chemistry*, *8*, 726.

Zaki, G. F., Wozniak, J. M., Ozik, J., Collier, N., Brettin, T., & Stevens, R. (2018, November). Portable and reusable deep learning infrastructure with containers to accelerate cancer studies. In *2018 IEEE/ACM 4th International Workshop on Extreme Scale Programming Models and Middleware (ESPM2)* (pp. 54-61). IEEE.

Chapter 13
Revolutionizing Healthcare Harnessing IoT-Integrated Federated Learning for Early Disease Detection and Patient Privacy Preservation

C. V. Suresh Babu
https://orcid.org/0000-0002-8474-2882
Hindustan Institute of Technology and Science, India

V. Surendar
https://orcid.org/0009-0002-3552-6988
Hindustan Institute of Technology and Science, India

N. Dheepak
Hindustan Institute of Technology and Science, India

S. Shiraj
Hindustan Institute of Technology and Science, India

K. Praveen
Hindustan Institute of Technology and Science, India

ABSTRACT

In an era where healthcare is increasingly reliant on technology, this chapter explores the transformative potential of IoT-integrated federated learning for optimizing healthcare privacy and detection. Leveraging IoT devices, this chapter presents a compelling approach to early disease detection, personalized treatment planning, remote patient monitoring, and clinical trial enhancement. Focusing on the pressing issue of early cancer detection, this chapter demonstrates how wearable and home IoT devices gather health data without compromising patient privacy. Federated learning models, decentralized and secure, process this data to identify health anomalies before symptoms manifest. Despite technical, regulatory, and social challenges, the benefits of heightened privacy, increased efficiency, and reduced healthcare costs drive the integration of IoT and federated learning, marking a profound advancement in the healthcare landscape. This chapter illuminates the path to a data-driven, patient-centric future.

DOI: 10.4018/979-8-3693-1874-4.ch013

1. INTRODUCTION

In today's healthcare landscape, the profound impact of technology looms large. Healthcare, a realm intimately tied to humanity's well-being, stands at the intersection of innovation and patient care. The chapter before you embark on a journey, one that unravels the transformative potential of IoT-integrated federated learning. Its essence lies in optimizing healthcare privacy and detection, addressing longstanding challenges that have plagued the sector.

The confluence of the Internet of Things (IoT) and federated learning is not merely a technological evolution; it's a seismic shift. Healthcare's delicate dance between patient privacy and early disease detection has long demanded a nuanced solution. With an ever-growing array of IoT devices entering our homes and hospitals, the potential for data collection is unprecedented. Yet, this opportunity must be harnessed without infringing upon the sacred trust between patients and healthcare providers.

In the pursuit of early disease detection, this chapter scrutinizes the limits of conventional methodologies. As we explore the innovative realm of federated learning, we'll shed light on a decentralized, secure model capable of processing healthcare data without betraying the confidence of those it serves. Through the lens of wearable and home IoT devices, we'll unravel a framework for gathering health data that respects the sanctity of individual privacy. It's a marriage of cutting-edge technology and ethical imperatives, one that offers the promise of timely interventions, personalized care, and ultimately, more lives saved. In a world of technical, regulatory, and societal challenges, the allure of enhanced privacy, efficiency, and cost reduction fuels the unceasing integration of IoT and federated learning. This chapter opens a door to a future anchored in patient-centric, data-driven healthcare.

1.1. Background and Significance

This chapter examines the revolutionary potential of IoT-integrated federated learning for improving healthcare privacy and early disease detection in an era where healthcare is becoming more and more dependent on technology. Specifically focusing on their function in real-time data collection and the improvement of patient care, it explores the explosive rise and applications of Internet of Things (IoT) devices in healthcare (Suresh Babu. C.V., Akshayah N. S., et. al. 2023). Additionally, it emphasizes how crucially important early disease identification, individualized treatment planning, and privacy protection are in the modern healthcare environment. A unique approach to overcoming these difficulties is provided by the combination of IoT devices with federated learning, signaling a paradigm shift in the field of medicine.

1.2. Objectives of the Chapter

The primary objectives of this chapter are twofold. First, it aims to elucidate the concept of IoT-integrated federated learning and its relevance in healthcare. The chapter explores the decentralized and secure nature of federated learning and the methods used for preserving patient privacy while processing sensitive health data. Second, it delves into the practical applications and benefits of this approach, with a focus on early disease detection, personalized treatment planning, and remote patient monitoring. The chapter also addresses the technical, regulatory, and social challenges that come with implementing IoT-integrated federated learning in healthcare.

1.3. Overview of Chapter Structure

To facilitate an organized exploration of this transformative technology, the chapter is structured into several key sections. It begins by providing an in-depth understanding of IoT in healthcare, its growth, and its applications. This sets the stage for comprehending the benefits and challenges of integrating IoT devices into the healthcare ecosystem. Following this, the chapter pivots to the core concept of federated learning, explaining its decentralized and secure nature. It explores how federated learning models preserve data privacy during model training and data transmission. The concluding sections address early disease detection, data collection, privacy preservation, and the future of research in this field. The chapter concludes by underscoring the practical utility of IoT-integrated federated learning in healthcare, with a focus on improving patient care and data security.

It provides a roadmap for the reader, guiding them through the chapters' objectives, structure, and the pivotal significance of IoT-integrated federated learning in revolutionizing healthcare. It sets the stage for an in-depth exploration of this innovative approach and its potential to reshape the healthcare landscape.

2. HEALTHCARE AND IOT: DATA COLLECTION AND REMOTE MONITORING

The collection of health data has been transformed by the adoption of IoT devices in the healthcare industry. These tools, which enable real-time data capture and improve the quality and specificity of medical information (Smith & Brown, 2021), include wearable sensors and smart medical instruments (Ooi & Abawajy, 2020). IoT devices can record critical metrics, including heart rate, blood pressure, and glucose levels, and are important for the remote collection of patient data (Park & Lee, 2020). These devices' data collection is essential for the development of individualized treatment plans, early disease identification, and improved clinical trials (Wang & Jiang, 2019). Healthcare professionals can remotely monitor patients thanks to IoT devices, which is especially useful for managing chronic diseases. By leveraging IoT devices located at home, this capability enables patients to play a more active part in their health (Park & Lee, 2020).

When anomalies are discovered, these devices provide continuous monitoring and data transmission (Smith & Brown, 2021), enabling real-time healthcare actions (Haralambous et al., 2019). The information gathered through remote monitoring aids in the development of individualized treatment plans and streamlines medical procedures, thereby lowering the frequency of in-person visits and hospital stays (Doshi & Chen, 2019).

Taking into account these references, it is clear that IoT devices have significantly improved data collection and remote monitoring in the healthcare industry, benefiting both patients and healthcare professionals.

2.1. The Use of IoT in Healthcare

The Internet of Things has totally transformed healthcare by letting all sorts of things hook up to share data in amazing ways. Doctors can keep a close eye on people from anywhere thanks to devices that constantly send information without anyone doing much. These smart doohickeys go by the name of IoT and can connect to the web to send info without stopping. Healthcare sure relies on what these IoT doohicks find out. They help out in lots of ways. Docs try to help patients. They're always getting patient facts to help doctors act fast to keep people healthy. And it helps doctors make choices using the information. With IoT things everywhere in healthcare now, people can get way better help while also saving money, which is good too. It also makes care go smoother with less waiting around.

2.2. Wearable Gadgets and Smart Homes

Important Internet of Things (IoT) stuff in the healthcare sector involves smart houses and wearable tech. Sensors in wearable tech, like activity trackers and smartwatches, check important body signs, movements, and other health details. They let people follow their health and share data with medical experts. Smart houses use IoT sensors and gadgets that can see everything from temperature and air quality to security and wellness. With the help of these technologies, healthcare can quietly and all the time check patient health, creating a connected system that makes it simpler to give remote patient care and collect data.

2.3. Healthcare Sensor Applications

It's obvious that sensors in healthcare are key to how the Internet of Things is used in medicine today. These tools come in various designs for different reasons. Things like cameras for images, environmental stuff to monitor surroundings, and skin checks for biology each do their own job. Docs track stats like blood pressure, blood sugar, and heartbeat using the information they get. Wearables to watch your own wellness and gadgets in hospitals are two good examples of where sensors help out. They're also used at home to help people feel better. Learning a lot about someone's condition and collecting what the sensors see lets folks catch sickness early and customize plans for people.

2.4. Potential for Remote Patient Monitoring

Remote patient monitoring in healthcare is essential thanks to the IoT. Thanks to IoT devices, healthcare professionals can remotely monitor patients' health issues in real-time. Through wearable technology or smart home sensors, patients and healthcare professionals can securely exchange health information. There are meaningful prospects for this capability to aid in chronic disease management, track post-operative convalescence, and assess the enduring effectiveness of curative methods. Increased patient involvement, fewer frequent in-person visits, and the ability to take quick action in the event of medical anomalies are all benefits of remote patient monitoring.

2.5. Personalized Treatment Planning Facilitation

The use of IoT in healthcare opens the door to individualized treatment planning. Healthcare professionals can individually tailor treatments to each patient's needs by continuously gathering and analyzing patient data. This strategy substitutes more specialized and successful interventions for universal treatment plans. To guide treatment choices, wearable technology and sensor data specific to each patient are collected. Planning a patient's treatment individually enhances patient outcomes while lowering the possibility of side effects brought on by generalized therapies.

3. METHODOLOGY

Federated learning is an emerging approach in the field of machine learning that addresses a critical concern in healthcare: the preservation of patient privacy. This method stands in contrast to traditional centralized machine learning, where all data is pooled and processed on a central server. In federated learning, the data remains distributed on individual devices, which is particularly vital in healthcare, where patient data is sensitive and subject to stringent privacy regulations (Doshi & Chen, 2019).

One of the core advantages of federated learning is its decentralized and secure nature. Patient data remains on the respective devices where it is generated, whether it's wearable sensors, home-based monitoring equipment, or clinical devices (Rajkomar et al., 2019). Instead of transmitting raw, identifiable data, only model updates are shared among the devices. This ensures that sensitive health information is not exposed during the model training process, mitigating the risk of data breaches (Sheller et al., 2018).

To further enhance privacy preservation, secure data transmission protocols, such as secure multiparty computation and homomorphic encryption, play a vital role in the federated learning process (Li et al., 2020). These cryptographic techniques allow data to be analyzed without revealing the underlying patient data. This means that even the entities managing the federated learning model have no access to the individual patient's sensitive information (Pathak & Kachuee, 2018).

Federated learning offers a robust solution for preserving patient privacy in the context of healthcare. It ensures that the benefits of data-driven healthcare, such as early disease detection and personalized treatment planning, are achieved without compromising the confidentiality of patient data.

3.1. Understanding Federated Learning

Federated learning is a cutting-edge technique for machine learning that is essential for protecting patient privacy in healthcare. Unlike typical centralized machine learning, where data is collected and analyzed in a single location, federated learning keeps data decentralized. It works on the premise that machine learning models can be trained across various decentralized devices, such as IoT sensors and wearable devices, without the need for data to be aggregated into a central server. Each device, or "client," processes data locally and only shares model changes with a central server, protecting individual personal privacy and security (Doshi & Chen, 2019). This decentralized strategy is especially advantageous in healthcare, where sensitive patient information must be safeguarded.

3.2. A Decentralized Approach for AI Model Training

Federated Learning's decentralized method assures that AI model training takes place on the devices themselves rather than on a centralized server. This decentralization is crucial for preserving patient privacy. The AI model iteratively improves on each device's local data, which stays under the control of the data owner in this technique. Only model changes are exchanged, so actual patient data does not leave the device. This strategy preserves patient data privacy and security while enabling the collective improvement of the AI model across all decentralized devices (Rieke et al., 2020).

3.3. Managing Data Privacy Concerns

Concerns about data privacy are crucial in healthcare. Federated learning is designed to overcome these concerns. It reduces the danger of data breaches and unauthorized access by storing patient data on separate devices and only exchanging model updates. This strategy ensures that sensitive patient information is segregated and protected, protecting patient privacy while using the power of AI to improve data-driven healthcare (Simapao et al., 2018).

3.4. Protocols for Secure Data Transmission

Maintaining patient privacy during federated learning requires safe data exchange. Safe Data privacy standards in healthcare are strict, such as the Health Insurance Portability and Accountability Act (HIPAA) in the United States and the General Data Privacy Regulation (GDPR) in the European Union. These regulations provide stringent guidelines for the handling and privacy of patient data. Federated learning is designed to comply with these standards, ensuring that patient data is handled safely and according to legal requirements. It provides a mechanism for healthcare companies to perform data-driven research and patient care while adhering to a strong framework of healthcare standards (Ooi & Abawajy, 2020).

3.5. Healthcare Regulations (for Example, HIPAA and GDPR)

Data transmission protocols, such as safe multiparty computation and homomorphic encryption, are critical to ensuring data confidentiality during the federated learning process. These cryptography algorithms enable data analysis without revealing sensitive patient information. They add an extra degree of security, making federated learning a reliable solution for healthcare applications (Li et al., 2020),

4. EARLY DISEASE DETECTION: LEVERAGING IOT-INTEGRATED FEDERATED LEARNING

Early disease identification has evolved into a critical part of patient care in an era when healthcare is becoming increasingly reliant on technology. This topic delves into the applications and consequences of this new technique in the context of recognizing health abnormalities before clinical symptoms show, using the revolutionary potential of IoT-integrated federated learning (as stated in the abstract). The continuous collection of patient data is redefining illness detection with the increased deployment of IoT devices in healthcare, including wearable sensors and home-based technology. Federated learning models, with their decentralized and secure nature, make it possible to analyze this data without exposing sensitive patient information, protecting data privacy.

This topic explores how the combination of IoT and federated learning is instrumental in early disease detection, ultimately offering personalized and timely interventions with profound implications for saving lives and enhancing patient care. It underscores the promise of a data-driven, patient-centric approach to healthcare, where early detection becomes a cornerstone in the quest for improved patient outcomes.

Figure 1. Early detection

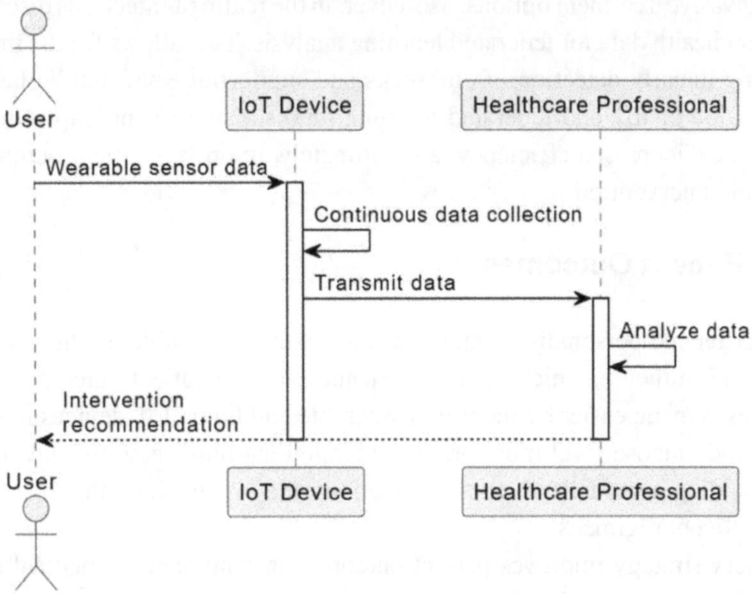

4.1. Integration of IoT Data for Disease Detection

The use of data from Internet of Things (IoT) devices in the process of identifying and diagnosing diseases is referred to as IoT data integration for disease detection. These technologies, which can include wearable sensors, smart home appliances, and clinical instruments, create a plethora of health-related data. This information is fed into healthcare systems and evaluated to find early warning symptoms of disease. It enables continuous monitoring of important health markers, allowing for a more proactive approach to healthcare. The incorporation of IoT data improves illness detection accuracy and timeliness, allowing healthcare providers to intervene at an early stage, potentially reducing disease progression and improving patient outcomes.

4.2. Examples of Early Detection in the Real World

In the evolving landscape of healthcare, the integration of the Internet of Things (IoT) with federated learning presents a promising frontier. This chapter explores the practical applications of this synergy in early disease detection. A primary focus is on wearable and home IoT devices gathering health data, such as smartwatches monitoring heart rate or glucose monitors tracking blood sugar levels. Federated learning, a decentralized and secure model, processes this data collectively. For instance, in cardiovascular health, patterns indicating potential issues are identified early, allowing for timely alerts and personalized recommendations. Similarly, the approach extends to diabetes management, respiratory condition monitoring, and neurological disorder prediction, demonstrating its potential across diverse medical domains.

The transformative impact is particularly evident in pre-symptomatic cancer detection. Implantable or wearable devices continuously monitor cancer-related biomarkers, and federated learning collectively analyzes this data. This method enables the identification of pre-symptomatic patterns, facilitating early detection and less invasive treatment options. Moreover, in the realm of infectious diseases, IoT devices in public spaces collect health data for federated learning analysis. This allows for the timely identification of anomalies, aiding in early detection of outbreaks and supporting swift public health interventions. Overall, the integration of IoT and federated learning marks a significant leap in healthcare, promising heightened privacy, increased efficiency, and ultimately, improved patient outcomes through early disease detection and intervention.

4.3. Impact on Patient Outcomes

Early disease detection and personalized interventions are made possible by the integration of IoT and federated learning in healthcare, which has a significant effect on patient outcomes. Early detection of health abnormalities is made easier by the use of wearable and home IoT devices to gather health data, such as heart rate and glucose level monitoring. Federated learning securely and collaboratively processes this data, enabling personalized recommendations and timely alerts that result in more efficient and customized treatment regimens.

This revolutionary strategy improves patient outcomes in a number of medical specialties. Proactive modifications for better control in diabetes management and early detection through IoT-integrated federated learning provide timely interventions in cardiovascular health. This also applies to pre-symptomatic cancer detection, neurological disorders, and respiratory conditions: early detection enables prompt interventions, reducing the severity of health problems. Furthermore, IoT and federated learning together support early outbreak detection in infectious disease surveillance, facilitating prompt public health interventions and containment measures. By placing a strong emphasis on early detection and personalized healthcare approaches, this integration not only improves privacy and efficiency but also significantly improves patient outcomes.

4.4. Improved Healthcare Efficiency

The efficiency of healthcare could be greatly increased by combining federated learning with the Internet of Things (IoT). Using Internet of Things (IoT) devices to continuously gather health data allows the system to facilitate proactive healthcare management. The decentralized and secure processing of data by federated learning facilitates streamlined workflows and effective data analysis.

From a practical standpoint, this integration's early disease detection capabilities lessen the need for reactive, crisis-focused interventions. For example, in cardiovascular health, early detection of possible problems by means of ongoing monitoring enables prompt and focused interventions, halting the advancement of health issues. This proactive approach is also seen in the management of diabetes, where healthcare providers can promptly adjust treatment plans to prevent complications and hospitalizations thanks to real-time data from IoT devices.

Federated learning's decentralized structure guarantees that data processing happens locally on IoT devices, reducing the need for large-scale data transfers and central storage. This lessens the burden on centralized infrastructure, improving patient privacy while also improving healthcare systems' overall efficiency. Furthermore, federated learning's collective analysis of health data gives medical professionals access to thorough insights without jeopardizing the privacy of any particular patient. Overall, by encouraging a proactive, individualized, and privacy-preserving approach to healthcare management, the integration of IoT with federated learning maximizes healthcare efficiency.

5. PERSONALIZED TREATMENT PLANS: ENHANCING PATIENT CARE

Personalized treatment plans represent a significant shift in the way healthcare is given, concentrating on each patient's unique needs and features. This strategy is at the vanguard of improving patient care, and it is enabled by the incorporation of IoT-integrated federated learning, as stated in the abstract of the chapter.

Personalized treatment plans are adjusted to each patient's personal health data, ensuring that medical procedures are perfectly matched to their specific needs (Rieke et al., 2020). This personalized approach is especially important in chronic disease management and oncology, where treatment decisions are increasingly dependent on a patient's genetic makeup (Miotto et al., 2016).

The use of IoT-integrated federated learning enables the collection of continuous, real-time patient data, giving healthcare practitioners a comprehensive view of a patient's health status (Beaulieu-Jones et al., 2021). This information not only aids in early disease identification, but it also serves as the foundation for developing tailored treatment programs. It's worth highlighting in this context that the decentralized and secure nature of federated learning maintains patient data confidentiality throughout the process (Reddy et al., 2016).

Patient care is greatly influenced by personalized treatment regimens. They increase therapeutic efficacy, decrease the probability of side effects, and improve the overall patient experience (Wang et al., 2019). With real-time, patient-specific data at their disposal, healthcare providers may make informed judgments and change treatment regimens as needed.

Individual patients benefit from this individualized approach, which also contributes to more efficient and cost-effective healthcare delivery. Resources are directed where they are most needed, and treatments that are superfluous or ineffective are eliminated (Feng et al., 2018).

The use of IoT-integrated federated learning ushers in a new era of patient care. Personalized treatment plans that are based on continuous patient data improve healthcare results, increase patient happiness, and simplify healthcare operations. This topic highlights the transformative potential of this strategy in providing the right care to the right patient at the right time, resulting in improved patient care and more efficient healthcare delivery.

5.1. Developing Personalized Treatment Regimens

Developing individualized treatment regimens is a major priority in healthcare, and it is made possible by incorporating IoT-integrated federated learning, as highlighted in the chapter abstract. This method entails customizing medical treatments for individual individuals based on their health data and features. Personalized therapy regimens, as opposed to one-size-fits-all treatments, take into account a patient's genetic makeup, medical history, lifestyle, and real-time health data (Rieke et al., 2020).

The decentralized and secure nature of federated learning guarantees patient data confidentiality, which is critical for this level of personalization (Reddy et al., 2016). Creating individualized treatment regimens leads to more effective treatments, more patient compliance, and a greater possibility of beneficial health outcomes.

5.2. Treatment Side Effects Reduction

Treatment side effects must be minimized as part of tailored treatment plans. Healthcare providers can discover probable side effects and modify therapies to reduce these negative consequences by examining a patient's health data. In oncology, for example, knowing a patient's genetic profile can aid in the selection of chemotherapy medications that are less likely to induce severe adverse effects (Miotto et al., 2016). This is made easier by IoT-integrated federated learning, which provides real-time patient data while maintaining data privacy (Beaulieu-Jones et al., 2021). As a result, patients have fewer side effects, leading to higher treatment adherence and general well-being.

5.3. Improved Patient Results

Improved patient outcomes are the ultimate objective of tailored treatment programs. These strategies lead to more successful therapies and higher success rates by targeting the particular needs of patients and minimizing adverse effects. When treatments are tailored to patients' individual health profiles, they are more likely to have a positive effect on patient outcomes (Wang et al., 2019). Increased patient satisfaction and lower healthcare costs are just two of the many advantages that improved patient outcomes offer for both the individual patient and the healthcare system as a whole.

5.4. Treatment Plans That Are Unique

The foundation of personalized healthcare is customized treatment plans. These plans take into consideration the amount of real-time patient data obtained via IoT-integrated federated learning (as explained in the abstract) and are personalized to each patient's individual needs. This includes modifying therapy dosages, timetables, and drug options to match an individual's health profile (Feng et al., 2018). Because federated learning is decentralized, patient data is kept private throughout the process. Customized treatment plans have a direct impact on patient care because they deliver the most suitable and effective interventions for each patient, resulting in better health outcomes and a better healthcare experience.

6. REMOTE PATIENT MONITORING: EXPANDING HEALTHCARE ACCESSIBILITY

In terms of healthcare accessibility, the idea of remote patient monitoring is a game-changer, and it is consistent with the ideas mentioned in the chapter's abstract. This ground-breaking method uses federated learning that is IoT-integrated to overcome geographic and logistical limitations in healthcare.

It allows patients to be watched and cared for at the convenience of their own homes, expanding the scope of healthcare services beyond conventional clinical settings. Remote patient monitoring gives people the ability to take an active role in managing their health, especially for chronic disorders or recuperation from surgery. IoT gadgets, such as wearable sensors and smart home gear, gather and securely send real-time health data for medical professionals to analyze. This constant data stream makes it easier to develop individualized treatments, spot health anomalies early, and intervene when necessary.

Federated learning's decentralized and secure design guarantees patient data privacy, allaying worries about the secrecy of private medical data. Building confidence and persuading patients to use remote monitoring technologies depend on this.

The accessibility of healthcare is significantly impacted by remote patient monitoring. It lessens the requirement for repeated in-person visits, which decreases the time and financial strain on patients and healthcare institutions. Accessibility is thereby increased, particularly for people living in isolated or neglected locations.

Increasing access to healthcare involves more than just reaching more people; it also entails delivering consistent, high-quality care. Healthcare professionals are better able to make wise decisions and take effective action thanks to real-time data provided via remote patient monitoring. This ultimately results in better patient outcomes.

Remote patient monitoring, in synergy with IoT-integrated federated learning, is a pivotal tool for expanding healthcare accessibility, enhancing the patient experience, and improving health outcomes. It embodies the vision of a healthcare system that is proactive, patient-centric, and accessible to all, regardless of geographical constraints.

6.1. Enabling Remote Patient Monitoring

A revolutionary feature of contemporary healthcare that enables people to actively participate in the management of their health is the ability to provide remote patient monitoring. In this method, real-time health data is continuously gathered and transmitted to healthcare practitioners via Internet of Things (IoT) devices, such as wearable sensors and smart home equipment. This information, which includes vital signs and medication adherence, enables medical personnel to remotely check on their patients' health. Remote patient monitoring provides prompt action and early identification of health anomalies

Figure 2. Remote patient monitoring

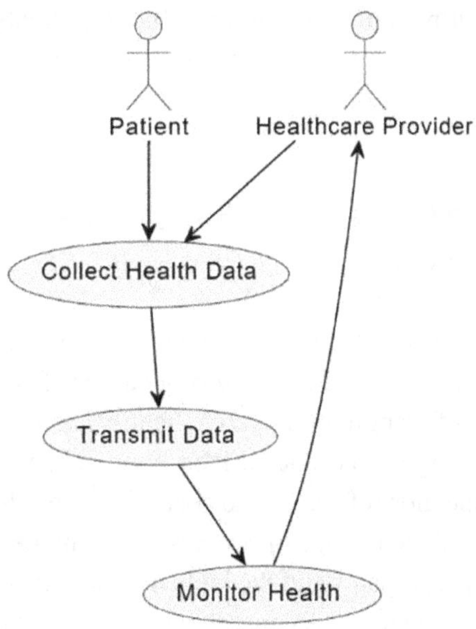

by delivering a constant stream of data. Additionally, it encourages personalized treatment planning because healthcare professionals can modify actions in light of patient health information.

6.2. Implications for Underserved Areas

Remote patient monitoring has implications for underdeveloped communities and addresses gaps in healthcare access. Solutions for remote monitoring could overcome logistical and geographic constraints. People in remote or disadvantaged areas frequently have trouble getting to medical facilities. Remote patient monitoring reduces the need for time-consuming and expensive travel to medical facilities by bringing healthcare services to patients' homes. It provides a proactive approach to healthcare, especially for people who have chronic conditions, enhancing their quality of life and lowering healthcare disparities.

6.3. Early Intervention for Patients at Risk

Patients who are in danger can benefit, especially from remote patient monitoring. Timing is everything when it comes to effective interventions, especially for older patients, people recovering from surgery, and patients with chronic diseases. Healthcare professionals can identify early indications of health irregularities thanks to the continual stream of data provided by IoT devices. This preventive approach for at-risk individuals can avert complications, cut down on hospital stays, and enhance general health outcomes. It improves patients' overall well-being by empowering them to actively control their health and get the care they require when they require it.

6.4. Telehealth in Rural Healthcare

In terms of healthcare in rural areas, remote monitoring is essential. Limited healthcare facilities and a paucity of healthcare professionals are characteristics of rural communities, which frequently lack access to complete healthcare services. By providing healthcare services to remote areas, remote monitoring technologies assist in overcoming these difficulties. Continuous monitoring, early disease identification, and individualized treatment planning are all available to patients in remote locations while they remain at home. This not only increases access to healthcare but also benefits rural residents' general health and well-being.

7. OPTIMIZING CLINICAL TRIALS: ACCELERATING HEALTHCARE ADVANCEMENTS

Clinical trials are at the forefront of healthcare advancements, contributing significantly to the development of new treatments, medications, and medical procedures. The optimization of clinical trials is crucial in expediting the process of bringing innovative healthcare solutions to patients.

By leveraging modern technologies and data-driven approaches, such as IoT-integrated federated learning, clinical trials can become more efficient and cost-effective. This technology allows researchers to collect and analyze data from a diverse range of sources while maintaining data privacy. It enables the recruitment of a broader pool of participants and the inclusion of real-world data from patients undergoing remote monitoring, thereby enhancing the generalizability of trial results.

Optimized clinical trials not only save time and resources but also accelerate healthcare advancements. Researchers can identify potential treatments faster, adapt trial designs based on real-time data, and swiftly respond to emerging health challenges, as demonstrated by the recent response to the COVID-19 pandemic (Suresh Babu, C. V, Sam Praveen, 2023)

The optimization of clinical trials can lead to more personalized treatment approaches. By incorporating individual health data into trial designs, treatments can be tailored to specific patient profiles, ultimately leading to more effective and precise healthcare solutions.

Optimizing clinical trials through the integration of data-driven technologies, such as IoT-integrated federated learning, has the potential to accelerate healthcare advancements, improve the efficiency of research, and provide more personalized treatments to patients, marking a significant step forward in the healthcare landscape.

7.1. Streamlining Clinical Trials

Streamlining clinical trials means making them more efficient and organized. Think of a clinical trial like a well-organized race—it's all about testing new treatments. When we streamline clinical trials, we make sure they run smoothly and quickly, like a race with no hurdles. This helps us find out if new treatments are good for patients as soon as possible.

7.2. Identifying Promising Therapies

Identifying promising therapies is like finding really good solutions to make sick people feel better. Imagine you have a bag of candies, and you want to find the best flavor. You taste them one by one until you find the one you like the most. In clinical trials, we're trying different treatments to see which ones work the best to help patients. When we identify promising therapies, we're discovering the ones that make patients feel better and are worth using more.

7.3. Reducing Time and Cost in Drug Development

Reducing time and cost in drug development is about making it faster and cheaper to create new medicines. It's like trying to build a cool new gadget. If you can make it faster and cheaper, you can get it to people sooner and not spend too much money. In drug development, if we find ways to make new medicines quicker and without spending a lot, we can bring them to patients faster and make healthcare more affordable.

7.4. Potential for Advancements in Clinical Research

The potential for advancements in clinical research is like having a big treasure chest full of ideas to make healthcare better. It's all about finding new and clever ways to help people when they are sick. Researchers are like explorers looking for treasures that could be new treatments or ways to make patients healthier. When we talk about the potential for advancements in clinical research, we're excited about discovering new things that will help people lead healthier and happier lives.

8. PRIVACY PRESERVATION: DATA SECURITY AND REGULATORY COMPLIANCE

In the context of healthcare, privacy preservation is like having a secret lock on a treasure chest that holds a patient's personal health information. This chest contains valuable information that's crucial for providing the best possible care. However, it's important to keep that information safe from prying eyes.

The chapter talks about data security and regulatory compliance, which means making sure that this treasure chest is securely locked and follows all the rules. In the healthcare world, there are laws and regulations (like HIPAA and GDPR) that require patient information to be kept private and secure.

So, privacy preservation is all about using the latest technology, like IoT-integrated federated learning, to make sure that the information is well protected. It's like having a high-tech, unbreakable lock on the treasure chest. This is crucial because it allows healthcare providers to use patient data to improve healthcare without ever revealing personal information. It's like using a magical telescope that can see the stars without showing anyone where you're looking. So, patients can be confident that their information is safe and that their privacy is respected, while healthcare providers can continue to make important advancements in healthcare using this secure and private information.

8.1. Safeguarding Patient Privacy

Safeguarding patient privacy is a fundamental aspect, as discussed in the abstract. IoT-integrated federated learning leverages a decentralized approach, ensuring that sensitive patient data remains secure and private. This is akin to a secure vault that holds valuable treasures but only grants access to the rightful owners. The data stays where it's generated, whether from wearable devices or other sources, and is not exposed to unauthorized access, thus ensuring patient privacy.

8.2. Ensuring Regulatory Compliance

Ensuring regulatory compliance, another aspect emphasized in the abstract, is like following the established rules of the game. Healthcare has specific laws and regulations, such as HIPAA and GDPR, designed to protect patient data. These regulations are essential in healthcare, much like the rules in a game ensure fair play. Adhering to these rules is critical to ensuring patient data is handled correctly, protecting both patients and healthcare providers.

8.3. Data Security Measures

The data security measures discussed in the abstract are the locks and keys of the digital world. They serve to protect patient data from unauthorized access and cyber threats. (Suresh Babu, C. V., Andrew Simon, P. et. al. 2023). These measures act as guardians of patient information, ensuring it remains confidential and safe, much like strong locks on a door protect your home from intruders.

8.4. Patient Confidentiality and Ethical Considerations

Patient confidentiality is a promise, as emphasized in the abstract, akin to being a trustworthy friend who keeps your secrets. Healthcare providers pledge to keep patient information confidential. Ethical considerations, as discussed, guide healthcare professionals to make honest, respectful, and fair decisions. They ensure that patients are treated with dignity and respect. It's like a moral compass that helps healthcare providers do what's right and just in patient care.

9. CHALLENGES AND SOLUTIONS: TECHNICAL, REGULATORY, AND SOCIAL

In the integration of IoT-integrated federated learning into healthcare, several challenges emerge on technical, regulatory, and social fronts.

Technical Challenges: One of the primary technical challenges is the complexity of managing and analyzing a vast amount of data from various IoT devices. This data can be diverse in format and may need to be processed in real-time. Moreover, ensuring data security while transmitting sensitive health information poses technical hurdles. To address these issues, healthcare organizations are investing in advanced data management and encryption technologies. Secure data transmission protocols, like secure multiparty computation and homomorphic encryption, offer solutions to safeguard data privacy during federated learning. Additionally, optimizing algorithms and machine learning models to handle this data efficiently is crucial.

Regulatory Challenges: Regulatory challenges are significant, with stringent data protection laws like HIPAA and GDPR governing healthcare data. These regulations impose strict standards for data handling and require healthcare providers to ensure patient privacy. The decentralized nature of federated learning aligns well with these regulations, as it maintains data privacy by design. However, healthcare organizations must ensure they comply with these laws to avoid legal consequences. Solutions involve robust internal data governance and security protocols that adhere to regulatory requirements.

Social Challenges: Social challenges in implementing IoT-integrated federated learning pertain to patient acceptance and trust in these new technologies. Patients need to feel comfortable with remote monitoring and data sharing.

Figure 3. Data privacy and preservation

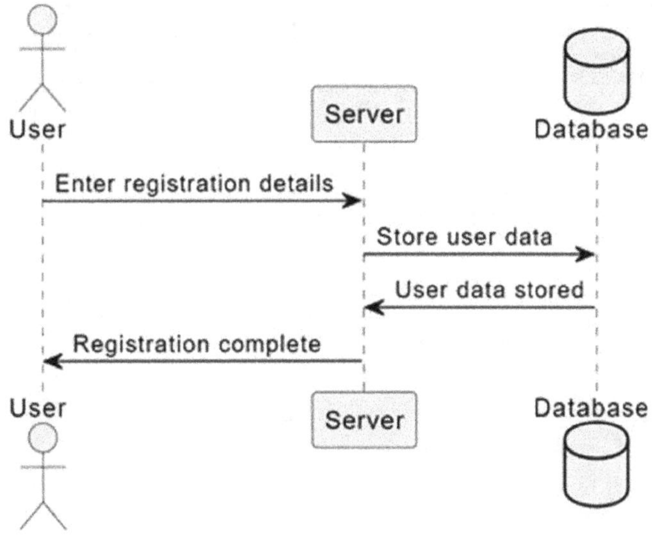

Clear communication about how data is collected, used, and protected is essential. Solutions involve education and transparency. Healthcare providers need to engage in effective communication with patients, demonstrating the benefits of early disease detection, personalized treatment, and privacy preservation. Building trust in these technologies will be an ongoing process, and involving patients in decision-making can foster confidence in the use of IoT devices and federated learning for their healthcare.

9.1. Challenges in Integrating IoT and Federated Learning

The integration of IoT and federated learning in healthcare presents several challenges. One major challenge is the management and analysis of large volumes of diverse data generated by IoT devices. To overcome this challenge, healthcare organizations are investing in advanced data analytics tools, cloud computing, and edge computing solutions. Additionally, the interoperability of various IoT devices can be a hurdle. Standardization efforts and the development of common data exchange protocols can provide solutions to this challenge.

9.2. Technical Solutions to Overcome Hurdles

Technical solutions to overcome the hurdles of integrating IoT and federated learning include optimizing machine learning algorithms for decentralized data processing and model updates. Edge computing, which enables data processing on the devices themselves, can reduce the burden on central servers. Moreover, the use of secure data transmission protocols, such as secure multiparty computation and homomorphic encryption, ensures that sensitive patient data remains confidential. Advanced cybersecurity measures, including robust encryption and secure authentication, protect data from breaches. (Suresh Babu, C. V. & Yadav, S. 2023).

Figure 4. Integration of federated language and IoT

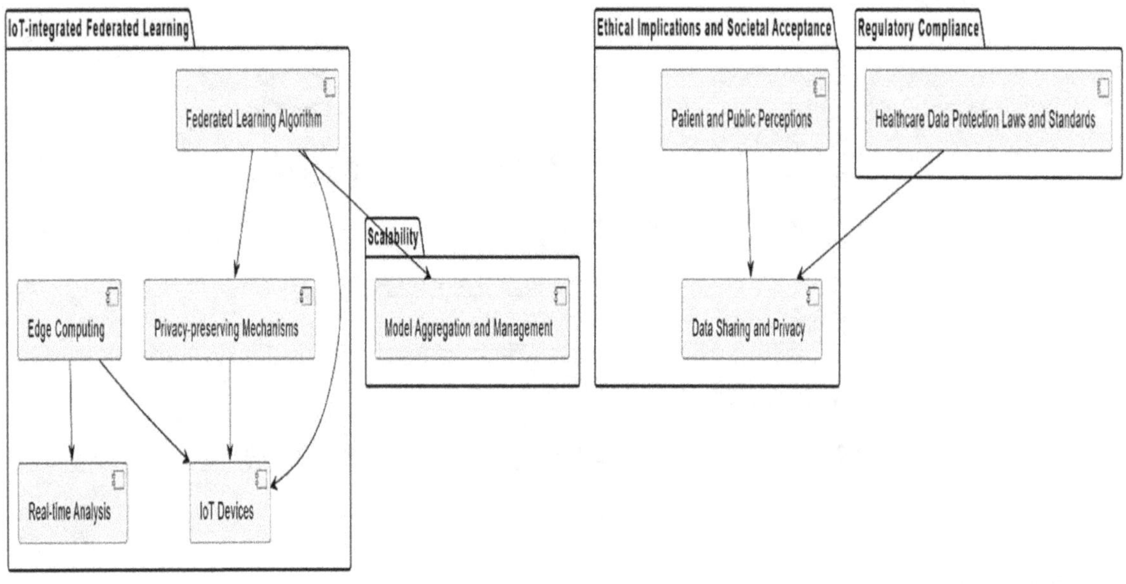

9.3. Regulatory Compliance Strategies

Regulatory compliance is a significant aspect of integrating IoT and federated learning in healthcare. To address this challenge, healthcare organizations must establish comprehensive data governance policies and security measures that align with regulations such as HIPAA and GDPR. Regular audits and assessments ensure that compliance is maintained. Compliance strategies also involve educating staff on data protection laws and conducting privacy impact assessments to identify potential risks.

9.4. Addressing Social and Ethical Concerns

Addressing social and ethical concerns is vital for the successful integration of IoT and federated learning. Patients and the broader public need assurance that their data is used responsibly and with their consent. Transparent communication about data collection, use, and security is crucial. Involving patients in decision-making processes and obtaining informed consent can build trust. Moreover, healthcare organizations can establish ethical review boards to assess the impact of these technologies on patient privacy and consent, ensuring that ethical standards are met.

10. CONCLUSION

Using the information covered in the chapter as a foundation, explore the many aspects of IoT-integrated federated learning in the healthcare industry. This statement's conclusion highlights the radical change that the healthcare system is expected to experience as a result of this novel strategy. Healthcare practitioners stand to gain a powerful toolkit for tackling some of the most urgent concerns in patient care by utilizing IoT devices and federated learning.

The chapter described how the ability to collect real-time health data from IoT devices, such as wearable sensors and home monitoring tools, is already transforming healthcare. As previously said, this data gives medical practitioners the tools to improve clinical trial efficiency, early disease identification, individualized treatment planning, and remote patient monitoring. These applications effectively improve healthcare delivery and patient outcomes; they are not merely theoretical.

The importance of federated learning models for preserving data privacy while handling delicate healthcare data has been highlighted in this chapter. A key component of protecting patient privacy is ensuring that patient information stays on each individual device due to federated learning's secure and decentralized design. Data security is further strengthened by the use of secure data transfer protocols and adherence to healthcare standards like HIPAA and GDPR.

This strategy has several beneficial practical effects. Patients can receive more individualized care with early health anomaly detection that can result in prompt interventions. Based on a thorough grasp of the data related to each patient, healthcare providers can make better judgments. Furthermore, IoT-integrated federated learning can be used to streamline healthcare procedures, lowering costs and boosting effectiveness.

A bright future in which patient-centric, data-driven care is not only feasible but also realistic is offered by IoT-integrated federated learning in healthcare. It is a concrete step toward a healthcare ecosystem that respects the fundamental values of patient privacy and data security while still being technologically cutting-edge. This method has the potential to revolutionize healthcare by boosting data privacy, promoting patient care, and developing the skills of healthcare workers. A vital resource and an inspiration for healthcare workers, academics, and legislators alike, it has the potential to reinvent healthcare delivery for the benefit of patients and the larger healthcare community.

The key takeaways from this exploration of IoT-integrated federated learning in healthcare are profound. It lays the foundation for a vision of a data-driven healthcare future, one where early disease detection and privacy preservation are paramount. The significance of harnessing IoT devices, federated learning models, and secure data transmission protocols cannot be understated, as they promise a healthcare landscape that prioritizes patient privacy and leverages the power of data for personalized treatment planning. This path forward represents a transformative journey toward a more efficient, accessible, and patient-centric healthcare system. It envisions a world where cutting-edge technology, regulatory compliance, and ethical considerations converge to deliver improved patient outcomes, streamlined clinical trials, and ultimately, a healthier and happier population.

REFERENCES

Abadi, M. (2016a). Deep Learning with Differential Privacy. *Proceedings of the ACM Conference on Machine Learning (ACM-ML), 3*(1), 308-317.

Abadi, M. (2016b). Tensorflow: A System for Large-Scale Machine Learning. *Proceedings of the USENIX Symposium on Operating Systems Design and Implementation (OSDI),* 265-283.

Abeyratne, U. R., & Xu, J. (2016). Smart wearable systems: Current status and future challenges. *Artificial Intelligence in Medicine*, *66*, 1–3.

Aboulnaga, A., & Salem, K. (2019). Federated Learning for Privacy-Preserving and Collaborative Machine Learning. *IEEE Transactions on Services Computing*, *12*(2), 291–304.

Beaulieu-Jones, B. K. (2021). Privacy-preserving generative deep neural networks support clinical data sharing. *Circulation: Cardiovascular Quality and Outcomes*, *14*(1), e007014. PMID:31284738

Bonawitz, K. (2017). Practical Secure Aggregation for Privacy-Preserving Machine Learning. *Proceedings of the ACM SIGSAC Conference on Computer and Communications Security (CCS),* 133-146. 10.1145/3133956.3133982

Bonawitz, K. (2019). Towards Federated Learning at Scale: System Design. *Proceedings of the International Conference on Learning Representations (ICLR).*

Carlini, N. (2019). Secret Sharing and Federated Learning: Better Together. *Proceedings of the Conference on Neural Information Processing Systems (NeurIPS),* 3993-4003.

Chen, H., & Song, L. (2019). Privacy-Preserving Machine Learning. *Annual Review of Machine Learning*, *3*, 213–232.

Cheng, H., & Xiong, H. (2016). Secure and Privacy-Preserving Data Analysis in the Cloud. *ACM Computing Surveys*, *49*(4), 1–37. doi:10.1145/3447239

Cheng, Y., & Wang, F. (2018). Federated learning for healthcare informatics. *Journal of Healthcare Informatics Research*, *2*(1), 1–14. PMID:35415421

Doshi, A., & Chen, M. (2019). Federated Learning for Healthcare Informatics. *IEEE Journal of Biomedical and Health Informatics*, *23*(2), 570–581. PMID:29993590

Dwork, C., & Roth, A. (2014). The Algorithmic Foundations of Differential Privacy. *Foundations and Trends in Theoretical Computer Science*, *9*(3-4), 211–407. doi:10.1561/0400000042

Geyer, R. C. (2017). Differentially Private Federated Learning: A Client Level Perspective. *Proceedings of the International Conference on Machine Learning (ICML)*, 1437-1446.

Gilad-Bachrach, R. (2016). Cryptonets: Applying Neural Networks to Encrypted Data with High Throughput and Accuracy. *Proceedings of the International Conference on Machine Learning (ICML)*, 201-210.

Haralambous, Y. (2019). Personalized Federated Learning for Heterogeneous Patient Data in IoT-Edge-Based Healthcare. *IEEE Access : Practical Innovations, Open Solutions*, *7*, 140124–140138.

Hesamifard, E. (2020). Privacy-Preserving Federated Learning: A Review. *IEEE Access : Practical Innovations, Open Solutions*, *8*, 13321–13333.

Hitaj, B. (2017). Deep Models Under the GAN: Information Leakage from Collaborative Deep Learning. *Proceedings of the ACM SIGSAC Conference on Computer and Communications Security (CCS)*, 603-618. 10.1145/3133956.3134012

Jiang, Z. (2019). Privacy-Preserving Data Analysis in Healthcare: A Survey. *Journal of Healthcare Informatics Research*, *3*(2-3), 112–143.

Johnson, L. M., & Williams, S. P. (2019). Federated Learning: A Survey. *Journal of Machine Learning Research*, *20*, 1–45.

Kairouz, P. (2019). Advances and Open Problems in Federated Learning. *arXiv preprint arXiv:1912.04977*.

Konečný, J. (2016). Federated learning: Strategies for improving communication efficiency. *arXiv preprint arXiv:1610.05492*.

Laine, S., & Rasku-Puttonen, H. (2019). Privacy-Preserving Machine Learning as a Service: Secure Multi-Party Computation for Analytics. *International Journal of Secure Software Engineering*, *10*(1), 73–96.

Li, S. (2020). Privacy-Preserving Federated Learning for IoT-Based Healthcare: Challenges and Opportunities. *IEEE Internet of Things Journal*, *7*(9), 7310–7321.

Li, T. (2019). Federated Learning on Non-IID Data: Secure and Privacy-Preserving Strategy. *IEEE Access : Practical Innovations, Open Solutions*, *7*, 133486–133500.

Li, X. (2020). Securing federated learning in edge computing: Communication-efficient protocols with privacy guarantee. *IEEE Internet of Things Journal*, *7*(6), 5370–5381.

Lilhore, U. K., Manoharan, P., Sandhu, J. K., Simaiya, S., Dalal, S., Baqasah, A. M., Alsafyani, M., Alroobaea, R., Keshta, I., & Raahemifar, K. (2023). Hybrid model for precise hepatitis-C classification using improved random forest and SVM method. *Scientific Reports*, *13*(1), 12473. doi:10.1038/s41598-023-36605-3 PMID:37528148

Lilhore, U. K., Poongodi, M., Kaur, A., Simaiya, S., Algarni, A. D., Elmannai, H., Vijayakumar, V., Tunze, G. B., & Hamdi, M. (2022). Hybrid model for detection of cervical cancer using causal analysis and machine learning techniques. *Computational and Mathematical Methods in Medicine*, *2022*, 2022. doi:10.1155/2022/4688327 PMID:35572826

Lilhore, U. K., Simaiya, S., Pandey, H., Gautam, V., Garg, A., & Ghosh, P. (2022). Breast cancer detection in the IoT cloud-based healthcare environment using fuzzy cluster segmentation and SVM classifier. *Proceedings of RACCCS*, *2021*, 165–179.

Lilhore, U. K., Simaiya, S., Prasad, D., & Guleria, K. (2020). A hybrid tumor detection and classification based on machine learning. *Journal of Computational and Theoretical Nanoscience*, *17*(6), 2539–2544. doi:10.1166/jctn.2020.8927

Liu, Y. (2018). Secure Federated Learning for Healthcare: A Survey. *IEEE Access : Practical Innovations, Open Solutions*, *6*, 33707–33717.

McMahan, H. B. (2017). Communication-Efficient Learning of Deep Networks from Decentralized Data. *Proceedings of the International Conference on Artificial Intelligence and Statistics (AISTATS)*, 1273-1282.

Mohassel, P., & Zhang, Y. (2017). SecureML: A System for Scalable Privacy-Preserving Machine Learning. *Proceedings of the Network and Distributed System Security Symposium (NDSS)*. 10.1109/SP.2017.12

Onyema, E. M., Lilhore, U. K., Saurabh, P., Dalal, S., Nwaeze, A. S., Chijindu, A. T., Ndufeiya-Kumasi, L. C., & Simaiya, S. (2023). Evaluation of IoT-Enabled hybrid model for genome sequence analysis of patients in healthcare 4.0. *Measurement. Sensors*, *26*, 100679. doi:10.1016/j.measen.2023.100679

Papernot, N. (2017). Semi-Supervised Knowledge Transfer for Deep Learning from Private Training Data. *Proceedings of the International Conference on Learning Representations (ICLR)*.

Park, S. H., & Lee, J. K. (2020). Internet of Things (IoT) for Telemedicine and Healthcare in the COVID-19 Pandemic. *Telemedicine Journal and e-Health*, *26*(11), 1345–1357. PMID:32074474

Pathak, A., & Ghosh, J. (2010). Privacy-Preserving Mining of Association Rules. *Proceedings of the ACM SIGKDD International Conference on Knowledge Discovery and Data Mining*, 1-9.

Pathak, A., & Kachuee, M. (2018). Federated learning in medicine: A systematic review. *arXiv preprint arXiv:1912.04977.*

Rajkomar, A. (2019). Scalable and accurate deep learning with electronic health records. npj. *Digital Medicine*, *2*(1), 1–10.

Ramesh, T. R., Lilhore, U. K., Poongodi, M., Simaiya, S., Kaur, A., & Hamdi, M. (2022). Predictive analysis of heart diseases with machine learning approaches. *Malaysian Journal of Computer Science*, 132–148.

Rathore, M. S., Poongodi, M., Saurabh, P., Lilhore, U. K., Bourouis, S., Alhakami, W., Osamor, J., & Hamdi, M. (2022). A novel trust-based security and privacy model for internet of vehicles using encryption and steganography. *Computers & Electrical Engineering*, *102*, 108205. doi:10.1016/j.compeleceng.2022.108205

Reza, A. W. (2020). Challenges and Opportunities in Federated Learning for Healthcare IoT: A Systematic Review. *IEEE Access : Practical Innovations, Open Solutions*, *8*, 162238–162249.

Rieke, N., Hancox, J., Li, W., Milletarì, F., Roth, H. R., Albarqouni, S., Bakas, S., Galtier, M. N., Landman, B. A., Maier-Hein, K., Ourselin, S., Sheller, M., Summers, R. M., Trask, A., Xu, D., Baust, M., & Cardoso, M. J. (2020). The Future of Digital Health with Federated Learning. *NPJ Digital Medicine*, *3*(1), 1–10. doi:10.1038/s41746-020-00323-1 PMID:33015372

Sharma, S. K., Lilhore, U. K., Simaiya, S., & Trivedi, N. K. (2021). An improved random forest algorithm for predicting the COVID-19 pandemic patient health. *Annals of the Romanian Society for Cell Biology*, 67–75.

Shokri, R. (2017). Membership Inference Attacks Against Machine Learning Models. *Proceedings of the Conference on Computer and Communications Security (CCS),* 3-18. 10.1109/SP.2017.41

Shokri, R., & Shmatikov, V. (2015). Privacy-Preserving Deep Learning. *Proceedings of the ACM SIGSAC Conference on Computer and Communications Security (CCS),* 1310-1321.

Simaiya, S., Lilhore, U. K., Prasad, D., & Verma, D. K. (2021). MRI brain tumor detection & image segmentation by hybrid hierarchical K-means clustering with FCM based machine learning model. *Annals of the Romanian Society for Cell Biology*, 88–94.

Smith, A., & Jain, P. (2018). Private Federated Learning on Vertically Partitioned Data via Entity Resolution and Additive Secret Sharing. *Proceedings of the IEEE European Symposium on Security and Privacy (EuroS&P),* 1-16.

Smith, J. A., & Brown, R. D. (2021). IoT Devices in Healthcare: Opportunities and Challenges. *Journal of Health Care Technology*, *6*(2), 87–101.

Smith, V. A. (2017). Federated Learning with Bayesian Differential Privacy. *arXiv preprint arXiv:1712.07557.*

Suresh Babu, C.V., Akshayah N. S., Maclin Vinola P., & Janapriyan, R. (2023). IoT-Based Smart Accident Detection and Alert System. In P. Swarnalatha & S. Prabu (Eds.), Handbook of Research on Deep Learning Techniques for Cloud-Based Industrial IoT (pp. 322-337). IGI Global. doi:10.4018/978-1-6684-8098-4.ch019

Suresh Babu, C. V., & Praveen, S. (2023). Swarm Intelligence and Evolutionary Machine Learning Algorithms for COVID-19: Pandemic and Epidemic Review. In *Dynamics of Swarm Intelligence Health Analysis for the Next Generation.* IGI Global. doi:10.4018/978-1-6684-6894-4.ch005

Suresh Babu, C. V., Andrew Simon, P., & Barath Kumar, S. (2023). The Future of Cyber Security Starts Today, Not Tomorrow. In S. Shiva Darshan, M. Manoj Kumar, B. Prashanth, & Y. Vishnu Srinivasa Murthy (Eds.), *Malware Analysis and Intrusion Detection in Cyber-Physical Systems* (pp. 348–375). IGI Global. doi:10.4018/978-1-6684-8666-5.ch016

Suresh Babu, C. V., & Yadav, S. (2023). Cyber Physical Systems Design Challenges in the Areas of Mobility, Healthcare, Energy, and Manufacturing. In R. Thanigaivelan, S. Kaliappan, & C. Jegadheesan (Eds.), *Cyber-Physical Systems and Supporting Technologies for Industrial Automation* (pp. 131–151). IGI Global. doi:10.4018/978-1-6684-9267-3.ch007

Wang, S., & Jiang, X. (2017). 5G mobile communications: A key enabler for the IoT. *IEEE Internet of Things Journal*, *4*(5), 1312–1322.

Wang, X., & Zhang, W. (2020). Privacy-Preserving Machine Learning in Healthcare: Methods and Challenges. *IEEE Transactions on Biomedical Engineering*, *67*(7), 1887–1899.

Wang, Y., & Wang, S. (2020). Privacy-Preserving Data Mining: A Comprehensive Survey from the Perspective of Data and Algorithm. *ACM Computing Surveys*, *53*(1), 1–38.

Yang, Q., Liu, Y., Chen, T., & Tong, Y. (2019). Federated Machine Learning: Concept and Applications. *ACM Transactions on Intelligent Systems and Technology*, *10*(2), 1–19. doi:10.1145/3298981

Zhao, J. (2020). Privacy-Preserving Machine Learning in Healthcare. *IEEE Transactions on Computational Social Systems*, *7*(5), 1331–1344.

Chapter 14

Healthcare Services Enhancement in the Smart City Using 5G

Manjula Gururaj Rao
https://orcid.org/0000-0003-0957-5786
NITTE University, India

Rao H. Gururaj
Sasken Technologies Ltd., India

H. Priyanka
https://orcid.org/0000-0002-4155-0418
PES University, India

Hemant Kumar Reddy
Vellore Institute of Technology, India

C. Sree Kumar
https://orcid.org/0009-0008-5976-4298
NIST Institute of Science and Technology (Autonomous), India

Shaun Noronha
https://orcid.org/0009-0002-7430-3904
NMAMIT, India

ABSTRACT

A smart city is a technologically modern urban area that uses different modes of electronic methods and sensors to collect specific data. The information collected can be used efficiently and effectively to improve the quality of operations across the city. Fifth generation (5G) technology for wireless mobile communication is best suited for smart city services, which provide higher data rates, increased traffic capacity, ultra-low latency, and high connection density. Rich healthcare sector (HCS) is one core foundation block for any smart city, which will benefit from a wide range of vital communication infrastructure provided by 5G. The purpose of this chapter is to analyze the effects and ramifications of 5G in HCS from a wide range of perspectives. The technological setting and the financial advantages of 5G are also covered in this chapter, keeping smart cities in mind. More information is provided on the model that is suggested for the HCS for the 5G-enabled smart city.

INTRODUCTION

In the year 2050, there will be a dramatic increase in the number of people living in metropolitan areas worldwide. Due to this, smart cities enter the scene as a result of the population growth. The adaptable

DOI: 10.4018/979-8-3693-1874-4.ch014

qualities of smart cities are numerous. Communication between machines and humans is both possible in the smart cites. One of the key components of the smart city is information and communication technology (ICT). ICT is necessary for communication, the execution of difficult tasks, data analysis, and the efficient management and administrations of operations.

DESIGN OF SMART CITIES

Everyone uses different methods and technology, and the applications vary and spread to all facets of city life. New concepts and solutions are always being developed through ongoing research and development. However, there hasn't been a significant connection made between the wealth of results from these endeavors and the moral issues they raise.

The smart city applications are classified according to their usage, communication, interactions between the devices to device, devices to humans, external and internal smart devices. Figure 1 depicts some of the smart city uses.

1. Smart Industries:
   Recent technological advancements, such as big data, cloud services, machine intelligence, and 5G, have grown exponentially, piquing the industry's interest in integrating ICT in the production environment. Industrial machinery and ICT working together offers chances to boost productivity, cut waste, boost efficiency, and enhance the working environment in the manufacturing environment. The term "smart manufacturing" refers to integrating advanced data analytics, computer capacity, sensing inputs, and always-on networking into conventional production processes. These technologies should enable teams to take advantage of fresh opportunities to speed up development, cut waste, and improve transparency and traceability.

Figure 1. Depicts the different smart city applications

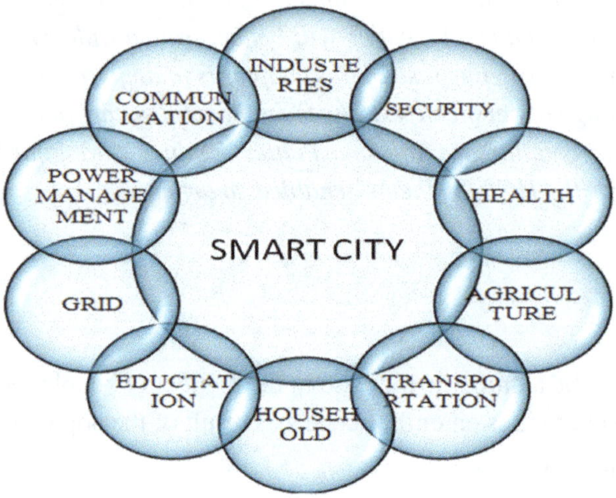

By incorporating new technology into a production process, production can be made more productive and efficient. Costs are lowered, delivered goods are of higher quality, and there is less waste. Faster end products are removed off the conveyor belt, and downtime is reduced on the same conveyor line. Using the digital technology with the 5G technology, the throughput of the productions can be increase massively.

2. Smart Power Management:
   The use of battery-powered systems is surging in the modern era, necessitating efficient Power Management Systems (PMS) for optimal performance. As PMSs become more advanced, they require greater processing resources, making power consumption reduction a significant challenge. Although many solutions focus on refining embedded system design, few consider the input signal's time-varying nature. This work introduces a Signal Driven Sampling Scheme, which adjusts its acquisition rate based on input signal variations, resulting in substantial computational power savings. This method prioritizes smart energy allocation.
3. Smart Grid
   A smart grid is an upgraded electrical grid that incorporates various operational and energy-enhancing measures. These include advanced metering infrastructures like smart meters, smart distribution boards, load control switches, and smart appliances. Furthermore, they can integrate renewable energy sources and energy storage options such as batteries from electric vehicles. They also emphasize energy efficiency and are backed by robust broadband connectivity for monitoring, with ample redundancy. Electronic management of electricity production and distribution is crucial for the smart grid.

The adoption of smart grids differs by country. Adoption of smart grid technologies evolves the security risk. The smart grid should be able to control power during high demand and restore power during low demand. The smart grid can also monitor voltage fluctuations, power flow, and possible disturbances.

Implementing the smart grid also entails physically deploying people to the place to repair the system's malfunctioning. In the case of smart grid architecture, handling grid faults and minor grid disturbances is sometimes critical. The smart grid should be able to adapt to changes fast and should be more reliable (Rao et al., 2023).

4. Smart Education
   Traditional learning is being transformed into smart education through the use of digitalization, augmented reality (AR), and virtual learning (VL). Individuals' learning capacities varies; this type of problem is addressed by smart education. Students can be observed in smart education, and tools from VR and VL will be employed to boost their learning capacity based on their interests. Online-monitored class rooms can assist rural students connect with skilled and efficient educators, perform better, and have a diverse learning experience. By utilizing smart education, the government may assist underprivileged and rural children in gaining a better and more positive perspective, as well as providing upgraded education to them.
5. Smart Logistics:
   Traditional warehouses can be transformed into revolutionized automated warehouses by utilizing AI, automated robotics, and intelligent transportation systems (ITS). Because of the usage of AI and ITS with minimal or no human intervention, smart logistics will complete the work with minimal time and errors, completing the work on time (Rao, Gagan, Nikhil et al, 2022).

Drone delivery is available in smart logistics, which will help to deliver items at the last moment and in congested areas where distribution takes a long time. This form of smart logistics will be useful in delivering drugs to those in need. Smart logistics is also more dependable, transparent, and secure for customers.

6. Smart Household:
   IoT and furniture can work together to transform a regular house into a smart house or smart household. With the help of AI technology, the furniture may be created in such a way that it can make sensible decisions. Cabinets and furniture can be personalized to meet the needs of the user and can alter intelligently when new perspectives emerge in the smart home. Adding the content of the security for home objects might lead to the creation of a safety design. The furniture in the smart home can be altered based on the user's entertainment needs, which leads to changes in the speakers and monitors with regard to VR and AR.
7. Smart Transport:
   Smart vehicles necessitate high-performance computation and rapid decision-making power on the vehicle board (Rao, Gagan, Nikhil et al, 2022; Rao, Pawar, Priyanka et al, 2022). The vehicle's cost will be quite expensive in order to attain this feature. The typical guy cannot buy a smart automobile because it is too pricey. To address this issue, a smart transport system is being built using IoT and cloud computing. The IoT not only collects information, but also communicates it with other gadgets on the road or in other vehicles, as well as with other devices connected to the internet. Vehicle-to-Everything (V2X), Vehicle-to-Vehicle (V2V), 5G-Network, AR-assisted navigation, and intelligent traffic planning all contributed to the development of the smart transportation system, which can be achieved through self-drive / remote drive (Rao, Reddy, Ahamed et al, 2022).
8. Smart Security:
   Smart security includes some technology, such as drone patrolling, robot patrolling, and the use of IoT and Cloud Computing technology. The adoption of 5 G, in conjunction with AR-mobile policies, helped to improve security by identifying better coordinates and positions. UHD (Ultra-High-Definition) real-time monitoring aids in policing and security. In addition, wearable security devices assist in alerting and identifying the victim's whereabouts.
9. Smart Agriculture:
   The Internet of Things holds great promise for revolutionizing agriculture. Farmers can improve crop growth while using less water and fertilizer by combining sensors with wireless internet in crop fields. Remote monitoring of livestock and agricultural machinery simplifies operations even further, resulting in more cost-effective production. likewise, 5G technology enables improved water body monitoring, allowing for multi-dimensional management and raising agricultural efficiency (Sharma & Singh, 2021).
10. Smart Health:
    Because of the internet revolution, the medical industry is now able to provide services in a highly timely and efficient manner. The adoption of 5G and IoT helps to transform the medical field's perspective into a smart one. Telemedicine, remote surgery, home assistant services, remote health monitoring, and health-bands are all part of the smart health sector. Smart health also contributes to a better understanding of pandemic circumstances. Monitoring and remote operations are now available thanks to UHD. Patients receive better treatment

on time because to the deployment of smart ambulances and smart hospitals (Lilhore et al., 2024; Lilhore et al., 2023).

11. Smart E-Governance:
    Smart E-Governance assists in providing governmental services to all people, regardless of location, gender, cast, or other characteristics. Because of smart E-Governance, the government can handle events such as epidemics, terror attacks, and natural catastrophes while also ensuring public safety. Smart E-Governance informs citizens about policies and advantages, and it is visible to everybody. Video conferencing enables public officials to understand the situation of people living in rural areas and to manage it effectively. E- Governance can also help educate individuals about new technologies, rules, and benefits.
12. Smart Environment Control:
    Environmental infrastructure management improves a city's resilience. This includes managing natural resources, energy, pollution management, and sewage and green space upkeep. It also involves grid management, lighting, and renewable energy sources. Environmental monitoring is critical, with developments such as smart garbage cans helping to improve urban management.
13. Smart Entertainment
    The use of internet bandwidth, IoT, VR, AR help the entertainment to convert into smart. In the future, 5G promises to add a new sensory dimension to entertainment advertising and online gaming, transforming traditional banner-based ads into immersive moving images. Real-time dynamics will be measured through technologies like eye surveillance and biometrics. Beyond improved streaming and downloading, companies are exploring how 5G can fundamentally alter entertainment. For instance, live concerts could be broadcast globally through augmented reality and edited in real-time. The possibilities for 5G applications in the entertainment industry are vast and diverse.
14. Smart Disaster Management
    5G city networks offer a robust foundation for enhancing emergency responses. The rapid spread of the coronavirus in Wuhan, accelerated by the Chinese New Year migrations, presented significant containment challenges. Effective pandemic control requires swift screening, diagnosis, and isolation of urban cases. Additionally, this data should be promptly sent to command centers for analysis and strategizing. A city-wide 5G network can enable real-time sensing and monitoring of a pandemic, facilitating coordinated and efficient responses. Such a system shifts the focus from mere reactive measures to proactive early warning and management.

Numerous obstacles remain in contemporary healthcare systems, and this debate focuses on a few significant issues. The most notable of them is the impact of urbanization and population increase, which has resulted in a major decrease in the effective use of healthcare resources. This drop can be ascribed to a variety of issues, including limited resources such as medical practitioners, facilities, drug availability, increased patient waiting times, long travel distances, and the availability of home healthcare services for continuous patient monitoring and elder care.

Patient data is restricted to specific hospital clusters, limiting access for other medical practitioners and impeding efficient utilization during emergency situations. This problem causes patients to undergo repeated testing, wasting time and money. As a result of this time waste, the condition may be diagnosed later and develop consequences.

The HCS addresses the aforementioned difficulties by integrating smart ambulances, telemedicine, smart hospitals, wearable IoT devices for patients, and implementing various monitoring systems for both patients and their environment. Effective data sharing, while maintaining privacy, makes it easier to get patient data during an emergency. Furthermore, robot-assisted surgery is used for essential and emergency procedures, whether in cities or rural places.

BACKGROUND

Numerous studies on smart health have been conducted in various countries. This section discusses some of the related research on the topic.

Yu et al (2020) discussed the plant Spike is an affordable, wireless sensor system designed for urban soil health monitoring. Easily implantable, it tracks soil moisture, temperature, and light intensity using advanced power management and Bluetooth for data transmission. The system's efficient power usage extends its battery life beyond two years, and its total cost is under $10 per module. Tested at Columbia University and in Morningside Heights, NYC, Plant Spike reliably captures data reflecting New York's climate zone conditions.

Buttazzoni et al (2020) discussed about Urban infrastructure systems significantly influence health and health equity. The term "smart city" encompasses various urban governance concepts that aim to achieve public health goals. This systematic review studied the inclusion of equity considerations in smart city health interventions, examining 28 articles from multiple databases. Results showed a varied focus on equity dimensions, with some aspects like residence and socio-economic status being more prevalent than others, like gender or religion.

Wu et al (2022) proposes Big data and IoT significantly influence urban residents' health within smart cities. Using data from the CHARLS survey, the study investigated the impact of smart city development on residents' health. Findings indicate that smart city construction enhances health, leading to decreased outpatient visits and increased inpatient services. Notably, rural residents exhibited more pronounced behavioral shifts in medical service use due to smart city influences.

The Internet of Things (IoT) allows organizations to automate processes and enhance service delivery by transferring data to the cloud is proposed by Gavrilović et al (2021). However, IoT requires specific software architectures tailored to users' needs in various fields. This paper examines the software architectures used in IoT systems for smart cities, healthcare, and agriculture. It offers suggestions for improvements, emphasizing the interactions between software architecture elements for enhanced performance. The research uniquely analyses layered, service-oriented, and cloud-based IoT architectures, recommending the most suitable architecture based on the application area.

The COVID-19 outbreak has led to city lockdowns, impacting global economies and health systems. As the virus spreads, there's an emphasized need for health data sharing. Allam et al (2020) suggests that smart cities should standardize data sharing protocols for better global management during such cases.

Smart Cities use advanced technology to enhance urban living, but their structures require regular maintenance, which is time-consuming and costly. Remote Structural Health Monitoring (RSHM) using IoT sensors offers a solution, especially for structures with bolted joints. M. Sidorov et al(2019) introduces Ten Sense M30, an IoT sensor using Long Range (LoRa) communication, designed for monitoring bolted joints, boasting precise monitoring, an 800-meter communication range, and a lifespan of over 5 years on coin cell batteries.

The recent pandemic underscores the need for advanced healthcare systems that can efficiently monitor patients and address disease outbreaks. Smart healthcare cyber-physical systems, integrating technologies like IoT, Machine Learning, and AI, bridge the physical and digital worlds for improved medical processes and patient monitoring. Verma et al (2022) delves into healthcare cyber-physical systems, discussing their features, the technologies driving them, and challenges in their implementation.

Smart city initiatives through e-government construction influence firms to reduce their environmental pollution behavior. Liu et al (2021), study of 16,347 Chinese industrial firms across 322 cities found that companies in regions with advanced e-government structures have lower environmental pollution levels. Moreover, the impact is even more pronounced for firms with higher artificial intelligence-related information processing capabilities.

The Internet of Health Things (IoHT) and 5G enable efficient connected health monitoring using deep learning to process vast amounts of data for decision-making. Yet, challenges like data security, privacy, and social acceptance of deep learning remain. Rahman et al (2021) proposes a framework addressing these issues by ensuring data privacy, using blockchain for trustworthiness, and adding explain ability to the deep learning process for societal acceptance.

S. Gera et al (2021) The Internet of Things (IoT) enhances healthcare through remote monitoring and expanding telemedicine capabilities. The proposed system aims to support patients in remote areas by analyzing data from wearable IoT sensors and facilitating interactions between patients, physicians, pharmacists, and diagnosticians. This interface streamlines traditional healthcare processes and bolsters decision-making.

Trencher et al (2019) Smart cities, often focused on economic and environmental goals, can center on social aims by integrating a health and well-being agenda. Technologies like wearable health monitors and open data platforms can enhance urban residents' lives. A case study in Kashiwanoha Smart City, Japan, demonstrates the potential for smart cities to address social issues and create more equitable, sustainable urban environments.

RICH HEALTH CARE SECTOR (HCS): COMPONENTS

In a smart city, the Health Care Sector is revolutionized by the integration of advanced technologies, digital infrastructure, and data analytics. HCS different sectors are as shown in the Figure 2. Here's how the Health Care Sector evolves in the context of a smart city:

1. ***Remote Patient Monitoring (RPM):*** With wearable devices and IoT, patients' health can be monitored in real-time, allowing for timely interventions and reduced hospital admissions. The term "remote patient monitoring" (RPM) describes the use of digital technologies to collect medical and other health data from patients in one area and electronically send that information securely to healthcare providers in another location for evaluation and suggestions. This kind of service enables a clinician to keep track of a patient's medical information after they are released, lowering the likelihood of readmission. RPM can improve the management of diseases like diabetes, hypertension, and heart failure. It is crucial for the management of chronic diseases. RPM enables medical personnel to keep an eye on vital signs, body weight, blood pressure, blood sugar, blood oxygen levels, and heart rate, ensuring that any possible problems are found before they have a serious impact. Furthermore, patients gain from more regular check-ins as opposed to waiting

Figure 2. Shows HCS-COMPONENTS

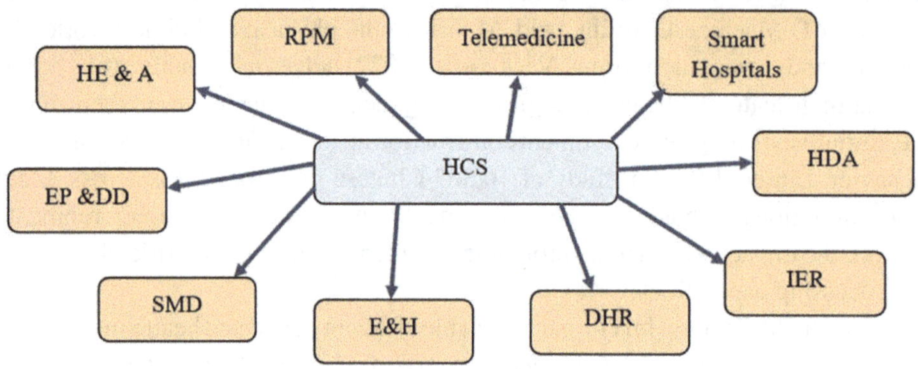

for in-person visits. With the use of technology, exacerbations may be detected early, allowing for speedier and more targeted therapy. RPM also strengthens the bonds between patients and their medical professionals, fostering real-time communication and better health results. RPM is positioned to become the norm in patient care as telehealth services are more in demand and technology develops.

2. ***Telemedicine:*** Leveraging 5G and broadband connectivity, doctors can consult with patients virtually, breaking the barriers of distance and ensuring timely healthcare access. When a patient and a practitioner are not physically present with one another, this practice is known as telemedicine. It makes use of contemporary communication technology to give patients quick, convenient, and non-travel access to medical knowledge. For people who live in remote locations where specialized medical care could be scarce, telemedicine has been very helpful. Doctors may diagnose and cure illnesses through real-time video conversations, including consultations and follow-up meetings. It can also help with prescription management so that a patient can get the drugs they need without having to go to the doctor in person. During the pandemic period telemedicine helped lot. Usages of telemedicine is cheaper and faster and patients can directly connect with the health professional easily and at any time the rural area people can get better services.
3. ***Smart Hospitals (SH):*** Integrating IoT, AI, big data and Cloud help to build a smart hospital. The smart hospitals will hold the information of the patients in the small chip or a card. It also helps to provide the monitoring of each and every parameter of the patients using the IoT and cloud. The smart hospital will have the information regarding the patients' health status and will prioritizes if any surgery or any other actions are required immediately. The smart hospital will help to manage resource efficiently. The smart hospital will also ensure to securing of the patients' data (Ahmad et al., 2022; Balyan et al., 2022).
4. ***Health Data Analytics (HDA):*** HDA refers to the systematic use of data to develop insights and improve outcomes for patients, research, and healthcare delivery. Analytics can detect patterns and trends in health and disease through analyzing massive amounts of patient data, such as data from wearable devices and electronic health records. This strategy assists medical practitioners in anticipating patient health risks, improving hospital operations, and personalizing treatment strategies. Deeper dataset research is enabled by cutting-edge approaches such as machine learning and artificial intelligence, which typically discover links that would not

be obvious from human study alone. Furthermore, health data analytics fosters evidence-based decisions, ensuring that therapies and interventions are both cost-effective and effective in terms of both cost and benefit.

5. ***Integrated Emergency Response (IER):*** Real-time data exchange, GPS tracking, and predictive analytics are examples of these. An integrated approach enables long-term relief and recovery for afflicted communities by considering post-emergency procedures in addition to the immediate crisis. The IER deals with how fast the responders get the service during the emergencies. IER is mainly deals with the integration of different sectors together and handle the situation within a time duration and provide the efficient solutions to the needy one. IER is very helpful during the disasters and pandemic situations (Sharma & Singh, 2021).
6. ***Digital Health Records (DHR):*** The patients health history is stored in the central server; such a data is called DHR or HER. This will help to diagnosis, treatments and also help to keep track of the patient's health from anywhere. This facility will help the rural patients to get the best services from their place without travelling. The DHR records have the security, reliability and help to reduce the wastage of the papers.
7. ***Environment & Health (E&H):*** Some of the patient's health is mostly affected by environmental variables. Some allergies are primarily influenced by environmental variables such as pollination, water pollution, and air pollution. Using the built-in smart IoT devices and the environment smart IoT devices help to track the patients' health and alert them to be more cautious about their health in a smarter way (Lilhore et al., 2024).
8. ***Smart Medical Devices (SMD):*** Medical gadgets are becoming more accurate and personalized, from smart insulin pumps to AI-driven diagnostic tools. Smart medical gadgets, which provide improved monitoring, diagnosis, and therapies, symbolize the confluence of technology and healthcare. These devices provide real-time data that may be necessary for patient treatment and are frequently linked to the internet or other devices. They meet a wide range of medical needs, from wearable fitness trackers that monitor heart rates to insulin pumps that modify dosages automatically.
9. ***E-Pharmacies and Drone Deliveries (EP & DD):*** Prescriptions can be ordered via the internet and delivered quickly by drones, ensuring that patients receive their medications on time. E-pharmacies have transformed the healthcare industry by offering simple online platforms for prescription renewals and medication purchasing. They bridge the gap among patients and drugs by providing timely and discrete deliveries, sometimes at low cost.
10. ***Health Education & Awareness (HE & A):*** Digital platforms in smart cities provide regular health updates, advisories, and educational content to residents, promoting preventive care and well-being. Making informed judgements regarding one's well-being is greatly facilitated by health education and knowledge. It promotes a proactive attitude towards one's own health by educating people on illness prevention, healthy lifestyles, and recent medical developments. Online portals, webinars, and mobile apps have improved accessibility to health information for a range of people in the digital age. Community outreach and awareness initiatives can also challenge false information and promote behaviors that stop the spread of disease. Continuous education is still crucial in promoting healthier communities around the world as health concerns change.

HCS RELATIONSHIP AND 5G

The advent of 5G technology promises to revolutionize many sectors, and among the most impacted are health care and urban development, as seen in the rise of smart cities. Figure 3 shows the relationship between the HCS, 5G and clients. The advent of 5G technology is poised to revolutionize healthcare systems in various ways (Guevara & Auat Cheein, 2020). With faster, more reliable, and low-latency communication offered by 5G, real-time telemedicine and remote patient monitoring become more feasible, leading to more timely interventions and better patient outcomes. Patients can now interact with their healthcare providers from the comfort of their homes, bridging the gap between rural and urban medical services. Wearable devices, which continuously monitor vital signs, can transmit large volumes of data in real-time due to 5G's high bandwidth. The monitoring will help the patients to face the crucial and emergency conditions (Haque et al., 2022).

The reliable benefits of the HCS model is mainly depends upon the following equation1.

$$S = D + T + H \quad (1)$$

Where S is the success of HCS, D is the data availability of the patient, it mainly depends upon equation 2.

$$D = P_H + P_C + A_T \quad (2)$$

Where P_H, P_C states the patient's history and patients' current data. A_T States the correct analysis of the patients made by the medical professionals.

T states the transportation of the patient to the hospital or medical professional to the patient's location (Lilhore et al., 2023; Qadir et al., 2021). T can also state transmission of data, this can be stated in the equation 3.

$$T = T_P + T_{PC} + T_{CH} + D_L \quad (3)$$

Where T_P, T_{PC}, T_{CH} are the time taken by the patients' devices to collect the data, transmit it to cloud and from cloud to smart hospital devices. D_L is the total delay during all the above process.

Figure 3. Shows the relationship between HCS and 5G and clients

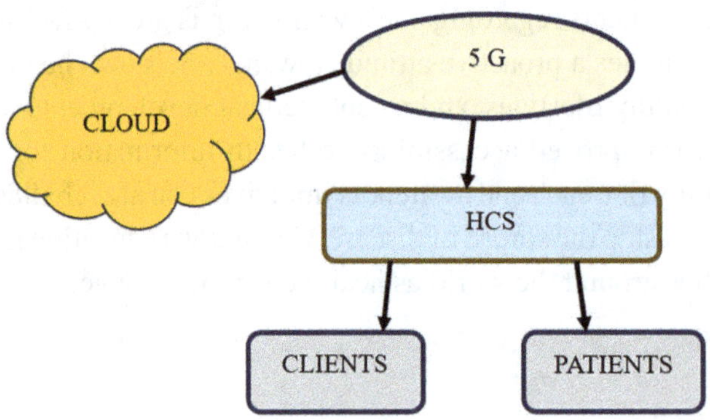

By optimizing patient care while ensuring data accessibility and security, the combination of 5G and cloud storage has the potential to launch healthcare systems into a new era. Advantages of using 5G in HCS include improved connectivity in smart cities, remote surgery and diagnosis, IoT and health monitoring systems, AI integration, emergency response, and VR in healthcare.

5G ARCHITECTURE AND ITS BENEFITS WITH HCS

5G network architecture has been developed with adaptability, rapidity, and links in mind, making it extremely suitable for HCS and smart city infrastructure. The following are some of the ways 5G can help the HCS succeed.

1. ***URLLC (Ultra-Reliable Low Latency Communication):*** 5G has ultrareliable and low latency in the communications. This feature helps the telemedicine consultant and the remote surgery in the case of HCS.
2. ***Enhanced Mobile Broadband (eMBB):*** the data rate offered by the 5G is massive, due this the applications such as AR, HD video surveillance, ITC is possible.
3. ***Massive Machine Type Communication (mMTC):*** Large connectivity of the devices is possible in the case of 5G. this helps the HCS to connect many sensor devices to many numbers of patients and monitor them without any interruptions.
4. ***Network Slicing:*** For a specific need the 5G is able to create a slice. For HCS, a dedicated slice ensures that critical health data and applications always have priority and guaranteed resources. Smart cities can allocate different slices for services like public safety, transportation, and utilities (Yang et al., 2021).
5. ***Edge Computing Integration:*** 5G architecture often integrates edge computing, allowing data processing closer to the data source. This is crucial for HCS as it enables faster diagnostics and patient care by processing health data on-site. Local data processing in smart cities can reduce latency in systems such as traffic control, trash management, and public security.
6. ***Enhanced Security Protocols:*** As cyber dangers have increased, 5G networks have been constructed with advanced security measures. This is critical for safeguarding sensitive health data in HCS. It is critical for smart cities to ensure the security of interconnected systems ranging from traffic lights to water supply systems (Rao, Reddy, Ahamed et al, 2022; Yang et al., 2021).

Health care system will combine following some features to become an HCS. They are:

1. ***Automatic Data gathering of Health Data:*** With the introduction of wearables and IoT devices, automatic data gathering monitors important information such as heart rate, blood pressure, and sleep habits in real-time. Continuous health monitoring can discover irregularities more quickly, forecasting possible health risks and allowing for timely actions. Smartwatches, diabetes monitors, and implanted gadgets that transmit health data to doctors or cloud-based health records.
2. ***Remote surgery***: Often known as telesurgery, is the practice of performing surgical procedures from a distance utilizing robotic equipment that are controlled by doctors. Removes geographic restrictions, allowing patients to receive specialized surgical skills without travelling.

3. ***Remote Diagnosis and Treatment:*** Using telemedicine platforms, clinicians can diagnose and treat patients in remote areas. Increases access to healthcare, particularly in rural or underdeveloped areas. It also helps to prevent hospital overcrowding and the transmission of contagious diseases. Platforms for virtual consultations, digital stethoscopes, and smartphone apps that transmit health data for remote analysis.
4. ***Super Ambulance:*** These are ambulances outfitted with cutting-edge medical technology that allows for on-the-spot diagnosis and treatment even before arriving at the hospital. By providing immediate medical measures, the odds of patient survival and recovery are increased. Ambulances outfitted with telemedicine capabilities that allow paramedics to communicate in real time with hospital-based doctors, improved life-support systems, and mobile diagnostic tools such as portable ultrasound machines.

5G NETWORK OVERVIEW

The 5G network is the next step in mobile communication, providing unprecedented speed and efficiency. The 5G base station is at the heart of this network, connecting devices to the network and managing resources to optimize data transfer speeds (Hassan et al., 2021). Multi-access Edge Computing (MEC) systems are implemented within or near these base stations, moving computational duties closer to the source of data, lowering latency and ensuring speedy real-time replies. The 5G Customer Premises Equipment (CPE) acts as a gateway, allowing users and devices in homes and businesses to connect to the 5G network easily.

Figure 4 shows the technical framework of 5G. The command center stands as the nexus, overseeing the entire network's operations, managing traffic, ensuring security, and optimizing the performance of both smart devices and ground stations (Lilhore et al., 2024). Together, these components drive the transformative potential of 5G, weaving a web of interconnected systems that promise to reshape our digital experiences. Form the command center data actions will take place, the data will be collected from the smart device or the ground station (Hassan et al., 2021). Because of the technicality benefits

Figure 4. Technical framework of 5G

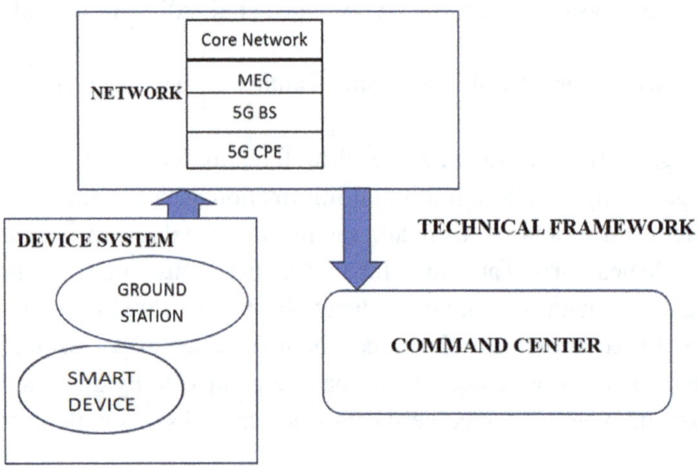

of the 5G network the HCS is improved, reliable and fast (Qadir et al., 2021). The comparison of the 5G HCS and Pre-5G HCS is tabulated in the Table I.

COMPARISON OF HCS WITH DIFFERENT FEATURES AND THE NETWORK

It's essential to recognize that the adoption, coverage, and performance of each network generation will vary based on a country's infrastructure, regulatory environment, and the specific carriers.

PROPOSED SYSTEM

The proposed 5G-HCS has the 3 modules which contains the 5G module, where the actual communication takes place, module data processing and storage and last, I/O accessories module. The proposed framework is as depicted by the Figure 5. The I/O accessories module will have the interaction with the 5G module or Data processing and storing module. I/O (Input/Output) accessories, such as sensors, play a pivotal role in modern technology by capturing real-world data and converting it into digital signals that computers can interpret and process.

The proposed 5G-HCS has the 3 modules which contains the 5G module, where the actual communication takes place, module data processing and storage and last, I/O accessories module. The I/O accessories module will have the interaction with the 5G module or Data processing and storing module. I/O (Input/Output) accessories, such as sensors, play a pivotal role in modern technology by capturing real-world data and converting it into digital signals that computers can interpret and process.

The use of IoT sensors, which will be marketed as wearable technology or highly advanced implants in them, significantly alters medical care. Health professionals, people, and family members can personally check each other's well-being. This administration is carried out from many locations. Smart homes and smart health are achievable with the use of sensors, and by connecting multiple modules to one another, improved outcomes can be achieved. The use of technology will change sectors, particularly the health sector, and contribute to security and adaptability.

The data is received by the stationary modules from a variety of input devices, specifically sensors. The pre-processing step will be completed after the data is received. After that, the pre-processed data

Table 1. Comparison of 5G in HCS and Pre-5G HCS

Features	5G in HCS	General Healthcare Systems (Pre-5G)
Latency Limitations	5G networks can achieve latency as low as 1 millisecond, enabling real-time remote consultations and surgeries	Older network technologies like 4G and 3G have higher latency, making real-time telemedicine less feasible
Data Transfer Speeds	With peak data rates exceeding 10 Gbps, 5G enables high-definition video streaming and large medical data transfers	Data transfer speeds in older networks may be insufficient for high-quality video consultations or transferring large medical images
IoT Constraints	5G supports massive IoT device connections, facilitating remote patient monitoring and data collection from wearable health devices.	Connectivity limitations may hinder the widespread use of IoT devices for remote patient monitoring
Telemedicine Challenges	5G contributes to the growth of telemedicine, making healthcare more accessible to remote and underserved areas	Telemedicine adoption may be slower due to network limitations, impacting healthcare access

Table 2. Comparison of the different networks

Features	2G	3G	4G/LTE	5G
Speed	Up to 64 Kbps	Up to 2 Mbps for non-moving users. In most conditions, speeds ranged from 144 Kbps to 2 Mbps	Up to 100 Mbps (real-world average speeds often range between 20 to 50 Mbps).	Up to 10 Gbps (peak data rate). In real-world conditions, often between 100 Mbps to 1 Gbps depending on the type of 5G being used
Latency	Higher than 3G, not typically quoted for data since 2G was more voice-centric.	Around 100 milliseconds	Between 30 to 50 milliseconds	As low as 1 millisecond
Frequency Bands	Primarily below 1 GHz	Below 3 GHz	Typically, below 6 GHz	Sub-6 GHz and mm Wave (24 GHz to 100 GHz)
Device Density	Much lower than 3G	Lower than 4G	Around 2,000 devices per square kilometer	Up to 1 million devices per square kilometer
Energy Efficiency	More power-intensive relative to the amount of data it could transmit.	Consumes more power than 4G for the same data transmission.	Less efficient than 5G but an improvement over 3G	Designed to be more energy-efficient with features like network slicing.

Figure 5. Framework of proposed 5G-HCS

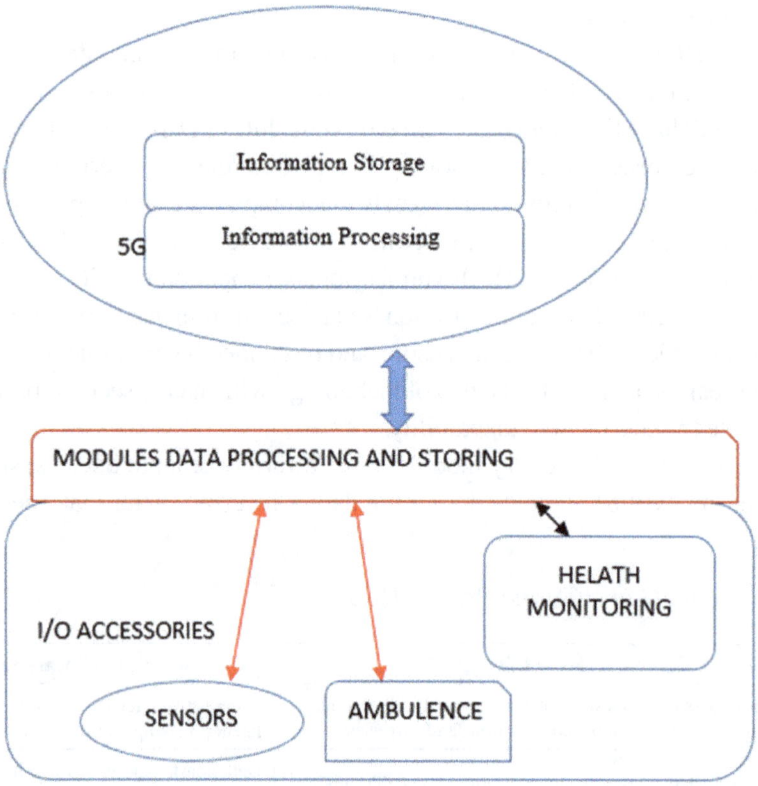

will either be sent to a professional for additional processing or transferred to the cloud. The data stored in the stationary module is large size and it should be reliable, fault tolerance, disaster management, access the data quickly and concurrency. The more crucial requirements are that the data be scalable and coordinated. In terms of communication, dependability, and time orientation, highly quick technology is needed to have the qualities in health care data. 5G has these qualities as well. In addition to its incredibly quick speeds and low latency, 5G offers increased mobile broadband capacity. Specific sections of the network can be allocated to specific tasks via 5G network slicing, ensuring optimized processing and prioritized storage for key applications. The rise of edge computing in the 5G era enables data to be processed closer to its source, reducing the need to send all data to centralized servers and improving storage efficiency and access times. The integration of 5G with advanced AI and machine learning tools facilitates smarter data processing, enabling devices to make more informed decisions based on the voluminous data stored and processed in real-time.

To perform the proposed model depending upon the priority of the task the data will be processed in the stationary station or it will be sent to the 5G module, where actual processing and the storing of the medical data into the cloud will take place. To perform the real time surgery the data bandwidth required is very high and it should be uninterrupted. The telemedicine also requires the multimedia data, which should be very fast. For some data i.e., health monitoring, where continuous data is not required and only after time duration data can be collected and processed will be stored in the data processing and storing. Implementation of the proposed module require very much precondition set with respect to processing and storing and taking action.

ETHICAL CONSIDERATION IN THE IMPLEMENTATION OF HCS

Some of the key factors should be included during the implementation of the HCS. They are as follows:

1. ***Data Security and Privacy:*** It should be made clear how patients' data is stored, shared, and accessed. Also, it should be apparent when obtaining patient data via telemedicine and preserving electronic health.
2. ***Informed Consent:*** Patients should be informed in their native language well in advance about the adoption of new technologies, the placement of wearable devices, and the implementation of monitoring devices in their surroundings. Patients should be able to control the dissemination.
3. ***Equality Access:*** All individuals should have equitable access to the facilities of the health care systems, regardless of any human race or socioeconomic standing.
4. ***Algorithmic Prejudice and Fairness:*** AI and ML approaches can sometimes lead to biases. Therefore, it should be transparent, accountable, and fair. This will benefit individuals regardless of their demographic reputation.
5. ***Human-Machine Collaboration:*** When humans collaborate with machines or robots, the ethical consideration ought to focus on the monitoring, responsibility, and accountability of the human operator or medical experts.
6. ***Quality of Care:*** During the deployment of modern technology on the patient, the patients' health should be prioritized, and ethical considerations should be focused on the ongoing monitoring of the influence of patient outcomes.
7. ***End-of-Life Care:*** Technologies used to improve health care may have an impact on end-of-life care decisions. Ethical principles should address autonomy, dignity, and the right use of technology in decisions about life-sustaining procedures.

8. ***Accountability and Transparency:*** Patients and their families should be able to see how health-care choices are made when AI and machine learning are used. Medical personnel should be held accountable for their use of technology and the outcomes of improved health-care systems.

CONCLUSION

This study delves into the expected evolution of urban areas into smart cities by 2050, driven by projected population surges. It emphasizes the profound influence of Information and Communication Technology (ICT), particularly in areas like manufacturing, entertainment, and notably, the Health Care Sector (HCS). The HCS's progression is articulated through its symbiotic relationship with technologies such as the Internet of Things, offering advancements like telemedicine and remote monitoring. Central to the smart city concept is the adoption of 5G technology, renowned for its high-speed, low latency, and vast connection capabilities, laying the foundation for an enriched HCS. This chapter further elaborates on the multi-faceted impact of 5G on the HCS, the technological landscape, financial benefits, and proposes a model tailored for a 5G-enhanced smart city HCS.

REFERENCES

Ahmad, K. A. B., Khujamatov, H., Akhmedov, N., Bajuri, M. Y., Ahmad, M. N., & Ahmadian, A. (2022). Emerging trends and evolutions for Smart city healthcare systems. *Sustainable Cities and Society*, *80*, 103695.

Allam, Z., & Jones, D. S. (2020, February). On the coronavirus (COVID-19) outbreak and the smart city network: universal data sharing standards coupled with artificial intelligence (AI) to benefit urban health monitoring and management. In Healthcare (Vol. 8, No. 1, p. 46). MDPI.

Balyan, A. K., Ahuja, S., Sharma, S. K., & Lilhore, U. K. (2022, February). Machine learning-based intrusion detection system for healthcare data. In *2022 IEEE VLSI Device Circuit and System (VLSI DCS)* (pp. 290-294). IEEE.

Buttazzoni, A., Veenhof, M., & Minaker, L. (2020). Smart city and high-tech urban interventions targeting human health: An equity-focused systematic review. *International Journal of Environmental Research and Public Health*, *17*(7), 2325.

Gavrilović, N., & Mishra, A. (2021). Software architecture of the internet of things (IoT) for smart city, healthcare and agriculture: Analysis and improvement directions. *Journal of Ambient Intelligence and Humanized Computing*, *12*(1), 1315–1336.

Gera, S., Mridul, M., & Sharma, S. (2021, April). IoT based automated healthcare monitoring system for smart city. In *2021 5th International Conference on Computing Methodologies and Communication (ICCMC)* (pp. 364-368). IEEE.

Guevara, L., & Auat Cheein, F. (2020). The role of 5G technologies: Challenges in smart cities and intelligent transportation systems. *Sustainability*, *12*(16), 6469.

Haque, A. B., Bhushan, B., & Dhiman, G. (2022). Conceptualizing smart city applications: Requirements, architecture, security issues, and emerging trends. *Expert Systems: International Journal of Knowledge Engineering and Neural Networks*, *39*(5), e12753.

Hassan, A., Prasad, D., Khurana, M., Lilhore, U. K., & Simaiya, S. (2021). Integration of internet of things (IoT) in health care industry: An overview of benefits, challenges, and applications. *Data Science and Innovations for Intelligent Systems*, 165-180.

Lilhore, U. K., Dalal, S., Faujdar, N., Simaiya, S., Dahiya, M., Tomar, S., & Hashmi, A. (2024). Unveiling the prevalence and risk factors of early-stage postpartum depression: A hybrid deep learning approach. *Multimedia Tools and Applications*, 1–35.

Lilhore, U. K., Manoharan, P., Sandhu, J. K., Simaiya, S., Dalal, S., Baqasah, A. M., ... Raahemifar, K. (2023). Hybrid model for precise hepatitis-C classification using improved random forest and SVM method. *Scientific Reports*, *13*(1), 12473.

Liu, W., Xu, Y., Fan, D., Li, Y., Shao, X. F., & Zheng, J. (2021). Alleviating corporate environmental pollution threats toward public health and safety: The role of smart city and artificial intelligence. *Safety Science*, *143*, 105433.

Qadir, Z., Ullah, F., Munawar, H. S., & Al-Turjman, F. (2021). Addressing disasters in smart cities through UAVs path planning and 5G communications: A systematic review. *Computer Communications*, *168*, 114–135.

Rahman, M. A., Hossain, M. S., Showail, A. J., Alrajeh, N. A., & Alhamid, M. F. (2021). A secure, private, and explainable IoHT framework to support sustainable health monitoring in a smart city. *Sustainable Cities and Society*, *72*, 103083.

Rao, M. G., Gagan, G., Nikhil, T. C., & Pradeep, A. B. (2022, December). Authentication and Parking of the Vehicle Using License Plate Detection and Recognition in the Campus. In *2022 International Conference on Artificial Intelligence and Data Engineering (AIDE)* (pp. 74-79). IEEE.

Rao, M. G., Pawar, S., Priyanka, H., Reddy, K. H. K., & Divakarala, U. (2023). Minimize the Energy Consumption for Communication Protocol in IoT. In Energy Systems Design for Low-Power Computing (pp. 214-234). IGI Global.

Rao, M. G., Pawar, S., Priyanka, H., Reddy, K. H. K., & Divakarla, U. (2022, December). Novel approach of Using Periocular and Iris Biometric Recognition in the Authentication of ITS. In *2022 Fourth International Conference on Cognitive Computing and Information Processing (CCIP)* (pp. 1-6). IEEE.

Rao, M. G., Priyanka, H., Kumar, A. P., & Divakarla, U. (2022, September). A Deep Learning Approach Towards Building Intelligent Transport System. In *2022 Second International Conference on Computer Science, Engineering and Applications (ICCSEA)* (pp. 1-6). IEEE.

Rao, M. G., Reddy, K. H. K., Ahamed, A., & Shetty, A. (2022, December). Deploy the VNPDR to Provide Authenticated Parking for Vehicles on Hospital Premise. In *2022 International Conference on Artificial Intelligence and Data Engineering (AIDE)* (pp. 107-111). IEEE.

Sharma, A., & Singh, P. K. (2021). UAV-based framework for effective data analysis of forest fire detection using 5G networks: An effective approach towards smart cities solutions. *International Journal of Communication Systems*, 4826.

Sidorov, M., Nhut, P. V., Matsumoto, Y., & Ohmura, R. (2019). LoRa-based precision wireless structural health monitoring system for bolted joints in a smart city environment. *IEEE Access : Practical Innovations, Open Solutions*, *7*, 179235–179251.

Trencher, G., & Karvonen, A. (2019). Stretching "smart": Advancing health and well-being through the smart city agenda. *Local Environment*, *24*(7), 610–627.

Verma, R. (2022). Smart city healthcare cyber physical system: Characteristics, technologies and challenges. *Wireless Personal Communications*, *122*(2), 1413–1433.

Wu, W., Zhu, D., Liu, W., & Wu, C. H. (2022). Empirical research on smart city construction and public health under information and communications technology. *Socio-Economic Planning Sciences*, *80*, 100994.

Yang, D., Karimi, H. R., Kaynak, O., & Yin, S. (2021). Developments of digital twin technologies in industrial, smart city and healthcare sectors: A survey. *Complex Engineering Systems*, *1*(1), 3.

Yu, C., Kam, K., Xu, Y., Cui, Z., Steingart, D., Gorlatova, M., ... Kymissis, I. (2020). Plant spike: A low-cost, low-power beacon for smart city soil health monitoring. *IEEE Internet of Things Journal*, *7*(9), 9080–9090.

Chapter 15
Healthcare 5.0:
Unveiling the Future of Integrated Medicine

J. Shanthalakshmi Revathy
https://orcid.org/0000-0003-1724-7117
Velammal College of Engineering and Technology, India

J. Mangaiyarkkarasi
https://orcid.org/0000-0003-1431-9584
NMSS Vellaichamy Nadar College, India

ABSTRACT

The chapter explores the transformative shift from traditional to integrated healthcare. It delves into technology, patient empowerment, interdisciplinary collaboration, data-driven decision-making, and preventive healthcare. The role of AI in diagnostics and treatment, along with the use of big data for improved outcomes, resource allocation, and disease surveillance, is highlighted. The chapter advocates for a proactive healthcare model, emphasizing early intervention and ethical considerations. It explores virtual reality and augmented reality's potential in medical practices and discusses the impact of telemedicine on accessible and convenient patient care, especially in underserved areas. This concise overview provides insights into the future of integrated medicine in Healthcare 5.0.

1. INTRODUCTION

In an integrated medical future, individuals become active participants in their own health, and technology acts as an enabler rather than a replacement for interpersonal relationships. A different, innovative and empathetic approach that maintains the principles of Healthcare 5.0 seems, providing the prospect of a community that feels more peaceful, well-being, and joyful. "Healthcare 5.0" is the next stage in development in healthcare, indicating an evolution of paradigms from traditional approaches to a comprehensive, focused on patients approach. Addressing the mind, body, and spirit is vital since true healing extends beyond simply alleviating symptoms. The chapter analyses the core elements of healthcare

DOI: 10.4018/979-8-3693-1874-4.ch015

5.0 by examining the revolutionary roles that artificial intelligence (AI) and machine learning (ML) are playing in changing diagnosis and treatments. It also focuses at the promise of precision medicine, which uses genetic data to personalise care for patients and enhance outcomes (Vale, El-Sharif, and Ali 2022).

The chapter also highlights how important it is to encourage cooperation between technology experts, researchers, and healthcare professionals in order to establish a setting where knowledge and creativity are freely exchanged. Through shedding light on the importance of this cooperative framework, the story reveals how it acts as a driving force behind revolutionary developments in healthcare. By fostering a synergy that breaks through conventional silos, this integrated strategy pushes the sector towards new frontiers of discovery and application.

Furthermore, the investigation explores the crucial function that patient empowerment plays in the Healthcare 5.0 framework. The importance of increased health knowledge and patient involvement in treatment choices is emphasised. In this Healthcare 5.0 vision, the convergence of inclusivity, creativity, and compassion drives medical advancement while simultaneously establishing the groundwork for a society that is not just happier and healthier but also more intricately connected through shared information and well-being.

1.1 Evolution of Healthcare: From Traditional to Integrated Medicine

Strictly focusing on treating certain ailments or symptoms with accepted medical procedures—frequently involving drugs and surgery—was the hallmark of traditional healthcare. With little regard for their general health or lifestyle choices, individuals under this approach sought medical assistance for specific symptoms. An individual with persistent headaches, for example, may be prescribed painkillers by their physician. This treatment targets the symptoms rather than probing deeper into underlying issues like anxiety, inadequate sleep, or malnutrition (Lemmen, Simic, and Stock 2021).

An important trend towards integrated medicine evolved as medical knowledge grew and patient outcomes were examined. This method adopted a more holistic viewpoint, accounting for a patient's emotional health as well as lifestyle, heredity, environment, and other aspects. Rehabilitating individual illnesses became less significant than treating the individual's condition as a whole. A patient with chronic back pain may receive physical therapy, chiropractic care, and stress reduction using mindfulness methods as part of the growing approach. In order improve general well-being, this multifaceted strategy seeks to tackle the underlying causes of pain in addition to just relieving it.

This evolution in healthcare signifies a progression from conventional, isolated medical practices to a cohesive approach that integrates traditional and modern medicine, as depicted in Figure 1. The emphasis is now on a comprehensive understanding of patients and a commitment to addressing health issues at their roots, reflecting a more patient-centered and holistic paradigm.

Alternatively referred to as holistic or integrative medicine, integrated medicine is the combination of evidence-based complementary and alternative therapies with standard medical procedures. Personalised treatment plans, patient empowerment, and active involvement in the healing process are at the centre of this approach. Using cutting-edge diagnostics, genetics, and technology, integrated medicine precisely customises interventions to meet each patient's specific needs.

Imagine an instance in integrated medicine where a patient with cancer receives a customised treatment plan. It incorporates alternative methods like acupuncture, yoga, and meditation with conventional treatments like radiation or chemotherapy in an effortless way. This method places holistic nature seeks to enhance the patient's general state of life as well as their health throughout the duration of therapy, in

Figure 1. Evolution of healthcare: From traditional to integrated medicine

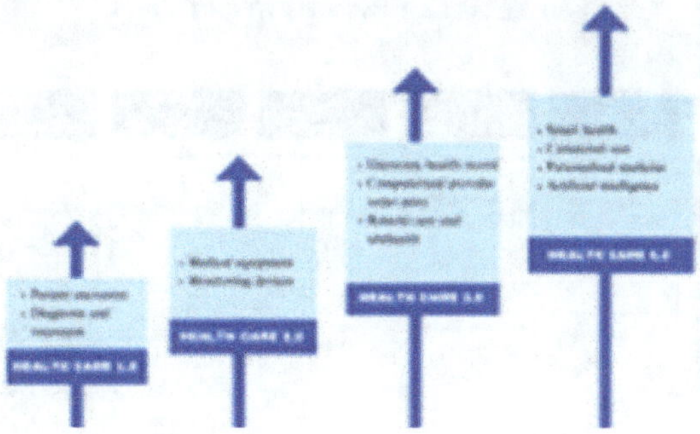

addition to fighting the illness. Thus, integrated medicine embodies a patient-centered philosophy that brings together the best aspects of complementary and traditional medicine to provide a more thorough and customised medical experience.

1.2. Definition and Concept of Healthcare 5.0

The healthcare industry has witnessed a significant and recent transformation as "Healthcare5.0." This places great emphasis on the patient, incorporating advanced technology, collaborative teamwork, and a comprehensive understanding of the patient's well-being. The goal is to seamlessly integrate data-driven technologies, personalized medicine, and patient empowerment to actively involve patients in their healthcare decisions (Seetharaman, Krishnan, and Schneider 2021). By utilizing wearable technology and medical monitoring apps, Healthcare 5.0 continuously collects data on various health indicators, sleep patterns, and activity levels. This data equips healthcare providers with a thorough understanding of the patient's condition, enabling them to tailor their plans accordingly by integrating it into the patient's digital health record.

Healthcare 5.0 is an evolving revolutionary change in the medical field, emphasising a patient-centric strategy that leverages advanced technologies, cooperative collaboration, and an in-depth understanding of the well-being of people. By integrating data-driven technologies, personalised medicine, and allowing patients to take an active role in their medical decisions, it aims to accomplish an easy transition. Employing wearable devices and medical monitoring apps, Health 5.0 gathers real-time data on the health of an individual, sleeping habits, and activity level. Since the fact because this data is integrated into the patient's electronic health record, physicians may use it to gain an in-depth understanding of the patient's condition and adjust their treatment plans accordingly. The idea of Healthcare 5.0 is an enhancement over past healthcare models, emphasising the significance of patient contribution, safeguarding, and welfare as a whole. It makes optimal use of the advantages of AI, ML, and big data in order to improve diagnosis, treatment, and care coordination while encouraging collaboration among healthcare professionals from various disciplines.

Through Healthcare 5.0, patients with chronic diseases such as diabetes can receive personalised treatment programmes that use lifestyle factors, genetic analysis, and data from wearable devices. The patient takes an active role in self-monitoring, makes informed decisions, and consults with physicians

Figure 2. Health industry revolution

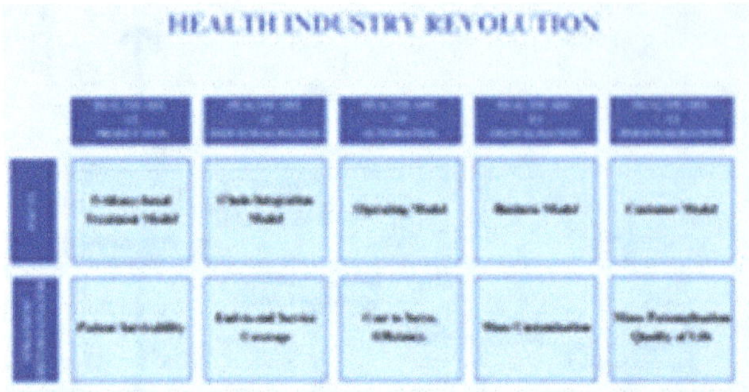

virtually through the use of virtual health platforms. Figure 2 illustrates the revolutionary changes and innovations that are reshaping healthcare delivery, technology, and services.

1.3 The Current Gaps in Knowledge or Limitations Identified in the Existing Research

Current healthcare systems often suffer from fragmented data across various platforms and institutions. Seamless data integration and exchange are crucial for comprehensive patient care and analysis but pose significant technological and policy challenges. While AI holds immense potential for personalized medicine and predictive analytics, ethical considerations regarding bias, transparency, and accountability require careful attention. Additionally, existing algorithms may not adequately capture the complexity of individual health factors and social determinants of health. The integration of technology should not overshadow the importance of human connection and patient-centered care. Building trust with patients and ensuring equitable access to these advancements remain crucial challenges. Successfully implementing Healthcare 5.0 requires adapting existing clinical workflows and training healthcare professionals on utilizing new technologies effectively. Resistance to change and the need for robust training programs hinder seamless integration.

Current legal and regulatory frameworks may not adequately address data privacy, ownership, and liability concerns with advanced healthcare technologies. Adapting these frameworks to ensure ethical and responsible implementation is essential. Implementing and maintaining sophisticated Healthcare 5.0 infrastructure and technologies can be expensive. Equitable access and affordability for resource-constrained settings require innovative solutions and partnerships. Many aspects of Healthcare 5.0 remain theoretical or in early stages of development. Rigorous research and robust clinical trials are necessary to validate the efficacy and safety of these technologies before widespread adoption. Healthcare 5.0 must go beyond individual-level interventions and address the broader social, economic, and environmental factors that impact health outcomes. Integrating social determinants of health into the framework is crucial for achieving true health equity. The healthcare landscape is constantly evolving, requiring Healthcare 5.0 systems to be adaptable and capable of learning from new data and emerging technologies. Building adaptive frameworks for continuous improvement is essential for long-term sustainability.

1.4 Purpose and Scope of the Chapter

This chapter's goal is to examine and clarify the healthcare industry's revolutionary transition from conventional methods to the integrated approach of Healthcare 5.0. The chapter seeks to emphasise the importance of patient-centric care, technological integration, and collaboration in influencing the future of healthcare by looking at the major turning points and conceptual framework.

Historical overview: This chapter will give a general account of how healthcare has changed throughout time, showing how old techniques gave way to integrated medicine.

Integrated Medicine: Extensive explanations of the ideas and methods of integrated medicine, emphasising its patient-centered methodology and providing instances of effective integrative treatment in the actual world.

The concept of Healthcare 5.0 and its essential components—such as the use of contemporary technologies, patient empowerment, and precision medicine—are described.

Applications in real time: demonstrating the impact of Healthcare 5.0 on patient outcomes and experiences while demonstrating its real-time use in a variety of healthcare contexts.

Future Consequences: talking about how Healthcare 5.0 might affect public health programmes, research, and healthcare delivery in the future.

Through an exploration of these facets, the chapter aims to offer a thorough comprehension of the development of healthcare and the revolutionary possibilities of Healthcare 5.0 in moulding a more effective, patient-focused, and cohesive healthcare framework.

2. FOUNDATIONS OF HEALTHCARE 5.0

Healthcare 5.0 denotes a revolutionary epoch in medical history, where patient-centered care, multidisciplinary collaboration, and state-of-the-art technologies combine to determine the future course of healthcare delivery. This chapter delves into the fundamental ideas of Healthcare 5.0, highlighting the significance of interdisciplinary collaboration and the transformative power of technological advancements in driving this ground-breaking paradigm shift.

2.1 Interdisciplinary Collaboration in Healthcare

The integration of various medical professions and specialists is depicted in Figure 3 as a means of improving patient care through all-encompassing and holistic approaches.

2.1.1 Collaborative Approach in Healthcare Delivery

Patient care was often fragmented in traditional healthcare since medical specialists typically worked independently in inflexible silos. Healthcare 5.0, on the other hand, encourages multidisciplinary cooperation and collaboration and brings together healthcare professionals from many specialties to work together to collaboratively address patient requirements. Dismantling divisions improves communication and information flow, which improves decision-making and patient outcomes (Johnson et al. 2021). An example of a collaborative healthcare setting involves a team of primary care physicians, endocrinologists, cardiologists, mental health specialists, and nutritionists treating a patient with multiple chronic

Figure 3. Multidisciplinary cooperation in the medical field

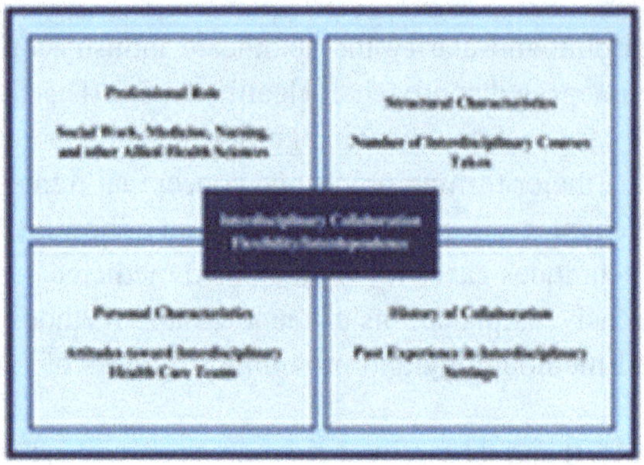

illnesses, such as diabetes, hypertension, and depression. The team works together to develop a comprehensive care plan that considers all aspects of the patient's health, leading to improved quality of life and more effective management.

2.1.2 Integration of Medical Disciplines for Comprehensive Care

Healthcare 5.0 places a strong emphasis on the integration of medical specializations in recognition of the human body's complexity as a networked system. This integration enables a comprehensive picture of a patient's condition, leading to more accurate diagnoses and customised treatment plans. Healthcare 5.0 integrates evidence-based alternative and complementary therapies with standard medicine to promote overall wellbeing and patient empowerment (Mehrabi et al. 2019). A patient with chronic pain may benefit from an integrated approach that combines pain management techniques like physical therapy and medicine with complementary therapies like acupuncture and meditation for stress reduction. This comprehensive therapy plan of action addresses emotional and psychological issues in addition to the physical causes of pain, leading to improved pain alleviation and general health.

2.2 Technological Advancements in Healthcare 5.0

2.2.1 Artificial Intelligence and Machine Learning

AI and ML, you know, are crucial elements in Healthcare 5.0 that change a lot of aspects of healthcare delivery. Therefore, these tools analyze massive amounts of data, identify patterns in the data, and provide meaningful information for customized treatment plans, early sickness detection, and improved patient outcomes. Additionally, AI-powered diagnostic tools and decision support systems have made it possible for healthcare workers to make clinical decisions more rapidly and accurately. For example, AI systems are completely capable of analyzing medical images, such as MRIs and X-rays, to assist radiologists in more precisely identifying irregularities. Additionally, medical teams can anticipate patient readmission risk by utilizing machine learning (ML) models.

2.2.2 Internet of Things (IoT) in Healthcare

The Internet of Things (IoT) consists of networked sensors and gadgets that gather and share data. IoT-enabled wearables and medical devices enable patients to track their health in real-time in Healthcare 5.0, enabling remote patient monitoring and early health issue detection. By giving medical professionals access to vital patient data, these gadgets enhance treatment efficiency and coordination (Beede et al. 2020). For instance, IoT-enabled glucose monitors can provide information to healthcare practitioners while continuously monitoring the blood sugar levels of diabetic patients. This makes it possible for medical staff to remotely track changes in blood sugar levels and promptly intervene or modify a patient's treatment regimen. The networked integration of medical systems and devices, shown in Figure 4, allows for data sharing and remote monitoring to enhance patient outcomes and healthcare productivity.

2.2.3 Big Data Analytics and Predictive Modelling

Large-scale databases are tapped into using big data analytics in Healthcare 5.0 to find trends, patterns, and correlations that guide evidence-based medical decisions. Forecasting illness patterns, identifying patient populations at high risk, and allocating resources optimally in healthcare institutions are all made possible by predictive modeling. For instance, big data analytics can forecast the occurrence of disease outbreaks, like flu epidemics, by analyzing demographic information, electronic health records, and environmental factors. Public health authorities can use this information to strategically allocate medical resources and put preventive measures into place.

2.2.4 Telemedicine and Virtual Care

In Healthcare 5.0, telemedicine and virtual care have become increasingly popular, particularly in the wake of the COVID-19 epidemic. By facilitating virtual diagnosis, digital health monitoring, and remote consultations, these technologies increase access to healthcare services while lessening the strain on traditional healthcare facilities. Example: Using a virtual telemedicine platform, a patient in a remote

Figure 4. Internet of things (IoT) in healthcare

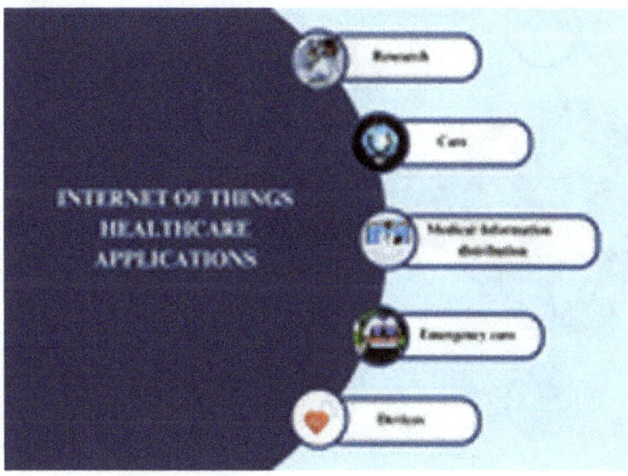

location can consult with a specialist in a nearby city. This eliminates the need for the patient to make lengthy trips by giving them rapid access to professional medical advice.

2.2.5 Wearable Devices and Remote Patient Monitoring

In Healthcare 5.0, wearable technology has gained popularity as it enables patients to continuously monitor their health parameters. By keeping an eye on vital signs, exercise, sleep habits, and other health indicators, these gadgets help patients and medical professionals address diseases early on. An illustration of this would be a patient with heart disease who wears a smartwatch to track heart rhythm and rate. The patient's medical team receives an alert from the gadget if it notices any abnormalities, which triggers timely follow-up care to avoid any complications.

These fundamental components spur innovation and revolutionize healthcare delivery as Healthcare 5.0 develops. While technological innovations empower patients and healthcare providers to make informed decisions, enhance outcomes, and build a more connected and patient-centric healthcare ecosystem, interdisciplinary teamwork assures a holistic approach to patient care (van Berkel, Sarsenbayeva, and Goncalves 2023). By embracing these pillars, Healthcare 5.0 has the ability to transform contemporary medicine and improve people's quality of life everywhere. In Figure 5, real-time medical data is provided and health metrics are tracked through the use of portable devices, which improves patient participation and allows for proactive healthcare management.

3. KEY COMPONENTS OF HEALTHCARE 5.0

Healthcare 5.0 embodies a patient-centric approach that leverages cutting-edge technology and interdisciplinary collaboration to transform the landscape of healthcare. This chapter delves into the core components of Healthcare 5.0, highlighting the significance of personalized and precision medicine, patient-centered care, prevention, and care coordination to optimize patient outcomes and improve overall well-being.

Figure 5. Wearable devices and remote patient monitoring

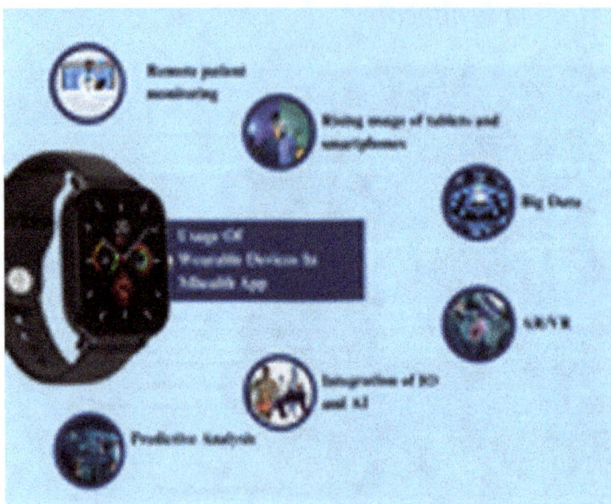

3.1 Personalized and Precision Medicine

3.1.1 Genomic Medicine and Targeted Therapies

In Healthcare 5.0, genomic medicine plays a pivotal role in tailoring treatments based on a patient's genetic makeup. Advancements in genomic sequencing enable healthcare providers to identify specific genetic variations that influence disease susceptibility, response to medications, and disease progression. Targeted therapies focus on addressing these genetic anomalies, maximizing treatment efficacy, and minimizing adverse effects. *Example:* In the case of certain cancers, genomic profiling of the tumor can reveal specific genetic mutations. Targeted therapies can then be prescribed to inhibit the growth of cancer cells with precision, sparing healthy cells and improving treatment outcomes (Wazid, Das, et al. 2022).

3.1.2 Biomarkers and Diagnostic Advancements

Healthcare 5.0 incorporates biomarkers as valuable tools for early disease detection, risk assessment, and treatment monitoring. Biomarkers are measurable indicators that provide insights into a patient's health status at the molecular level. Diagnostic advancements, such as liquid biopsies and novel imaging techniques, aid in the identification of biomarkers, enabling early interventions and personalized treatment strategies. *Example:* Biomarker testing in cardiovascular disease helps identify patients at high risk of heart attacks. This allows healthcare professionals to implement preventive measures, such as lifestyle modifications and medication, to reduce the risk of adverse cardiac events. Figure 6 involves tailoring medical treatments and interventions to individual characteristics, genetics, and health profiles, optimizing effectiveness and minimizing side effects.

3.2 Patient-Centered Care and Shared Decision-Making

3.2.1 Empowering Patients in Their Healthcare Journey

Healthcare 5.0 emphasizes the empowerment of patients as active participants in their healthcare journey. Patient-centered care recognizes the unique needs, values, and preferences of individuals, fostering a collaborative partnership between patients and healthcare providers. Patients are encouraged to take ownership of their health, make informed decisions, and actively engage in shared decision-making.

Figure 6. Personalized and precision medicine

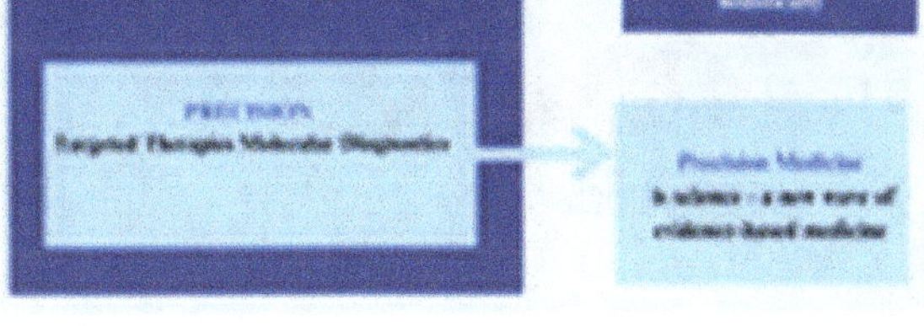

Example: Through patient-centered care, a diabetic patient is involved in setting personalized treatment goals, choosing appropriate medication options, and deciding on lifestyle modifications. This approach fosters adherence to the treatment plan and enhances overall treatment success (Wazid, Bera, et al. 2022).

3.2.2 Shared Decision-Making Tools and Patient Education

Healthcare 5.0 integrates shared decision-making tools and patient education resources to facilitate informed choices and enhance health literacy. Decision aids, educational materials, and interactive platforms empower patients to understand their health conditions, available treatment options, and potential risks and benefits, enabling them to make well-informed decisions. *Example:* A shared decision-making tool for prostate cancer treatment options presents patients with detailed information about surgery, radiation therapy, and active surveillance. With this knowledge, the patient can collaboratively decide on the most suitable treatment based on their preferences and priorities. Figure 7 illustrates the process of involving patients in medical choices by providing them with information, resources, and interactive tools to make informed decisions aligned with their preferences and values.

3.3 Prevention and Wellness Promotion

3.3.1 Focus on Proactive and Preventive Measures

Healthcare 5.0 shifts the focus from reactive treatment to proactive prevention. Preventive measures, such as vaccinations, screenings, and lifestyle interventions, are prioritized to identify and address health risks before they escalate into chronic conditions. By emphasizing prevention, Healthcare 5.0 aims to reduce the burden of disease and improve overall population health. *Example:* Immunization programs prevent the spread of infectious diseases, such as measles and influenza. By vaccinating individuals, Healthcare 5.0 contributes to herd immunity, protecting vulnerable populations and reducing the occurrence of outbreaks.

Figure 7. Shared decision-making tools and patient education

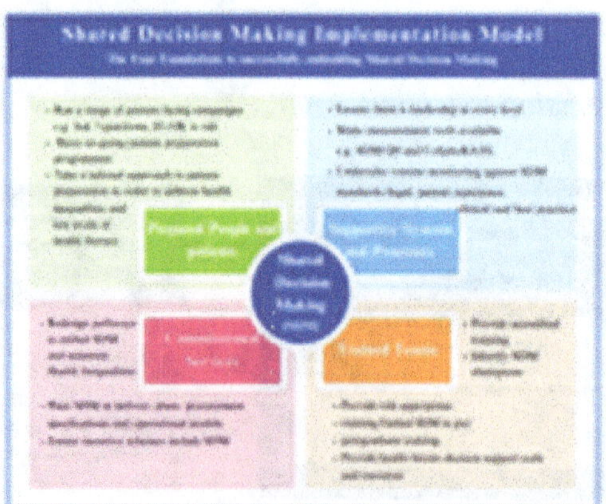

3.3.2 Integrating Lifestyle Medicine and Behavioural Health

Healthcare 5.0 recognizes the crucial role of lifestyle factors and behavioural health in maintaining overall well-being. Lifestyle medicine interventions, including nutrition counselling, exercise prescriptions, and stress management, are incorporated into patient care plans to support health promotion and disease prevention. *Example:* A patient at risk of developing type 2 diabetes receives lifestyle medicine counselling, including dietary recommendations and physical activity plans. These interventions empower the patient to make positive lifestyle changes, potentially preventing or delaying the onset of diabetes. Figure 8 outlines strategies, interventions, and education aimed at proactively maintaining and improving individuals' health, reducing the risk of diseases, and enhancing overall well-being.

3.4 Continuum of Care and Care Coordination

3.4.1 Seamless Transition Across Healthcare Settings

Healthcare 5.0 prioritizes the seamless transition of patients across different healthcare settings to ensure continuous and coordinated care. Effective care coordination involves clear communication between healthcare providers, smooth transitions from hospital to home or rehabilitation facilities, and the integration of services to avoid gaps in care (Rahman et al. 2023). *Example:* A patient undergoing hip replacement surgery receives coordinated care from the hospital team, the physical therapist, and the home health nurse during post-operative recovery. This integrated approach supports the patient's successful rehabilitation and reduces the risk of complications.

3.4.2 Integrated Electronic Health Records and Interoperability

Healthcare 5.0 leverages electronic health records (EHRs) to consolidate patient information, ensuring healthcare providers have access to comprehensive medical histories, test results, and treatment plans. Interoperability allows EHRs to seamlessly exchange information between different healthcare systems, enhancing care coordination and reducing redundancies. *Example:* With interoperable EHRs, a patient's

Figure 8. Prevention and wellness promotion

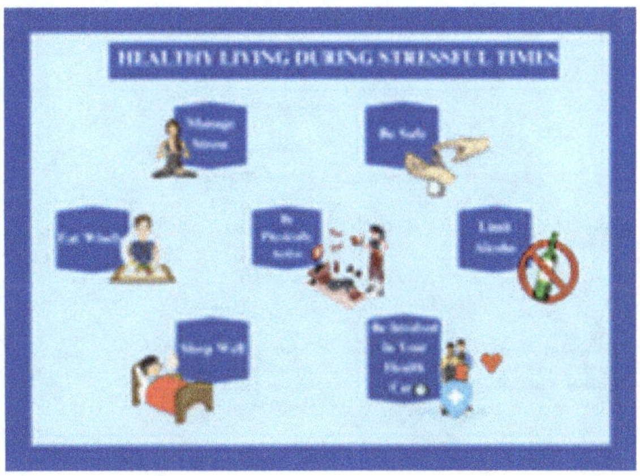

primary care physician can easily access the medical records from a recent hospital visit, facilitating informed decision-making and providing comprehensive care. Figure 9 depicts the seamless sharing and exchange of patient health information across different healthcare systems and providers, enabling comprehensive and coordinated care while maintaining data accuracy and privacy.

4. BENEFITS AND IMPACTS OF HEALTHCARE 5.0

Healthcare 5.0 represents a transformative approach to medicine, harnessing advanced technologies and patient-centered practices to revolutionize healthcare delivery. This chapter explores the far-reaching benefits and impactful outcomes of Healthcare 5.0, ranging from improved health outcomes and enhanced patient experiences to more efficient and cost-effective healthcare delivery. Figure 10 illustrates the transformative effects of the fifth wave of healthcare evolution, characterized by patient-centric care, advanced technologies, data-driven insights, and improved outcomes, ultimately leading to enhanced patient experiences and population health.

4.1 Improved Health Outcomes

4.1.1 Early Disease Detection and Prevention

One of the significant benefits of Healthcare 5.0 is the early detection and prevention of diseases. Through the integration of advanced diagnostics, predictive modelling, and patient monitoring technologies, Healthcare 5.0 enables healthcare providers to identify health risks and diseases at their earliest stages. Timely interventions allow for early treatment, preventing the progression of diseases and reducing long-term complications.

Impact: Early detection of conditions such as cancer, cardiovascular diseases, and diabetes can lead to more successful treatment outcomes, increased survival rates, and improved quality of life for patients.

Figure 9. Integrated electronic health records and interoperability

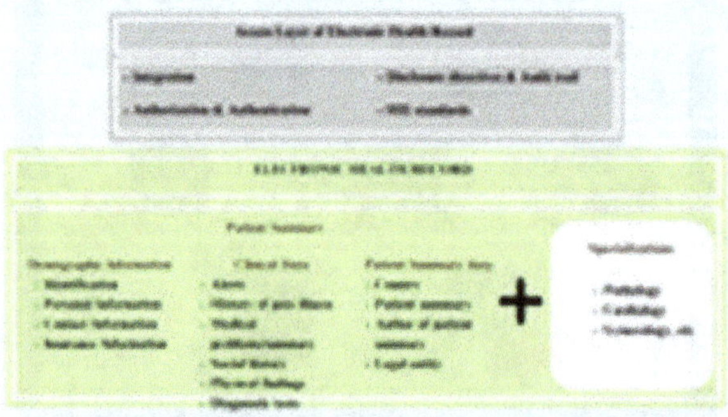

Figure 10. Benefits and impacts of Healthcare 5.0

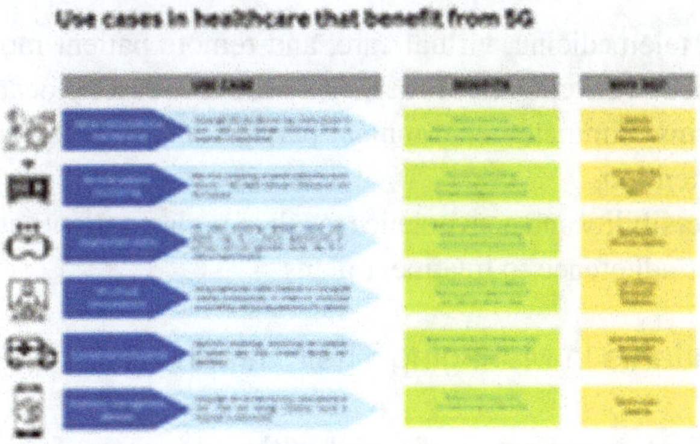

4.1.2 Enhanced Treatment Outcomes and Reduced Complications

Healthcare 5.0 leverages personalized and precision medicine to tailor treatments based on an individual's unique characteristics. By integrating genomic medicine, targeted therapies, and biomarker-driven approaches, Healthcare 5.0 optimizes treatment efficacy and minimizes adverse effects. Additionally, patient-centered care and shared decision-making ensure that treatment plans align with patients' preferences and needs, resulting in improved treatment adherence and outcomes (Paterick et al. 2017).

Impact: Enhanced treatment outcomes translate to reduced hospital readmissions, lower healthcare costs, and improved overall patient well-being.

4.2 Enhanced Patient Experience and Engagement

The table 1 outlines how modern healthcare practices and technologies contribute to improving the overall patient experience and engagement.

Table 1. Enhanced patient experience and engagement

Factors	Patient Engagement	Patient Experience
Goals	Drive better health and outcomes. Empower patients and loved ones to be active in their own care. Reduce costs.	Drive better health and outcomes. Exceed expectations. Reduce suffering. Brand differentiation.
Stakeholders	Patient, likely others.	Patient, likely others.
Context	Patient's own health.	All-encompassing (access communication, food, etc.)
Patent involvement (Behaviors and ownership)	Required	Not required (through in an ideal experience, patient are partners and co-designers)
Time	Patient, likely others	Transactional and Longitudinal
Use of health self-management tool/services	Yes	No
Validated measurement	Patient Activation Measure (PAM) PROMIS, Patient Health Engagement (PHE) Scale	HCAHPS, CGCAHPS, etc.

4.2.1 Accessible and Convenient Healthcare Services

Healthcare 5.0 embraces telemedicine, virtual care, and remote patient monitoring, enabling patients to access healthcare services conveniently from their homes or remote locations. Virtual consultations and digital health platforms eliminate geographical barriers and reduce wait times, ensuring patients receive timely medical attention.

Impact: Increased accessibility and convenience result in higher patient satisfaction, improved healthcare utilization, and better adherence to treatment plans.

4.2.2 Empowered Patients in Managing Their Health

Healthcare 5.0 places patients at the center of their healthcare journey, fostering patient empowerment and engagement. Through shared decision-making, patient education, and health monitoring tools, patients are actively involved in making informed choices about their health and treatment options. This collaborative approach promotes self-management and encourages patients to take ownership of their well-being.

Impact: Empowered patients are more likely to comply with treatment regimens, adopt healthier lifestyles, and proactively manage chronic conditions, leading to better health outcomes and reduced healthcare utilization.

4.3 Efficient and Cost-Effective Healthcare Delivery

4.3.1 Streamlined Care Processes and Reduced Inefficiencies

Healthcare 5.0 optimizes care delivery through interoperable electronic health records, AI-driven diagnostics, and care coordination platforms. These technologies streamline care processes, reducing administrative burdens and eliminating redundant procedures. Additionally, interdisciplinary collaboration promotes efficient communication among healthcare teams, ensuring a coordinated approach to patient care.

Impact: Streamlined care processes improve healthcare provider productivity, reduce wait times for patients, and enhance overall healthcare system efficiency.

4.3.2 Optimal Resource Utilization and Healthcare Expenditure

Healthcare 5.0 emphasizes prevention and proactive interventions, reducing the burden of disease on healthcare systems. By identifying high-risk populations and implementing preventive measures, Healthcare 5.0 reduces the need for costly treatments and hospitalizations. Moreover, personalized medicine and targeted therapies lead to better treatment efficacy, reducing wasteful spending on ineffective treatments (O'Regan et al. 2008).

Impact: Optimal resource utilization results in cost savings for healthcare institutions and payers, allowing for reinvestment in improved patient care and technological advancements.

In conclusion, the benefits and impacts of Healthcare 5.0 are far-reaching, transforming healthcare delivery across the globe. Improved health outcomes through early disease detection and precision medicine, enhanced patient experiences, and engagement through accessible healthcare services, and efficient, cost-effective care delivery are the hallmarks of Healthcare 5.0. By leveraging advanced technologies and patient-centric practices, Healthcare 5.0 represents the future of medicine, promising better health and well-being for individuals and societies as a whole.

5. CHALLENGES AND CONSIDERATIONS IN IMPLEMENTING HEALTHCARE 5.0

Healthcare 5.0 represents a promising future for healthcare, but its successful implementation comes with several challenges and considerations. This chapter explores the critical obstacles and factors that must be addressed to realize the full potential of Healthcare 5.0.

5.1 Ethical and Legal Implications

5.1.1 Privacy and Security of Patient Data

With the integration of advanced technologies and interconnected devices, patient data becomes more vulnerable to breaches and cyberattacks. Healthcare 5.0 must prioritize robust data security measures to protect sensitive patient information. Balancing data accessibility for medical research and treatment purposes with patient privacy rights poses a significant ethical challenge.

Consideration: Implementing strict data encryption, access controls, and regular security audits can safeguard patient data while complying with privacy regulations such as HIPAA.

5.1.2 Ethical Considerations in Using AI and IoT in Healthcare

Healthcare 5.0 relies heavily on AI and IoT, raising ethical concerns regarding algorithm transparency, bias, and accountability. Decisions made by AI systems in diagnosis and treatment plans must be explainable and understandable by healthcare professionals and patients. Ensuring that AI models are fair and do not perpetuate existing biases is crucial.

Consideration: Ethical frameworks and guidelines for the responsible use of AI and IoT in healthcare need to be established, and healthcare professionals should be involved in the development and validation of AI algorithms.

5.2 Workforce Readiness and Training

5.2.1 Preparing Healthcare Professionals for Integrated Care

Healthcare 5.0 demands a shift in the roles and responsibilities of healthcare professionals. Interdisciplinary collaboration and patient-centered care require effective communication and teamwork skills. Training healthcare professionals to work effectively in a multidisciplinary environment may pose challenges due to differing education backgrounds and institutional cultures (Mbunge, Jiyane, and Muchemwa 2022).

Consideration: Integrating interprofessional education into medical training and providing ongoing professional development opportunities can prepare healthcare professionals for collaborative care.

5.2.2 Upskilling and Adapting to Technological Advancements

As Healthcare 5.0 incorporates advanced technologies, the workforce needs to be proficient in leveraging these tools effectively. Some healthcare professionals may face challenges in adopting new technologies or may fear the displacement of traditional roles.

Consideration: Offering continuous training and support in using healthcare technologies can help healthcare professionals embrace innovations and enhance their technological fluency.

5.3 Infrastructure and Interoperability

5.3.1 Integration of Healthcare Systems and Data Sharing

Healthcare 5.0 requires seamless integration and interoperability among different healthcare systems, electronic health records, and medical devices. Legacy systems and proprietary formats may hinder data exchange and collaboration among healthcare providers.

Consideration: Investing in interoperable health IT solutions and fostering industry-wide data exchange standards can facilitate smoother data sharing and continuity of care.

5.3.2 Standardization and Interoperability Challenges

Healthcare 5.0 involves the integration of various technologies, which may use different data formats and standards. Achieving full interoperability among these technologies poses technical challenges and requires cooperation between vendors and healthcare institutions. Encouraging industry collaboration and promoting the adoption of international standards, such as HL7 and FHIR, can foster interoperability and data sharing (Maxhelaku and Kika 2019).

The implementation of Healthcare 5.0 faces several challenges, ranging from ethical and legal concerns surrounding data privacy and AI usage to the need for workforce readiness and training. Infrastructure and interoperability challenges also play a crucial role in realizing the full potential of integrated medicine and advanced technologies. Addressing these challenges requires a collaborative effort from healthcare stakeholders, policymakers, and technology providers to ensure that Healthcare 5.0 can effectively transform healthcare delivery, improve patient outcomes, and promote a more patient-centric and connected healthcare ecosystem.

6. CASE STUDIES AND EXEMPLARY MODELS OF HEALTHCARE 5.0

Healthcare 5.0 has witnessed successful implementations across various healthcare settings, showcasing the transformative power of integrated medicine and advanced technologies. This chapter examines exemplary models and real-world case studies that exemplify the principles and benefits of Healthcare 5.0.

6.1 Successful Implementations of Integrated Medicine

6.1.1 Collaborative Healthcare Networks and Accountable Care Organizations

Case Study: Geisinger Health System

Geisinger Health System, based in Pennsylvania, USA, is a pioneering example of an integrated health network that embodies the principles of Healthcare 5.0. Geisinger focuses on value-based care delivery through its ProvenCare® program, which utilizes evidence-based clinical pathways and interdisciplinary care teams to optimize patient outcomes(Lampley and Therrien 2023).

Impact: Geisinger's ProvenCare® program has shown remarkable results in reducing complications, readmissions, and overall healthcare costs for specific conditions, such as heart failure and joint replacement surgeries.

6.1.2 Integrated Health Systems and Population Health Management

Case Study: Kaiser Permanente

Kaiser Permanente, a large integrated health system in the United States, emphasizes population health management through its comprehensive approach to patient care. The organization leverages EHRs, data analytics, and care coordination to proactively identify health risks, manage chronic conditions, and promote preventive measures among its patient population (Nathaniel et al. 2021).

Impact: Kaiser Permanente's population health management approach has led to improved health outcomes, reduced hospitalizations, and better patient engagement, contributing to higher patient satisfaction rates.

6.2. Real-World Examples of Healthcare 5.0 in Action

6.2.1 Remote Patient Monitoring for Chronic Disease Management

Case Study: University of Mississippi Medical Center (UMMC)

UMMC implemented a remote patient monitoring program for patients with chronic conditions, such as hypertension, diabetes, and heart failure. Patients use wearable devices and IoT-enabled health monitoring tools to transmit vital data, such as blood pressure, blood glucose levels, and weight, to healthcare providers in real-time. Healthcare teams use this data to track patients' health status and intervene promptly if any abnormalities are detected (Peyroteo et al. 2021).

Impact: The remote patient monitoring program at UMMC has led to improved patient adherence to treatment plans, early detection of health issues, and reduced hospitalizations among chronic disease patients.

6.2.2 AI-Powered Clinical Decision Support Systems

Case Study: IBM Watson for Oncology

IBM Watson for Oncology is an AI-powered clinical decision support system that assists oncologists in formulating personalized cancer treatment plans. The system analyzes vast amounts of medical literature, clinical trial data, and patient records to provide evidence-based treatment recommendations aligned with the patient's specific cancer type, stage, and genetic profile (Somashekhar et al. 2017).

Impact: IBM Watson for Oncology has demonstrated its ability to assist oncologists in making more informed treatment decisions, potentially expanding treatment options, and improving patient outcomes.

These case studies and exemplary models demonstrate the successful implementation of Healthcare 5.0 principles in real-world healthcare settings. Collaborative healthcare networks, integrated health systems, remote patient monitoring, and AI-powered clinical decision support systems showcase the transformative potential of integrated medicine and technology in improving patient care, enhancing outcomes, and optimizing healthcare delivery. As more healthcare organizations and institutions embrace Healthcare 5.0, the potential for positive impact on patient well-being and the future of medicine continues to grow.

7. FUTURE DIRECTIONS AND OUTLOOK

Healthcare 5.0 holds immense potential to revolutionize the healthcare landscape and improve patient outcomes. As the field continues to evolve, several anticipated advancements and societal implications are likely to shape the future of Healthcare 5.0.

7.1 Anticipated Advancements in Healthcare 5.0

7.1.1 Genomic Medicine and Personalized Therapeutics

Genomic medicine is expected to become increasingly prevalent in Healthcare 5.0. Advancements in genetic sequencing technologies and bioinformatics will enable more comprehensive and affordable genome profiling. As a result, personalized therapeutics tailored to an individual's genetic makeup will become more commonplace, optimizing treatment efficacy and minimizing adverse effects(Streeter, Beron, and Iyer 2017).

Anticipated Impact: Personalized therapeutics will lead to more precise and targeted treatments for various diseases, increasing treatment success rates and enhancing patient quality of life.

7.1.2 Advancements in AI and Machine Learning Applications

AI and machine learning will continue to drive significant advancements in Healthcare 5.0. AI-powered diagnostic tools, predictive modeling, and decision support systems will become more sophisticated and accurate, empowering healthcare professionals with data-driven insights. Additionally, AI-driven robotics and automation may enhance surgical precision and streamline administrative processes.

Anticipated Impact: AI advancements will improve diagnostic accuracy, streamline healthcare workflows, and potentially alleviate healthcare workforce shortages, leading to more efficient and cost-effective healthcare delivery.

7.2 Societal Impact and Implications

7.2.1 Accessible Healthcare for Underserved Populations

Healthcare 5.0 has the potential to address healthcare disparities and improve accessibility for underserved populations. Telemedicine and virtual care platforms can bridge the gap between patients and healthcare providers in remote or rural areas. Moreover, AI-driven diagnostics and point-of-care technologies may enhance early disease detection and treatment in resource-limited settings.

Anticipated Impact: Improved accessibility to healthcare services can lead to better health outcomes and reduced healthcare disparities among marginalized communities.

7.2.2 Redefining the Role of Healthcare Professionals

Healthcare 5.0 will reshape the roles and responsibilities of healthcare professionals. With the integration of AI and automation, routine tasks may be delegated to technology, allowing healthcare professionals to focus on more complex and patient-centric aspects of care. Emphasizing patient education and empowerment will further shift the role of healthcare professionals from being purely authoritative to collaborative partners in patients' health journeys.

Anticipated Impact: Redefining the role of healthcare professionals will enhance patient engagement, improve communication, and foster stronger therapeutic relationships.

In conclusion, the future of Healthcare 5.0 holds exciting possibilities with anticipated advancements in genomic medicine, AI applications, and personalized therapeutics. As these technologies mature and become more accessible, healthcare delivery is expected to become more precise, efficient, and patient-centered (Xu, Wermus, and Bauman 2011). Moreover, the societal impact of Healthcare 5.0 is poised to extend accessibility to healthcare services for underserved populations and redefine the roles of healthcare professionals, enhancing patient care and well-being across the globe. By embracing the principles of integrated medicine and leveraging cutting-edge technologies, Healthcare 5.0 is poised to shape a more connected, efficient, and patient-centric healthcare ecosystem in the years to come.

8. CONCLUSION

This book chapter provides a comprehensive exploration of Healthcare 5.0, envisioning a transformative future for healthcare delivery through integrated medicine. The evolution from traditional practices to patient-centric care and interdisciplinary collaboration characterizes this paradigm shift. Anchored in personalized and precision medicine, patient-centered care, prevention, and care coordination, Healthcare 5.0 empowers patients, optimizes treatment outcomes, and enhances proactive health management. The paradigm offers numerous benefits, including improved health outcomes via early disease detection and precision medicine, enriched patient experiences, and efficient, cost-effective healthcare delivery. However, challenges such as ethical, legal, workforce, and infrastructure considerations must be navigated for successful integration. Real-world case studies showcasing collaborative networks, remote patient monitoring, and AI-driven clinical decision support systems underscore the potential of merging medicine and technology in Healthcare 5.0's success.

Envisioning the future of integrated medicine within the Healthcare 5.0 framework anticipates transformative advancements in healthcare. This future encompasses precise personalized treatments through genomic medicine and AI, patient empowerment fostering accessible care, collaborative healthcare professional efforts integrating AI, telemedicine, and data sharing, a holistic approach emphasizing well-being, and efficient, cost-effective healthcare via technology-driven solutions and coordinated care. Ultimately, Healthcare 5.0 embodies a patient-centered, collaborative, and technology-empowered paradigm poised to revolutionize healthcare, promising enhanced patient outcomes, inclusivity, and a more interconnected and streamlined healthcare landscape, with the potential to shape a healthier and empowered society.

REFERENCES

Beede, E. (2020). A Human-Centered Evaluation of a Deep Learning System Deployed in Clinics for the Detection of Diabetic Retinopathy. In *Proceedings of the 2020 CHI Conference on Human Factors in Computing Systems* (pp. 1–12). ACM. doi:10.1145/3313831.3376718

Johnson, K. B., Wei, W.-Q., Weeraratne, D., Frisse, M. E., Misulis, K., Rhee, K., Zhao, J., & Snowdon, J. L. (2021). Precision Medicine, AI, and the Future of Personalized Health Care. *Clinical and Translational Science*, *14*(1), 86–93. doi:10.1111/cts.12884 PMID:32961010

Lampley, K., & Therrien, N. (2023). *Geisinger Ambulatory Pharmacy Care Program Field Notes*. https://stacks.cdc.gov/view/cdc/126232

Lemmen, C., Simic, D., & Stock, S. (2021). A Vision of Future Healthcare: Potential Opportunities and Risks of Systems Medicine from a Citizen and Patient Perspective—Results of a Qualitative Study. *International Journal of Environmental Research and Public Health*, *18*(18), 9879. doi:10.3390/ijerph18189879 PMID:34574802

Lilhore, U. K., Dalal, S., Faujdar, N., Margala, M., Chakrabarti, P., Chakrabarti, T., Simaiya, S., Kumar, P., Thangaraju, P., & Velmurugan, H. (2023). Hybrid CNN-LSTM model with efficient hyperparameter tuning for prediction of Parkinson's disease. *Scientific Reports*, *13*(1), 14605. doi:10.1038/s41598-023-41314-y PMID:37669970

Lilhore, U. K., Dalal, S., Faujdar, N., Simaiya, S., Dahiya, M., Tomar, S., & Hashmi, A. (2024). Unveiling the prevalence and risk factors of early stage postpartum depression: A hybrid deep learning approach. *Multimedia Tools and Applications*, 1–35. doi:10.1007/s11042-024-18182-3

Lilhore, U. K., Manoharan, P., Sandhu, J. K., Simaiya, S., Dalal, S., Baqasah, A. M., Alsafyani, M., Alroobaea, R., Keshta, I., & Raahemifar, K. (2023). Hybrid model for precise hepatitis-C classification using improved random forest and SVM method. *Scientific Reports*, *13*(1), 12473. doi:10.1038/s41598-023-36605-3 PMID:37528148

Lilhore, U. K., Poongodi, M., Kaur, A., Simaiya, S., Algarni, A. D., Elmannai, H., Vijayakumar, V., Tunze, G. B., & Hamdi, M. (2022). Hybrid model for detection of cervical cancer using causal analysis and machine learning techniques. *Computational and Mathematical Methods in Medicine*, *2022*, 2022. doi:10.1155/2022/4688327 PMID:35572826

Lilhore, U. K., Simaiya, S., Pandey, H., Gautam, V., Garg, A., & Ghosh, P. (2022). Breast cancer detection in the IoT cloud-based healthcare environment using fuzzy cluster segmentation and SVM classifier. *Proceedings of RACCCS*, *2021*, 165–179.

Lilhore, U. K., Simaiya, S., Prasad, D., & Guleria, K. (2020). A hybrid tumor detection and classification based on machine learning. *Journal of Computational and Theoretical Nanoscience*, *17*(6), 2539–2544. doi:10.1166/jctn.2020.8927

Maxhelaku, S., & Kika, A. (2019). Improving interoperability in healthcare using HL7 FHIR. In *Proceedings of the 47th International Academic Conference*. International Institute of Social and Economic Sciences. doi:10.20472/IAC.2019.047.012

Mbunge, E., Sipho'esihle, J., & Muchemwa, B. (2022). Towards Emotive Sensory Web in Virtual Health Care: Trends, Technologies, Challenges and Ethical Issues. *Sensors International*, *3*, 100134. doi:10.1016/j.sintl.2021.100134

MehrabiN.2019). *A Survey on Bias and Fairness in Machine Learning*. http://arxiv.org/abs/1908.09635

Nathaniel, T. I., Goodwin, R. L., Fowler, L., McPhail, B., & Black, A. C. Jr. (2021). An Adaptive Blended Learning Model for the Implementation of an Integrated Medical Neuroscience Course During the Covid-19 Pandemic. *Anatomical Sciences Education*, *14*(6), 699–710. doi:10.1002/ase.2097 PMID:33915035

O'Regan, D., Shah, S., Mirsadraee, S., Al-Ruzzeh, S., Karthik, S., & Jarvis, M. (2008). Implementation of a Process-Orientated Multidisciplinary Approach (POMA), a System of Cost-Effective Healthcare Delivery within a Cardiac Surgical Unit. *Quality & Safety in Health Care*, *17*(6), 459–463. doi:10.1136/qshc.2006.021279 PMID:19064663

Onyema, E. M., Lilhore, U. K., Saurabh, P., Dalal, S., Nwaeze, A. S., Chijindu, A. T., Ndufeiya-Kumasi, L. C., & Simaiya, S. (2023). Evaluation of IoT-Enabled hybrid model for genome sequence analysis of patients in healthcare 4.0. *Measurement. Sensors*, *26*, 100679. doi:10.1016/j.measen.2023.100679

Paterick, T. E., Patel, N., Tajik, A. J., & Chandrasekaran, K. (2017). Improving Health Outcomes Through Patient Education and Partnerships with Patients. *Baylor University Medical Center Proceedings*, *30*(1), 112–13. https://www.tandfonline.com/doi/full/10.1080/08998280.2017.11929552

Peyroteo, M., Ferreira, I. A., Elvas, L. B., Ferreira, J. C., & Lapão, L. V. (2021). Remote Monitoring Systems for Patients With Chronic Diseases in Primary Health Care: Systematic Review. *JMIR mHealth and uHealth*, *9*(12), e28285. doi:10.2196/28285 PMID:34932000

Rahman, A., Hossain, M. S., Muhammad, G., Kundu, D., Debnath, T., Rahman, M., Khan, M. S. I., Tiwari, P., & Band, S. S. (2023). Federated Learning-Based AI Approaches in Smart Healthcare: Concepts, Taxonomies, Challenges and Open Issues. *Cluster Computing*, *26*(4), 2271–2311. doi:10.1007/s10586-022-03658-4 PMID:35996680

Seetharaman, M., Krishnan, G., & Schneider, R. H. (2021). The Future of Medicine: Frontiers in Integrative Health and Medicine. *Medicina, 57*(12), 1303. https://www.mdpi.com/1648-9144/57/12/1303

Somashekhar, S. P., Sepúlveda, M.-J., Norden, A. D., Rauthan, A., Arun, K., Patil, P., Ethadka, R. Y., & Kumar, R. C. (2017). Early Experience with IBM Watson for Oncology (WFO) Cognitive Computing System for Lung and Colorectal Cancer Treatment. *Journal of Clinical Oncology*, *35*(15, suppl), 8527–8527. doi:10.1200/JCO.2017.35.15_suppl.8527

Streeter, Beron, & Iyer. (2017). Precision Medicine. *Otolaryngologic Clinics of North America, 50*(4), 765–73. https://linkinghub.elsevier.com/retrieve/pii/S0030666517300609

Vale, D., El-Sharif, A., & Ali, M. (2022). Explainable Artificial Intelligence (XAI) Post-Hoc Explainability Methods: Risks and Limitations in Non-Discrimination Law. *AI and Ethics*, *2*(4), 815–826. doi:10.1007/s43681-022-00142-y

van Berkel, N., Sarsenbayeva, Z., & Goncalves, J. (2023). The Methodology of Studying Fairness Perceptions in Artificial Intelligence: Contrasting CHI and FAccT. *International Journal of Human-Computer Studies*, *170*, 102954. doi:10.1016/j.ijhcs.2022.102954

Wazid, M., Bera, B., Das, A. K., Mohanty, S. P., & Jo, M. (2022). Fortifying Smart Transportation Security Through Public Blockchain. *IEEE Internet of Things Journal*, *9*(17), 16532–16545. doi:10.1109/JIOT.2022.3150842

Wazid, M., Das, A. K., Mohd, N., & Park, Y. (2022). Healthcare 5.0 Security Framework: Applications, Issues and Future Research Directions. *IEEE Access : Practical Innovations, Open Solutions*, *10*, 129429–129442. doi:10.1109/ACCESS.2022.3228505

Xu, E., Wermus, M., & Bauman, D. B. (2011). Development of an Integrated Medical Supply Information System. *Enterprise Information Systems*, *5*(3), 385–399. doi:10.1080/17517575.2011.566630

Chapter 16
Overview of Federated Learning and Its Advantages

Alisha Kakkar
Banasthali Vidyapith, India

Sudesh Kumar
Banasthali Vidyapith, India

ABSTRACT

Federated learning (FL) is closely linked to decentralized education. A decentralized system primarily targets expediting the operation phase, whereas federated learning concentrates on constructing a cooperative prototype devoid of privacy disclosure. Some of the most notable and frequently utilized FL-driven applications include Android's Keyboard for smart typing assistance and Google Virtual Assistant. FL can address data distributed across rows based on specimens and data spread across columns based on features in a cooperative training environment. This chapter explores the fundamental principles of FL, elucidating its foundational technologies and structures. In this chapter, categorization and its utilization for market scenarios in the fields of data analytics, medical care, learning, and business are examined. This chapter also pinpoints research forefronts to tackle federated learning and contribute to progressing our comprehension of Federated Learning for forthcoming enhancement.

1. INTRODUCTION

With the continuous advancements in computing power and data retention capabilities, the importance of machine learning in the field of operations research becomes more apparent. The past years have witnessed the rapid growth of Machine Learning, Artificial Intelligence, and Intelligent Manufacturing in operational research (Lin, 2018). Still, two significant hurdles persist in this domain amidst machine learning advancements. Initially, data management stands out as the paramount factor. Certain information is deregulated due to legal considerations. The privacy and the legal protection provided by the EU Privacy Law ensures that individuals have authority over how their data is utilized. Breaking down information silos could lead to more effective instruction, but the existing compartmentalization

DOI: 10.4018/979-8-3693-1874-4.ch016

poses a barrier to achieving this improvement. AlphaGo, which relied on a large dataset of individual chess games and demonstrated the ability to outperform novice players, and Alpha Zero, which used significantly fewer human-generated chess records along with artificial data. Despite using less data, Alpha Zero achieved effortless victories against experienced opponents, showcasing advancements in AI capabilities and efficiency. Furthermore, data notation depends on proficient personnel in specific domains like the healthcare sector, which might result in a scarcity of reliable records. The insufficiency of annotated data also harms commercialized progress, but the rise of FL addresses these difficulties in this sector. FL is an emerging approach to artificial intelligence that addresses the issue of isolated records whilst safeguarding information confidentiality. It pertains to numerous users (like smartphones, entities, corporations, etc.) synchronized with one or more main servers for distributed cognitive computing configurations. In 2016, Google initially proposed anticipating user-generated text across numerous smartphones while retaining information on the gadgets (McMahan et al., 2017). This variant of the collaborative learning method is called the federated average. This forms the foundation of Federated Learning in numerous other studies. Initially, each gadget acquires a standard worldwide prototype for subsequent decentralized learning. Next, the installed prototype undergoes enhancements through various settings using records specific to each android phone. Subsequently, the relevant information is encrypted before being uploaded to the cloud. Then, the mean adjustment of local prototypes executed in the cloud is sent to the phone as an updated worldwide prototype.

In conclusion, the processes above iterate until the prototype attains a specific targeted efficiency or the ultimate time limit is met. The advent of this technique is poised to resolve the conflict associated with information security and information exchange for distributed gadgets because information remains undisclosed to a third party. Federated Learning is suitable for use in scenarios where information is confidential. In medical or android phones, legal constraints prevent the compilation of data, possibly for privacy or regulatory reasons.

2. ATTRIBUTES OF FEDERATED LEARNING

Federated Learning is closely linked to decentralized education. The classic scattered structure comprises scattered mathematics and scattered retention. The initial suggested Federated Learning of pattern revision for users is somewhat akin to dispersed arithmetic. Both Federated Learning and decentralized AI systems are strongly focused on ensuring the protection of privacy within decentralized systems. Dispersed handling involves linking numerous systems situated in various places through a network, all managed by a primary server. This enables each system to handle distinct segments of a shared work for completion. Consequently, a decentralized system primarily targets expediting the operation phase, whereas Federated Learning concentrates on constructing a cooperative prototype devoid of privacy disclosure.

2.1 Applicability in Inter-Entity Situations

Fundamentally, Federated Learning introduced by Google is a securely dispersed Artificial intelligence technique, enabling contributors to construct a collaborative learning prototype while retaining the foundational information on the device. It enables participants to collaboratively build a learning model while keeping the underlying data on their individual devices secure. Originally centered on security, Federated Learning has evolved to encompass any security-conscious, distributed, cooperative technology in artificial intelligence. The technique is capable of addressing data distributed across both rows based on samples and columns based on features in a cooperative training environment (Yang et al., 2019). It can also extend to incorporate collaborations between entities within a federal system. For example, when a financial institution possessing information on clients' purchasing capacity collaborates with a digital commerce system that holds data on product attributes. This collaboration allows the creation of a collective model that considers various organizations, diverse data sources, and distinct characteristics. The key outcome is the achievement of collaborative value across systems and locally while ensuring data privacy and security.

2.2 Highly Diverse Independent Allocation

In Federated Learning, information is distributed across numerous android phones. The amount of information that can be accessed or stored in any individual node is constrained by the overall count or quantity of nodes in the system or network. While the decentralized model aims for synchronization to alleviate the burden on the primary server, it may not have as many nodes as a Federated Learning system. The globe has ushered into a period of personal gadgets widely employed for health surveillance (Edwards, 2019). Every device solely produces a few data and cannot be juxtaposed with the overall count of gadgets. In this scenario, Federated Learning is better suited for enhancing prototypes. In contrast to the decentralized model, which operates mainly on evenly distributed and identically independent data, federated learning is focused on imbalanced and non-identically disconnected information due to diversity among gadget capabilities.

2.3 Distributed Technique

From a precisely technical perspective, distribution does not signify absolute distribution, but there is no conclusive epicenter. Dispersion is solely to diffuse the consciousness of the primary vertex. There is no central point or singular focus for understanding every customer. Instead, it implies that each customer has an impact on the overall or primary system. The impact among nodes produces an indirect association across the network that customers create. Parameter hub, a representative hybrid technique, primarily utilizes a primary server that controls the dissemination of information allocation and processing capabilities to achieve an effective collective system (Ho et al., 2013). This type of consolidated data handling approach leads to a dual messaging burden This occurs when specific data scattered across different databases is collected for learning purposes. The information must then be duplicated and transmitted to the primary server in the initial stages of the process. Subsequently, the main host will distribute data to each decentralized customer for decentralized processing. It introduces extra rigorous challenges to the system regarding processing capability, storage, and network speed. In scenarios within Federated Learning, every customer is entirely independent. A central entity does not assign data, and the host does not regulate the learning approach. Hence, Federated Learning is a comprehensive technique that merges computational learning and integrated data via distributed cooperation.

2.4 Uniformity of Condition for Each Intersection

Every participant experiences identical status and specific authority within this collaborative structure to attain shared success. Regarding parity, whoever possesses the vast majority of information takes the leading role in traditional decentralized collective learning. Therefore, the progress of cooperative training in the commercial sector might be adversely affected by the bias towards enterprises with an abundance of data or visuals featuring various classifications. In the realm of collaborative learning within Artificial intelligence, entities possessing substantial datasets could exert influence over the assuming framework, resulting in a lack of motivation for nano-scale enterprises to engage in collaborative learning. However, in Federated Learning, the elevation of customers with limited data would be fostered owing to parity among all stakeholders. In conclusion, Federated Learning is a distributed technique that facilitates dispersed customers or entities to train a collective system independently while maintaining data localization. This approach can assist corporate entities in exchanging collaborative frameworks without divulging unprocessed data.

3. COMMUNITY-DRIVEN SYSTEM

There are currently two prevalent community-driven systems for Federated Learning, and they are beginning to solidify. One is the TensorFlow Federated (TFF) model, which caters to the requirements of Artificial intelligence or other deep machine learning needs for distributed datasets. This represented the first standalone model designed for the manufacturing stage, specifically tailored for Android devices. Specifically, TFF incorporates FedAvg for modification and safe consolidation to address privacy considerations. The TensorFlow model encompasses the FL Application Programming Interface and the Federated Core (FC) Application Programming Interface. Specifically, the FL Application Programming Interface provides a suite of high-level junctions, enabling customers to apply the incorporated deep learning approach for Federated Learning. The FC Application Programming Interface and the foundational stratum for computational training functions in the decentralized system. Additionally, it has been effectively utilized in subsequent predictive typing or Emoji forecasting within a phone keypad (Ramaswamy et al., 2019). In actual deployment, it has realized execution across numerous gadgets, with the aspiration of achieving extensive growth to manage algorithms across multiple devices. The alternate framework is the Federated Artificial Intelligence Technique Enabler (FATE). Being the initial community-driven commercial-grade model, it predominantly caters to collaborative enterprise design. It ensures ample privacy for the customers through privacy-preserving encryption and collaborative computation. Additionally, diverse deep learning techniques like task transfer and logistic models can be constructed within this decentralized system. Moreover, with this pre-configured method, most conventional approaches can be adjusted to fit this federal framework. Webank Group has advanced the deployment of a range of FATE instances in credit threat management, product identification, and financial crime. Both models are widely adopted in practical scenarios for federated learning, and there are ongoing efforts to improve their methods.

4. CLASSIFICATION OF FEDERATED LEARNING

Federated Learning can be broadly classified into Vertical Federated Learning, Horizontal Federated Learning, and Federated Transfer Learning. As data housed in various nodes or organizations predominantly takes the form of a data matrix, it is typical for data to encompass numerous cases. Furthermore, the sheet's lateral axis is considered the user, with the perpendicular axis denoting the user attributes.

4.1 Vertical Federated Learning

Vertical Federated Learning is appropriate for scenarios where information is divided vertically based on the input space (Figure 1). Each involved participant possesses uniform data, signifying a partial intersection in specimen ID. However, they vary in dimensionality. As an illustration, consider a healthcare facility aiming to predict conditions like diabetes. As per investigations, individuals experiencing elevated hypertension and overweight might be susceptible to the onset of type 2 diabetes. Consequently, it could be examined considering specific approximate sizes including factors like age group and body weight alongside their health record. Suppose a youthful individual without hypertension or overweight exists but has a higher caloric consumption and a deficiency in exercise. He is also at risk of acquiring high blood sugar levels, yet forecasting and personalization remain challenging due to data gaps. With the advancement of Federated Learning, collaboration can be established with firms possessing data from mobile apps, including a step meter or nutritional framework. Additionally, they can collaborate seamlessly without the necessity of transmitting unprocessed information. Typically, researchers address this issue by extracting identical individuals involving diverse attributes to undergo collaborative learning. Compared to horizontal Federated Learning, this constitutes a more intricate task due to record linkage. It's not as straightforward as the scenario in horizontal Federated Learning. Pooling all data on a shared platform for learning within a global framework is ineffective in vertical Federated Learning, as the alignment between distinct data holders remains a significant issue yet to be resolved. Nock and co-authors devised a comprehensive plan for a straight-line model and employed privacy-preserving encryption to safeguard against a truthful yet inquisitive opponent in vertical federated learning (Nock et al., 2017). Reports indicated that existing uses for entities sharing a mutual event space, such as evaluations for driving offences and small business credit analysis, rely on FATE. However, these approaches are only applicable to basic deep learning techniques like machine learning (Cheng et al., 2019). As a result, there is considerable scope for enhancement in vertical federated learning to facilitate its application in more intricate algorithms.

4.2 Horizontal Federated Learning

In horizontal federated learning, there is a degree of overlap among the characteristics of the dataset distributed across different nodes, even though the data varies significantly in potential outcomes. Currently, the prevailing federated learning computations are predominantly designed for intelligent gadgets or appliances within the smart devices network. In these situations, federated learning is commonly categorized as horizontal federated learning. Since the dataset can markedly vary within the potential outcome but concurrently share analogous variable spaces. As previously noted, the resolution for updating smartphone devices proposed by Google generally constitutes a type of horizontal federated learning. In response to the constraint of a scarcity of marked objects, Gao and co-authors presented a layered, diverse, horizontal federated learning framework (Gao et al., 2019). The issue of label scarcity can be tackled through the iterative application of diverse transfer learning, using each party as the target space on each occasion. This would benefit the absence of data labeling in Neurological signal sorting. An extensive effort is indispensable for information gathering in practical instances like healthcare. Regarding inter-regional collaboration, it is nearly unfeasible for every medical centre to establish a data reservoir for collaboration. Therefore, federated learning could establish a nationwide network for inter-regional medical centres with comparable hospital data to enhance the collaborative frameworks (Figure 2).

Figure 1. Vertical federated learning

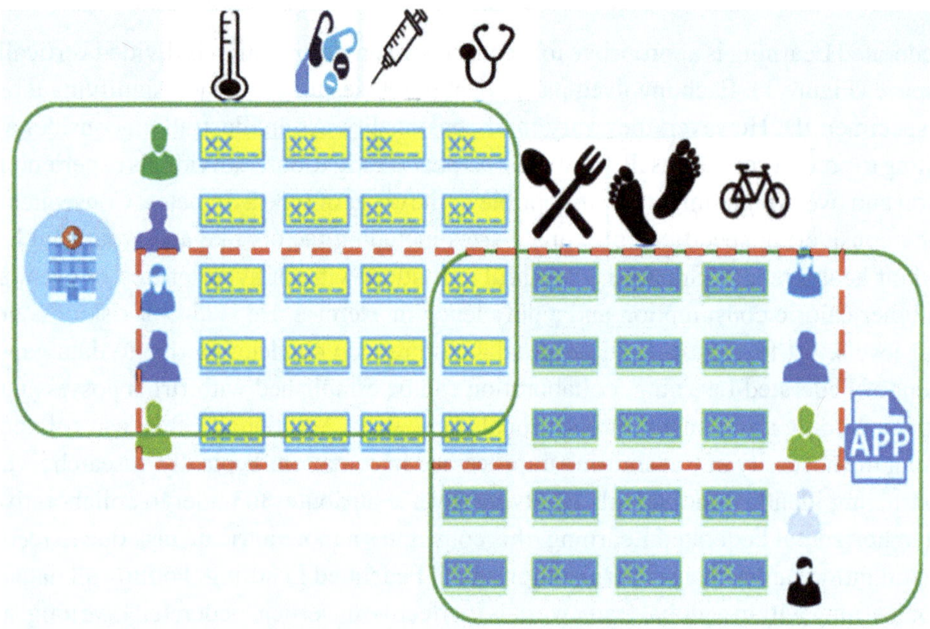

4.3 Federated Transfer Learning

Unlike the situations in horizontal and vertical federated learning, data commonly lacks outcome set and input space alignment in this context. Consequently, the primary challenge in this scenario revolves

Figure 2. Horizontal federal learning

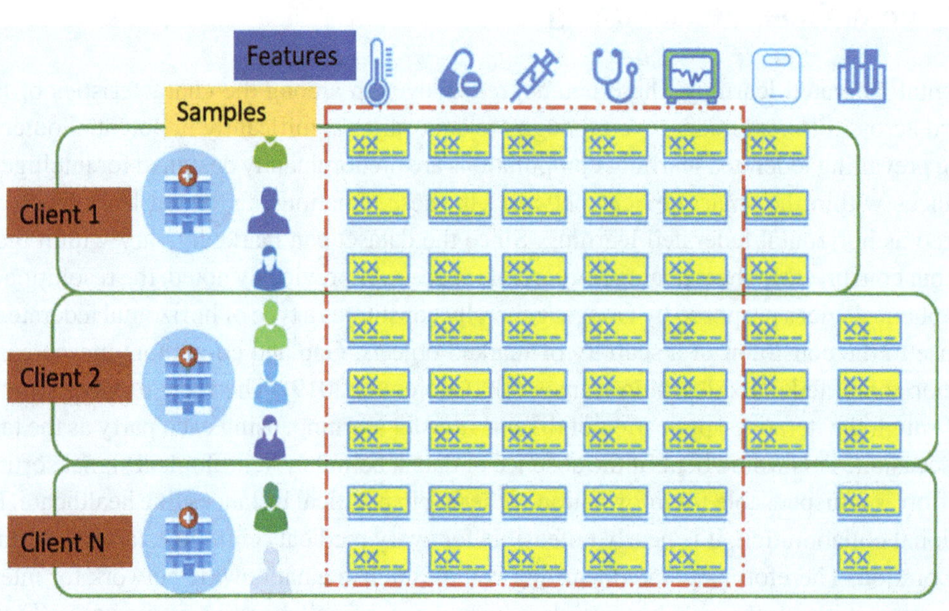

around inadequate data annotations coupled with suboptimal data accuracy. Transfer learning enables the transfer of information from one domain to a different domain or target space to achieve improved training outcomes, making it a suitable strategy for this particular situation. In this manner, Liu and co-authors formulated federated transfer learning to extend federated learning for more extensive usage, especially in situations involving shared entities with limited overlap (Liu et al., 2018). This signifies the first comprehensive framework for federated learning, constructed based on domain adaptation principles, covering both learning and assessment aspects. Furthermore, the deep learning models within this framework, incorporating privacy-preserving computation techniques, protect against privacy breaches and ensure accuracy comparable to conventional methods that do not prioritize privacy. However, the efficacy of exchanging thoughts still poses a challenge. Consequently, Sharma and co-authors strived to enhance federated transfer learning (Sharma et al., 2019). They leveraged distributed key generation techniques instead of homomorphic encryption to minimize operational costs without compromising correctness. Moreover, the potential extension could impede a nasty host. In contrast to prior research, where the assumption is that the framework is partially correct, Chen and co-authors devised a Fed-Health framework for practical usage that aggregates information from diverse bodies through federated learning and provides tailored medical facilities via adaptive learning (Chen et al., 2019). Specific ailment analyses and medical care details from a particular medical facility could be migrated to another medical facility (**Figure 3**), aiding in additional ailment analyses through federated transfer learning. The exploration of federated transfer learning is still in its early stages, indicating ample potential for advancement to enhance its adaptability to varying datasets. Challenges such as data silos and concerns related to safeguarding privacy remain in the ongoing extensive modernization of Artificial intelligence. Nonetheless, collaborative adaptive learning proves to be an efficient method to ensure the confidentiality of data and the security of clients.

5. ADVANTAGES

5.1 Smart Phones

Federated learning has received considerable focus from scientists since Google initially introduced the idea of forecasting client data from keyboards on smartphones. Moreover, emoji prognostication is also a focal point of investigation. Moreover, extending the Federated Learning framework to smart devices for predicting human trajectories or behavior is a potential application, despite the rapid growth in storage capacity and computational power of Android phones. Meeting the escalating quality requisites of smartphone users poses a challenge due to limitations on data transfer rates. Therefore, many comprehensive service providers choose to offer a facility setting at the periphery of the mobile communication system, close to the user, instead of consolidating distributed computing and cloud backup in the central network. This is done to mitigate bandwidth overload. This technique is called mobile periphery computation (MPC), but it also encounters heightened peril of data disclosure. One potential resolution is the fusion of adaptive learning and MPC. Qian and co-authors employed Federated Learning on MPC (Qian et al., 2019). They formulated a confidentiality-conscious facility arrangement strategy to deliver top-notch facilities by storing the sought-after service on the periphery host in proximity to the clients. In this context, portable gadgets not only refer to conventional smart devices but also encompass devices within Neural Network configurations. Brilliant residence stands out as a crucial applicable sector of

Figure 3. Federated transfer learning

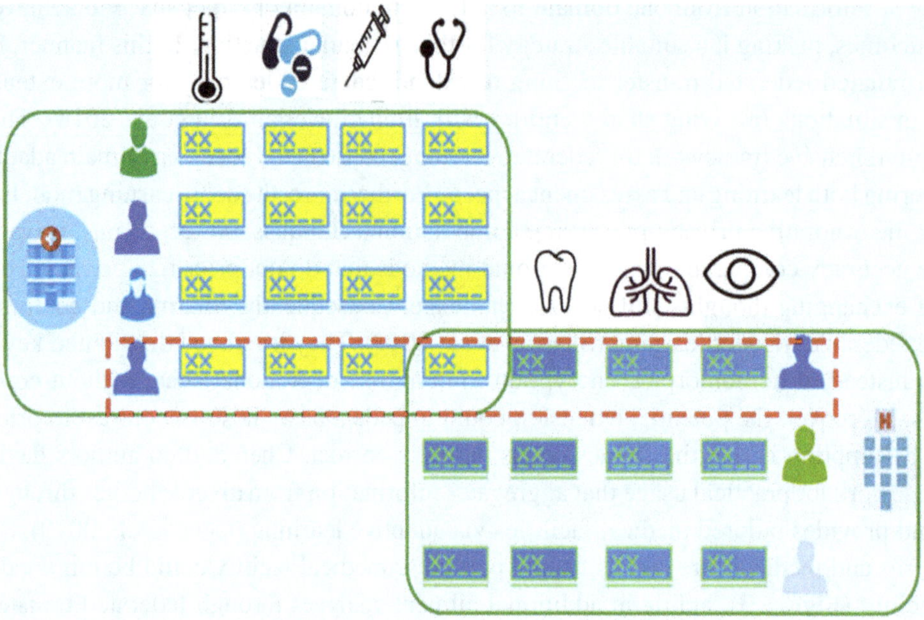

the Neural Network System. For an enhanced understanding of client's choices, gadgets within the intelligent abode framework might transmit pertinent data to a web host, potentially compromising data. Hence, Aïvodji and co-authors introduced an ample and safe federated structure to construct collaborative frameworks (Aïvodji et al., 2019). Likewise, Yu and co-authors established a distributed collective learning model for Intelligent Home Automation to comprehend clients' habits autonomously, aiming to identify potential safety risks proficiently (Yu et al., 2020). Moreover, Liu and co-authors suggested a data amalgamation strategy founded on Federated Learning for robotic mimicry learning in Automated Interaction (Liu et al., 2020). This approach could be utilized in autonomous vehicles to produce guiding frameworks and anticipate diverse crises.

5.2 Manufacturing Technology

Motivated by the success of federated learning in safeguarding data confidentiality, it is reasonable for manufacturing science to pursue it with the implementation of Federated Learning. As information in these domains is not accessible directly owing to certain legal and regulatory restrictions, we can only harness these scattered data to attain limitless advantages when federated learning is utilized in these domains. To our utmost understanding, accompanying the emergence and development of Federated Learning, it could potentially gain broad popularity and utilization in confidential sectors within process engineering. Using environmental preservation as an example, Hu and co-authors conceived an innovative ecological assessing model based on collaborative localized learning to address the challenges of substitutable display information (Hu et al., 2018). Therefore, overseeing information distributed from diverse detectors might be employed to enhance the cooperative framework's efficacy. Federated Learning is also utilized in visual examination assignments. It would assist in addressing the issue of insufficient imperfect specimens for identifying faults in manufacturing assignments and provide privacy assurances for producers. In visual domains, the convergence of sight and speech is also a focal point. Besides visual identification, Federated Learning is appropriate for identifying hostile assaults in an information network of Autonomous Flying Machines.

Considering that the characteristics of Autonomous Flying Machines, such as imbalanced information dispersion and uncertain transmission circumstances, closely mirror the challenges in Federated Learning. With the widespread adoption of sustainable transport, Saputra and co-authors formulated a federated approach for forecasting power requirements for diverse power points to avert power overload during communication (Saputra et al., 2019). In the realm of text analytics, Wang and co-authors utilized a commercial-scale federated system (Wang et al., 2020). It has undergone evaluation with authentic records for tasks like unsolicited content screening and emotional tone assessment. In summary, Federated Learning empowers dataset proprietors to expand the range of record uses and enhance framework efficiency using repeated engagement between various bodies. In the future, Federated Learning is poised to bolster additional sectors in attaining heightened smartness. Integrating Federated Learning into Machine Learning will construct a federated environment without information confidentiality issues.

5.3 Medical Sector

As an innovative approach to safeguard data confidentiality, Federated Learning holds tremendous potential in the medical sector. Every healthcare facility could possess abundant client information, which might be insufficient for developing their forecasting frameworks. Integration of Federated Learning and illness prognosis is a commendable resolution to dismantle the hindrances of examination across diverse medical institutions. Digital medical reports encompass numerous significant medical ideas. Kim and co-authors tried applying matrix decomposition frameworks for typing examination to extract insights hidden in medical data without disclosing client-specific information (Kim et al., 2017). This might be considered the inaugural endeavor for Federated Learning implementation in the health sector. Pfohl and co-authors investigated distinct personalized learning for digital medical data in a federated environment (Pfohl et al., 2019).

Moreover, they subsequently illustrated that efficiency is akin to learning in a unified environment. Huang and co-authors utilized digital health records distributed among medical centers to forecast the death rate for individuals with heart disease (Huang et al., 2019). Throughout the learning method, there was no exchange of information among the datasets of different hospitals. Moreover, information aggregated from numerous distant users into a primary host was pre-encoded, and the decoding mechanism was discarded upon completion of learning. Furthermore, Brisimi and co-authors also leveraged electronic medical data to assess whether a heart patient will be admitted to a hospital, employing a Federated Learning computation named cluster Primary Double Splitting (Brisimi et al., 2018). This forecasting task could be carried out on medical care surveillance gadgets or medical institutions storing this clinical data without any data disclosure. Using medical data, Lee and co-authors introduced a collaborative healthcare hashing model to identify comparable individuals distributed across various medical institutions without divulging client-specific details (Lee et al., 2018). This record linkage technique could assist healthcare professionals in summarizing common traits and guiding them to manage people with increased expertise.

Furthermore, Huang and co-authors utilized Gradient-boosted Federated Averaging with loss-based adaptation on medication utilization derived from the MIMIC-III repository to forecast the death rate of people (Huang et al., 2019). This investigation focused on mathematical intricacy, transmission expenditure, and precision for individual users, thus surpassing standard benchmarks. Research findings also illustrated that Federated Learning could be employed within Computational Linguistics to scrutinize accurate details from medical data. Liu and co-authors emphasized the necessity of handling random records within patient files (Liu et al., 2019). This marked the inaugural endeavor in utilizing Natural Language Processing grounded on Federated Learning. They executed a two-phase federated learning framework comprising a preliminary phase for forecasting a feature framework for every individual to investigate each type of ailment. Recently, Federated Learning has gained extensive application in medical visualization examination. Silva and co-authors introduced Distributed Principal factor examination to derive characteristics from magnetic resonance tomography from various hospitals (Silva et al., 2019).

Additionally, Gao and co-authors introduced a layered, diverse horizontal Federated Learning model for brainwave recording categorization to surmount the obstacle of restricted marked occurrences and confidentiality restrictions (Gao et al., 2019). To our current understanding, in tandem with the ascent and development of Federated Learning, there exists the potential for extensive adoption and utilization in privacy-conscious domains alongside the previously mentioned sectors. Table 1 illustrates the surge in the utilization of Federated Learning. Consequently, there is a positive outlook on the substantial potential of Federated Learning in upcoming progress. Federated Learning predominantly plays a role in horizontal cooperative learning for deploying uses. This implies that the event space of every dataset is comparable. In the prospective era, healthcare records within medical facilities might collaborate with external entities like insurance agencies to acquire equitable costs. Hence, Vertical Federated Learning presents a hopeful avenue for investigation. Additionally, a challenge lies in that current federated learning predominantly relies on a limited subset of firms and cannot expand to collective knowledge for many gadgets or firms. Consequently, the enhancement of examining smartphone data through efficient utilization of Federated Learning should lead to the generation of more meaningful insights.

5.4 Education

Guo and co-authors introduced a Learning Analytics System named Federated Education Data Analysis, which relies on Federated Learning. This framework aims to overcome the limitations posed by statistics silos when delving into the study of educational information in the pursuit of smart education transformation. Through the application of federated learning to address institutional apprehensions regarding scholar confidentiality, the researchers unlocked potential avenues for achieving extensive pedagogical examination, which was formerly unattainable. Balta and co-authors introduced compelling research that examined the responsibility of the Federated Learning procedure and its consequences on legal and regional matters that commonly emerge in government entities where a government-funded educational facility could be implicated. By scrutinizing the responsibility structure of Federated Learning, there is an enhanced sense of confidence in educational institutions fostering the realization of a smart learning transformation. Recyclable educational entities play a crucial role in enhancing the academic encounter. The recyclable educational entity enables the professional to express their perspectives regarding an educational asset by choosing one from the various alternatives within a provided educational framework.

Table 1. Applications of federate learning

Practical Sphere	Observation	Advantages	References
Mobile keypad	Emoji prediction	Outperform a centralized model	Ramaswamy et al. 2019
Cloud computing	Confidentiality-conscious service allocation	Suggest a confidentiality-sensitive service arrangement approach to fulfill client-centric services.	Qian et al., 2019
Connected home devices	Create a robust and secure networked intelligent home environment.	Integrates Federated Learning with protected data consolidation	Aivodji et al., 2019
Battery-powered automobiles	Collaborative energy consumption forecasting	Implement the cluster-oriented power requirement federated approach to enhance the forecasting precision	Saputra et al., 2019
Medical prognosis	Demonstrate the effectiveness of Federated Learning compared to unified and localized learning.	Conduct Federated Learning in a privacy-preserving way	Pfohl et al., 2019
Magnetic Resonance Imaging examination	Offer a decentralized system that aligns with the ENIGMA analytical workflows.	Effectively manage the diversity of complex attributes	Silva et al., 2019

6. FUTURE OUTLOOK

Federated Learning holds significant promise for eco-friendly advancement in implementing applicability within the manufacturing science and medical sector. It proposes stringent requisites for the architecture of federated systems to address the circumstances amidst the swift evolution of Artificial Intelligence and escalating privacy apprehensions. Numerous studies have yet to be investigated within the field of federated learning. Present primary directions are dedicated to implementing privacy standards, assault protection, efficacy enhancement, and handling diversities. In this segment, attention is directed toward noteworthy state-of-the-art outcomes to address persisting challenges for the improved establishment of Federated Learning in real-world production uses. Moreover, specific encouraging pathways to guide future advancements in this domain are also explained.

6.1 Uncoordinated Learning Approach

A fundamental decision in the worldwide framework training approach is opting for an uncoordinated or coordinated procedure. Lately, collaborative learning has emerged as the predominant form of Federated Learning owing to the enhanced efficiency of Stochastic Gradient Descent in primary host configurations compared to the uncoordinated approach. Previous optimization efforts in Federated Learning primarily centered on the coordinated development of FedAvg. Still, this approach depends on a robust prediction that is not pragmatic in real-world scenarios. The diverse material regarding distinct mathematical capabilities and varied Neural Network configurations, coupled with uneven data dissemination, can lead to disparate learning durations and unpredictable transmission expenses. Derived from prior research on uncoordinated descent optimization, Sprague and co-authors evaluated an independent aggregation strategy against FedAvg, yielding fundamentally acceptable outcomes (Sprague et al., 2019). The authors formulated an independent methodology for updating the user framework on the client end. Strata in computations were categorized into profound and superficial layers with varying alteration rates. On the server end, independent consolidation may be executed. For example, the uncoordinated digital federated learning model introduced by Chen et al. (2019) refreshes the core model independently by incorporating attribute training and adaptive learning rate. Wu and co-authors suggested a partially synchronized model that permits lagging users to not consistently synchronize with the primary host, considering the balance between the benefits of dependent refreshing and independent learning (Wu et al., 2019). The primary concept involved effectively incorporating laggers into the training regimen to expedite the learning method by leveraging their gradually updating frameworks. Drawing considerable insight from this partial independent approach, a fusion of synchronous and asynchronous models represents an encouraging avenue. Through this approach, it is possible to diminish undesired power load and provide minimal durability to laggers.

6.2 Slope Consolidation

Typically, during the gradient consolidation phase, the central framework's gradient is the summation of the scaled gradients generated by every individual. The sampling proportion determines the assignment of weights to every user. Still, there is no proof indicating that this weighted average slope obtained from regional users is identical to genuine central slope information owing to skewed analysis in regional users. Xiao and collaborators noted that as the iteration count increases and the parameter length expands, the shared data also rises, indicating a connection between users (Xiao et al., 2020). This investigation demonstrated that slope mean may not be an optimal approach for gradient consolidation. To eradicate slope skewness during the partial learning phase, Yao and co-authors monitored the delivered universal settings in every partial learning cycle (Yao et al., 2019). Given that the instantaneous slope update depends on versatile settings, the slope can be consolidated impartially. For enhanced comprehension of consolidation methods in federated learning, Ji and co-authors presented a temporal aggregator to derive an efficient approach for slope consolidation autonomously (Ji et al., 2019). Contemplating dependent data among users, slope consolidation through a straightforward mean method may not be an optimal selection. It could be more advantageous if scientists incorporated dynamic weights for every user or employed artificial intelligence techniques to understand how to combine these slopes effectively.

6.3 Rewards Structure

For enhancing efficiency, beyond optimizing material deployment or creating innovative design frameworks, establishing a motivational system to inspire more participants to engage in the learning process is also a highly efficient approach. The initial FedAvg utilized a random user-picking process. Every user appears to have an equal chance of participating in the learning process. In reality, specific inactive individuals with superior data quality or self-centered users concerned about energy usage might, with some likelihood, opt out of the entire learning procedure. Motivational systems might be implemented to inspire these participants. The virtual host would distribute rewards to every contributor based on their input level, and the participant would optimize their satisfaction to acquire increased earnings. Consequently, a favorable periodic influence would be developed to achieve a content model. Approaches like Stackelberg-oriented decision modeling are widely embraced in the design of incentive methods. Researchers investigated an innovative way within the Stackelberg framework to motivate employees to assign additional processing power resources for localized training. Khan and co-authors deliberated on a Stackelberg-oriented motivational system to adjust immediate recurrence durations dynamically for optimal effectiveness (Khan et al., 2019). The collective contribution structure embraced a two-phase

Stackelberg framework to optimize satisfaction between users and the host. In forthcoming research, additional systems such as pairing and bidding models could be incorporated to address the balance between the number of contributors and the modification lag.

6.4 Validation of Received Model

Many data security techniques in federated learning are built upon a robust presumption that participants are partially trustworthy, adhering to learning regulations while maintaining inquisitiveness about acquiring confidential information. Nonetheless, practical implementations often involve a different scenario. Whether knowingly or unknowingly, participants might transfer a faulty model, driving the worldwide model to diverge from its expected trajectory. For example, enemies could produce seemingly credible yet inaccurate information on mobile health devices to undermine the complete framework. This type of Byzantine issue is consistently faced in federated learning. Hence, a Byzantine resilient framework needs to be created, signifying that the cooperative learning approach remains effective even when specific participants don't adhere to the learning framework or act with malice to target the central model. To identify abnormal modifications in the model. Li and co-authors employed a self-encoding model that allows weights of the model to be substituted with simplified vectors, thereby uncovering irregularities in parameter modifications (Li et al., 2019). Munoz-Gonzalez and co-authors examined the use of adaptive Federated Learning to detect anomalous changes using a Hidden Markov prototype to assess its quality (Munoz-Gonzalez et al., 2019). Conventional Byzantine resilient systems rely on protective measures instead of identifying hostile users. Given the decline in correctness within the federated system, it is advisable to construct a more robust Byzantine resilient framework that relies on error identification to mitigate or minimize potential risks.

7. CONCLUSION

Federated learning facilitates collective learning of computational models for optimizing edge computing networks. This approach allows numerous points to collaboratively create a unified training model to tackle key issues like authorization, retrieval of diverse data, confidentiality, and protection. Recently, a decentralized system has attracted considerable interest from both the educational and commercial sectors. Numerous novel implementations are emerging, leveraging federated learning to enhance the excellence and confidentiality of data-centric uses. This chapter illustrates the framework of Federated Learning basics, factors to consider, and practical applications. Significantly, this undertaking focuses on spotlighting contemporary popular services and scenarios that employ federated learning in innovation and industries. It explored the applicability of federated learning in domains like medicine, education, industry, and smartphones. This examination additionally introduces remarkable cutting-edge results to address persisting challenges for the improved establishment of federated learning in real-world production uses. Various sectors, including FinTech, and the robotics sector can incorporate federated learning. However, difficulties in these sectors may include diversity in statistics, system disparity, skewed data distribution, resource distribution, and safety concerns. Using this inclusive chapter, this investigation serves as an expansive benchmark for forthcoming research in federated learning.

Conflict of Interest

Neither a technological nor a fiscal conflict of interest exists.

Research Funding

No research funding is available.

REFERENCES

Aïvodji, U. M., Gambs, S., & Martin, A. (2019). IOTFLA: A secured and privacy-preserving smart home architecture implementing federated learning. *IEEE Security and Privacy Workshops (SPW),* 175–180. doi:10.1109/SPW.2019.00041

Balta, D., Sellami, M., Kuhn, P., Schöpp, U., Buchinger, M., Baracaldo, N., ... (2021). Accountable federated machine learning in government: Engineering and management insights. In *International conference on electronic participation* (pp. 125–138). Springer.

Brisimi, T. S., Chen, R., Mela, T., Olshevsky, A., Paschalidis, I. C., & Shi, W. (2018). Federated learning of predictive models from federated Electronic Health Records. *International Journal of Medical Informatics, 112*, 59–67. https://doi.org/.ijmedinf.2018.01.007 doi:10.1016/j

Chen, Y., Ning, Y., & Rangwala, H. (2019). *Asynchronous online federated learning for edge devices.* ArXiv:1911.02134 [Cs]. Retrieved from http://arxiv.org/abs/1911.02134

Cheng, K., Fan, T., Jin, Y., Liu, Y., Chen, T., & Yang, Q. (2019). *SecureBoost: A lossless federated learning framework.* ArXiv:1901.08755 [Cs, Stat]. Retrieved from http://arxiv.org/abs/1901.08755

Edwards, J. (2019). Medicine on the Move: Wearable devices supply healthcare providers with the data and insights necessary to diagnose medical issues and create optimal treatment plans [Special Reports]. *IEEE Signal Processing Magazine*, *36*(6), 8–11. doi:10.1109/MSP.2019.2930767

GaoD.JuC.WeiX.LiuY.ChenT.YangQ. (2019). *HHHFL: Hierarchical heterogeneous horizontal federated learning for electroencephalography.* ArXiv: 1909.05784 [Cs, Eess]. Retrieved from http://arxiv.org/abs/1909.05784

Guo, S., Zeng, D., & Dong, S. (2020). Pedagogical data analysis via federated learning toward Education 4.0. *American Journal of Education and Information Technology*, *4*(2), 56.

Ho, Q., Cipar, J., Cui, H., Lee, S., Kim, J. K., Gibbons, P. B., ... Xing, E. P. (2013). More effective distributed ML via a stale synchronous parallel parameter server. In C. J. C. Burges, L. Bottou, M. Welling, Z. Ghahramani, & K. Q. Weinberger (Eds.), Advances in neural information processing systems (Vol. 26, pp. 1223–1231). Retrieved from http://papers.nips.cc/paper/4894-more-effective-distributed-ml-via-a-stale-synchr onous-parallel-parameter-server.pdf

Hu, B., Gao, Y., Liu, L., & Ma, H. (2018). Federated region-learning: An edge computing based framework for urban environment sensing. *IEEE Global Communications Conference (GLOBECOM),* 1–7. 10.1109/GLOCOM.2018.8647649

Huang, L., Shea, A. L., Qian, H., Masurkar, A., Deng, H., & Liu, D. (2019). Patient clustering improves efficiency of federated machine learning to predict mortality and hospital stay time using distributed electronic medical records. *Journal of Biomedical Informatics, 99,* Article 103291. https://doi.org/. jbi.2019.103291. doi:10.1016/j

Ji, J., Chen, X., Wang, Q., Yu, L., & Li, P. (2019). Learning to learn gradient aggregation by gradient descent. In *Proceedings of the twenty-eighth international joint conference on artificial intelligence* (pp. 2614–2620). 10.24963/ijcai.2019/363

Khan, L. U., Tran, N. H., Pandey, S. R., Saad, W., Han, Z., Nguyen, M. N. H., & Hong, C. S. (2019). *Federated learning for edge networks: resource optimization and incentive mechanism.* ArXiv:1911.05642 [Cs]. Retrieved from http://arxiv.org/abs/1911. 05642.

Kim, Y., Sun, J., Yu, H., & Jiang, X. (2017). Federated tensor factorization for computational phenotyping. In *Proceedings of the 23rd ACM SIGKDD international conference on knowledge discovery and data mining* (pp. 887–895). 10.1145/3097983.3098118

Lee, J., Sun, J., Wang, F., Wang, S., Jun, C.-H., & Jiang, X. (2018). Privacy-preserving patient similarity learning in a federated environment: Development and analysis. *JMIR Medical Informatics*, *6*(2), e20. Advance online publication. doi:10.2196/medinform.7744 PMID:29653917

LiT.SahuA. K.ZaheerM.SanjabiM.TalwalkarA.SmithV. (2019). *Federated optimization in heterogeneous networks.* ArXiv:1812.06127 [Cs, Stat]. Retrieved from http://arxiv.org/abs/1812.06127

Lilhore, U. K., Dalal, S., Faujdar, N., Margala, M., Chakrabarti, P., Chakrabarti, T., Simaiya, S., Kumar, P., Thangaraju, P., & Velmurugan, H. (2023). Hybrid CNN-LSTM model with efficient hyperparameter tuning for prediction of Parkinson's disease. *Scientific Reports*, *13*(1), 14605. doi:10.1038/s41598-023-41314-y PMID:37669970

Lilhore, U. K., Dalal, S., Faujdar, N., Simaiya, S., Dahiya, M., Tomar, S., & Hashmi, A. (2024). Unveiling the prevalence and risk factors of early stage postpartum depression: A hybrid deep learning approach. *Multimedia Tools and Applications*, 1–35. doi:10.1007/s11042-024-18182-3

Lilhore, U. K., Manoharan, P., Sandhu, J. K., Simaiya, S., Dalal, S., Baqasah, A. M., Alsafyani, M., Alroobaea, R., Keshta, I., & Raahemifar, K. (2023). Hybrid model for precise hepatitis-C classification using improved random forest and SVM method. *Scientific Reports*, *13*(1), 12473. doi:10.1038/s41598-023-36605-3 PMID:37528148

Lilhore, U. K., Poongodi, M., Kaur, A., Simaiya, S., Algarni, A. D., Elmannai, H., Vijayakumar, V., Tunze, G. B., & Hamdi, M. (2022). Hybrid model for detection of cervical cancer using causal analysis and machine learning techniques. *Computational and Mathematical Methods in Medicine*, *2022*, 2022. doi:10.1155/2022/4688327 PMID:35572826

Lilhore, U. K., Simaiya, S., Pandey, H., Gautam, V., Garg, A., & Ghosh, P. (2022). Breast cancer detection in the IoT cloud-based healthcare environment using fuzzy cluster segmentation and SVM classifier. *Proceedings of RACCCS, 2021*, 165–179.

Lin, K. (2018). User experience-based product design for smart production to empower industry 4.0 in the glass recycling circular economy. *Computers & Industrial Engineering, 125*, 729–738. doi:10.1016/j.cie.2018.06.023

Liu, B., Wang, L., Liu, M., & Xu, C.-Z. (2020). Federated imitation learning: A novel framework for cloud robotic systems with heterogeneous sensor data. *IEEE Robotics and Automation Letters, 5*(2), 3509–3516. doi:10.1109/LRA.2020.2976321

LiuY.ChenT.YangQ. (2018). *Secure federated transfer learning*. ArXiv: 1812.03337 [Cs, Stat]. Retrieved from http://arxiv.org/abs/1812.03337

Liu, Z., Li, T., Smith, V., & Sekar, V. (2019). *Enhancing the privacy of federated learning with sketching*. ArXiv:1911.01812 [Cs, Stat]. Retrieved from http://arxiv.org/abs/1911.01812.

McMahan, B., Moore, E., Ramage, D., Hampson, S., & Arcas, B. A. Y. (2017). Communication-efficient learning of deep networks from decentralized data. *Artificial Intelligence and Statistics*, 1273–1282. http://proceedings. mlr.press/v54/mcmahan17a.html.

Munoz-Gonzalez, L., Co, K. T., & Lupu, E. C. (2019). *Byzantine-robust federated machine learning through adaptive model averaging*. ArXiv:1909.05125 [Cs, Stat]. Retrieved from http://arxiv.org/abs/1909.05125

NockR.HardyS.HeneckaW.Ivey-LawH.PatriniG.SmithG.ThorneB. (2018). *Entity resolution and federated learning get a federated resolution*. ArXiv: 1803.04035 [Cs]. Retrieved from http://arxiv.org/abs/1803.04035

Pfohl, S. R., Dai, A. M., & Heller, K. (2019). *Federated and differentially private learning for electronic health records*. ArXiv:1911.05861 [Cs, Stat]. Retrieved from htt p://arxiv.org/abs/1911.05861

Qian, Y., Hu, L., Chen, J., Guan, X., Hassan, M. M., & Alelaiwi, A. (2019). Privacy-aware service placement for mobile edge computing via federated learning. *Information Sciences, 505*, 562–570. doi:10.1016/j.ins.2019.07.069

Ramaswamy, S., Mathews, R., Rao, K., & Beaufays, F. (2019). *Federated learning for emoji prediction in a mobile keyboard*. ArXiv:1906.04329 [Cs]. Retrieved from htt p://arxiv.org/abs/1906.04329

Saputra, Y. M., Hoang, D. T., Nguyen, D. N., Dutkiewicz, E., Mueck, M. D., & Srikanteswara, S. (2019). Energy demand prediction with federated learning for electric vehicle networks. *IEEE Global Communications Conference (GLOBECOM)*, 1–6. 10.1109/GLOBECOM38437.2019.9013587

SharmaS.ChaopingX.LiuY.KangY. (2019). Secure and efficient federated transfer learning. ArXiv:1910.13271 [Cs]. doi:10.1109/BigData47090.2019.9006280

Silva, S., Gutman, B. A., Romero, E., Thompson, P. M., Altmann, A., & Lorenzi, M. (2019). Federated learning in distributed medical databases: meta-analysis of largescale subcortical brain data. In *2019 IEEE 16th International Symposium on Biomedical Imaging (ISBI 2019)* (pp. 270–274). .8759317.10.1109/ISBI.2019.8759317

Sprague, M. R., Jalalirad, A., Scavuzzo, M., Capota, C., Neun, M., Do, L., & Kopp, M. (2019). Asynchronous federated learning for geospatial applications. In A. Monreale, C. Alzate, M. Kamp, Y. Krishnamurthy, D. Paurat, M. Sayed-Mouchaweh, ... R. P. Ribeiro (Eds.), *ECML PKDD 2018 Workshops* (pp. 21–28). doi:10.1007/978-3-030-14880-5_2

Wang, Y., Tong, Y., & Shi, D. (2020). Federated latent dirichlet allocation: A local differential privacy based framework. *AAAI 2020- AAAI Conference on Artificial Intelligence*, 6283–6290. 10.1609/aaai.v34i04.6096

Wu, W., He, L., Lin, W., Rui, M., & Jarvis, S. (2019). *SAFA: A semi-asynchronous protocol for fast federated learning with low overhead.* ArXiv:1910.01355 [Cs]. Retrieved from http://arxiv.org/abs/1910.01355

Xiao, P., Cheng, S., Stankovic, V., & Vukobratovic, D. (2020). Averaging is probably not the optimum way of aggregating parameters in federated learning. *Entropy (Basel, Switzerland)*, *22*(3), 314. doi:10.3390/e22030314 PMID:33286088

Yang, Q., Liu, Y., Chen, T., & Tong, Y. (2019). Federated machine learning: Concept and applications. *ACM Transactions on Intelligent Systems and Technology*, *10*(2), 1–19. doi:10.1145/3298981

YaoX.HuangT.ZhangR.-X.LiR.SunL. (2019). *Federated learning with unbiased gradient aggregation and controllable meta updating*. ArXiv:1910.08234 [Cs, Stat]. Retrieved from http://arxiv.org/abs/1910.08234

Yu, T., Li, T., Sun, Y., Nanda, S., Smith, V., & Sekar, V. (2020). Learning contextaware policies from multiple smart homes via federated multi-task learning. *IEEE/ ACM Fifth International Conference on Internet-of-Things Design and Implementation (IoTDI),* 104–115. 10.1109/IoTDI49375.2020.00017

Chapter 17
AI in Mental Health Federated Learning and Privacy

Shyelendra Madansing Pardeshi
Oriental University, India

Dinesh Chandra Jain
Oriental University, India

ABSTRACT

This chapter explores the integration of artificial intelligence (AI) in the realm of mental health, focusing on the application of federated learning to ensure privacy and confidentiality. The study delves into the challenges of implementing AI-driven solutions in mental health contexts while prioritizing the protection of sensitive patient information. By leveraging federated learning, a decentralized machine learning approach, the research aims to enhance the accuracy and efficacy of mental health diagnostics without compromising individual privacy. The chapter discusses the potential benefits and ethical considerations associated with the use of AI in mental health, emphasizing the importance of technological advancements.

INTRODUCTION

An essential component of healthcare is mental health assessment, which acts as a guide for understanding the complex web of human emotions and psychological well-being. Clinical interviews, self-reported surveys, and professional evaluations have traditionally been used in the quest to fully assess a person's mental health status. But as the digital era progresses, a new field has opened up, one that uses machine learning and sentiment analysis to reveal insights concealed in written text.

This chapter sets out on a transformational journey into the world of "The Use of Machine Learning for Sentiment Analysis in Mental Health Assessment." We are on the verge of a paradigm shift in the assessment of mental health thanks to the development of natural language processing (NLP) and machine learning techniques. The profound complexities of mental health are now within the scope of sentiment analysis, a branch of natural language processing (NLP) that was previously primarily used for marketing and social media analytics.

DOI: 10.4018/979-8-3693-1874-4.ch017

The purpose of this research is to clarify how machine learning and mental health assessment work together. We set out on a journey that travels through data collection, preprocessing, and the creation of reliable sentiment analysis models by dissecting the fundamental elements of sentiment analysis and machine learning. Through this journey, we demonstrate the potential of machine learning to improve our comprehension of emotional states, identify early indicators of mental health conditions, and precisely target interventions.

We explore the technical aspects of this combination while also navigating the moral concerns that have an important effect on how sensitive mental health data is handled. Through case studies from the real world, we highlight how machine learning-driven sentiment analysis is progressing in a variety of contexts, from interpreting social media sentiment to gleaning insights from medical records. With the ultimate goal of enhancing people's wellbeing, we invite individuals to collaborate with us on this exploration as we forge a link between technology and healthcare. This chapter provides a compass for controlling this exciting new frontier in mental health assessment that is poised at the nexus of sentiment analysis and machine learning.

Sentiment Analysis in Mental Health

Computing the sentiment of a piece of text, like a social media post, news article, or product review, is the process of sentiment analysis. Positive, negative, or neutral emotions can all be classified as sentiment. Figure 1 explains sentiment analysis uses in mental health assessment. In mental health, sentiment analysis can be used to spot individuals who might be experiencing mental health issues. A number of steps are performed before the actual processing begins, such as tokenization, part-of-speech tagging, stemming, noun extraction, and noun filtering (Kaur and Dutta, 2018; Asani, 2021). For instance, a study conducted by scientists at the University of Pittsburgh discovered that suicide risk could be determined using sentiment analysis. According to the study, those who were at risk of suicide used negative language more frequently in their social media posts. The development of those undergoing mental health treatment can also be monitored using sentiment analysis.

Early Detection

The timely detection of small changes or patterns in a person's emotional and psychological state is an important aspect of early detection in sentimental analysis throughout mental health. Sentiment analysis algorithms may recognize variations from a person's baseline sentiment, which might indicate the onset of mental health issues, by cautiously monitoring and analyzing textual data, such as social media posts, chat interactions, or clinical notes. A word's inflectional form can be reduced to its rootword, or "lemma," by the process of lemmatization. The lemmatization of the word "saw" results in the word "see," for instance. (Fung and Belaidan, 2021).

This early detection offers several advantages, including the opportunity for prompt interventions and support, which can be instrumental in preventing the exacerbation of mental health conditions. People in many nations have changed their habits in response to the fast global spread of COVID-19. This includes things like keeping social distance and wearing masks on public transit (Patel, 2017). Furthermore, it facilitates more efficient resource allocation within healthcare systems, directing attention and resources to those who may need them most urgently. Ultimately, early detection through sentimental analysis

Figure 1. Sentiment analysis in mental health

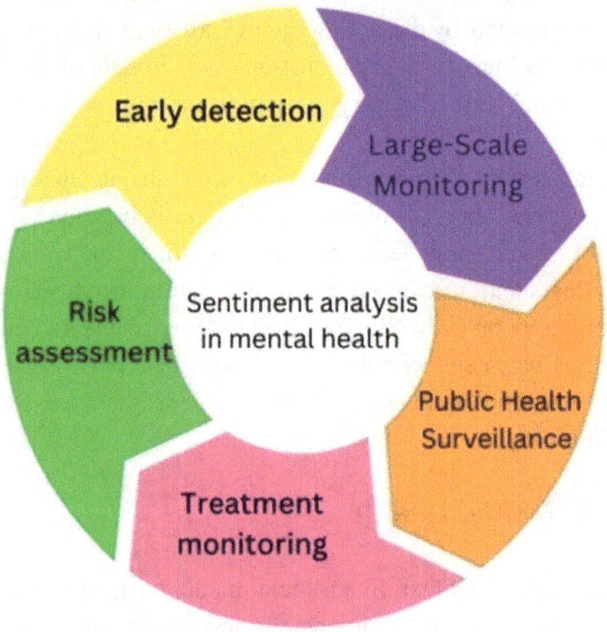

plays a vital role in improving mental health outcomes by enabling proactive and timely responses to individuals' emotional well-being.

Risk Assessment

Analyzing potential difficulties and pitfalls connected with the application of sentiment analysis techniques is a key component of risk assessment in sentimental analysis within the context of mental health. The accuracy of sentiment classification poses a serious risk because incorrect assessments and interventions can result from misclassifying emotional states or sentiments. The analysis frequently uses sensitive mental health data, so ethical issues like data privacy and informed consent pose another important risk. It is crucial to ensure that sentiment analysis models are impartial and equitable across various demographic groups because biased algorithms can worsen inequality. In order to ensure that sentimental analysis supports clinical judgment rather than substitutes for it, it is also important to carefully manage the potential for healthcare professionals to misinterpret results or to rely too heavily on automated assessments. Despite these dangers, a considerate and moral approach to sentimental analysis risk assessment can assist in easing these difficulties and maximizing its transformative potential in mental health assessment and support.

Public Health Surveillance

Machine learning algorithms for sentiment analysis have greatly aided public health monitoring. These algorithms can automatically assess public sentiment and emotional responses towards various health-related topics, such as vaccination campaigns, disease outbreaks, or healthcare services, by analyzing social media posts, online reviews, and other digital sources. Public health authorities can quickly detect and address emerging concerns thanks to this insightful information. They can also spot potential intervention areas and adjust communication strategies accordingly. Additionally, sentiment analysis aids in assessing public opinion, evaluating the success of health messaging, and better interacting with communities in order to encourage healthier lifestyles and enhance general public health outcomes.

Large Scale Monitoring

Large-scale monitoring in sentiment analysis using machine learning algorithms involves the automated analysis of vast amounts of text data from diverse sources such as social media, customer reviews, and news articles to extract valuable insights about public sentiment towards products, services, or topics. Machine learning algorithms play a pivotal role in this process by leveraging natural language processing techniques to classify and quantify sentiments as positive, negative, or neutral. One way to prepare data for analysis is to filter out irrelevant information from source texts. (Yamini, 2022). These algorithms are trained on labeled datasets and continuously fine-tuned to adapt to evolving language patterns and context. Scalability is a key consideration, with distributed computing and parallel processing facilitating the analysis of massive datasets in real-time or near-real-time. The results of such monitoring are invaluable for businesses, governments, and organizations to make informed decisions, identify emerging trends, and manage their reputation in the digital age.

Treatment Monitoring

In order to ensure that machine learning algorithms are effective at detecting and interpreting sentiment in textual data, treatment monitoring in sentiment analysis entails ongoing evaluation and modification of these algorithms. Prior to feeding data into a machine learning model, this step is essential. In order to improve the Machine's Learning and Performance, it eliminates extraneous data. Transforming raw data into a clean dataset is what this technique is all about (Aeri, 2022; Ng et al., 2022). The continuous collection of labeled data for training and retraining models, as well as the assessment of model performance metrics like accuracy, precision, recall, and F1-score, are typically part of this process. To adjust to changing data patterns and evolving sentiment expressions, machine learning algorithms may be adjusted, hyper parameters optimized, or even replaced with more sophisticated models. Detecting concept drift or sentiment shifts over time may also be a part of monitoring techniques, allowing for timely updates to the sentiment analysis system to keep it accurate and relevant across a range of domains and applications.

Machine Learning Techniques in Sentiment Analysis in Mental Health Assessment

Sentiment analysis for mental health assessment relies heavily on machine learning techniques like Support Vector Machines (SVM), Convolution Neural Networks (CNN), and Recurrent Neural Networks (RNN). Through their powerful classification abilities, SVMs excel at spotting sentiment patterns in textual data, helping in the early identification of mental health issues. Acquiring a dataset pertinent to the e-learning domain constitutes the initial and paramount component of the model (Almalki, 2022).

Actually, it's the other way around; this might make political bickering even worse and make it harder for the administration to rein in the spreading epidemic (Rezapour and Hansen, 2022; Ng et al., 2022). CNNs, on the other hand, are useful for analyzing multimedia content that might contain emotional cues because they are skilled at extracting spatial features from textual and visual data. RNNs, with their sequential modeling capabilities, are especially helpful in analyzing longer narratives or conversations because they can capture the temporal aspect of mental health expressions. In combination, these machine learning techniques offer a thorough method for sentiment analysis that enables mental health professionals to discover more about people's emotional well-being from a variety of data sources, resulting in more precise assessments and quick interventions.

Support Vector Machine (SVM) in Sentiment Analysis

SVMs, or support vector machines, are crucial in sentiment analysis for evaluating mental health. SVMs are incredibly good at identifying emotional states in textual data, allowing for the early identification of mental health problems. Figure 2 explains about SVM classification in sentiment analysis. SVMs can correctly classify sentiments expressed in text through a process of rigorous training involving parameter optimization, which is essential in determining a person's mental health. By analyzing written or spoken expressions, SVM-based sentiment analysis is able to spot possible indications of distress, depression, or anxiety in people. SVMs offer a useful tool for mental health professionals, assisting in the prompt identification and support of people who may be experiencing mental health challenges by providing a quantitative assessment of mental states.

Support Vector Machines (SVM) have been widely employed in sentiment analysis, including its application in mental health assessment. SVM is a supervised machine learning algorithm that can be effectively used for binary and multiclass sentiment classification tasks.

Figure 2. SVM classification for sentiment analysis

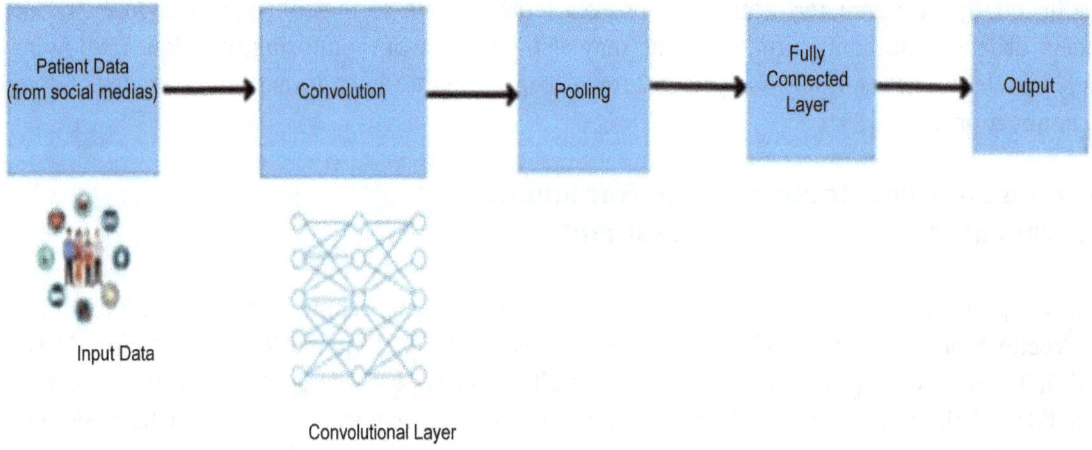

Data Preparation

Data Collection: Gather textual data from various sources, such as social media posts, patient forums, clinical notes, or therapy transcripts, containing expressions of emotional and mental states.

Data Preprocessing: Clean and preprocess the text data by removing noise, handling missing values, and tokenizing the text into words or phrases. Additionally, perform tasks like stemming or lemmatization to standardize text.

Feature Extraction

TF-IDF (Term Frequency-Inverse Document Frequency): TF-IDF Convert the preprocessed text data into numerical feature vectors .TF-IDF assigns weights to words based on their frequency in a document relative to their frequency across the entire corpus. This technique helps capture the importance of words in distinguishing sentiment.

Word Embeddings: Alternatively, you can use word embeddings (e.g., Word2Vec, GloVe) to represent words as dense vector representations. These embeddings capture semantic relationships between words, which can enhance the model's ability to understand context and sentiment.

SVM Model Construction

These models enable accurate sentiment classification by building a hyperplane that maximizes the margin between various sentiment classes. SVMs can be used to analyze text data, such as patient reviews or social media posts, in the context of mental health assessment in order to ascertain the sentiment expressed and gauge the individual's mental state. The SVM can be taught to distinguish between positive, negative, and neutral sentiments by being trained on labeled data. This helps in the early detection of mental health issues and gives healthcare professionals insightful information to use when providing timely support and intervention. SVMs are a good option for sentiment analysis in mental health assessment due to their robustness and ability to handle high-dimensional data.

Training and Evaluation

Hyper parameters like the selection of the kernel and regularization parameters must be optimized during training in order to increase SVMs' performance at accurately classifying sentiments, which is crucial for assessing mental health. SVM models have the ability to adapt to changing linguistic nuances and the dynamic nature of expressions related to mental health because they can evolve over time as they are exposed to more varied and extensive datasets. SVM-based sentiment analysis' adaptability enables more effective and timely assessments of people's mental health and interventions for their support. It can provide insightful information about people's mental health.

Interpretability: SVM models are known for their interpretability. You can identify support vectors (data points closest to the decision boundary), which can provide insights into the most critical features or words contributing to the sentiment classification.

Convolution Neural Network (CNNs) in Sentiment Analysis in Mental Health Assessment

Convolution Neural Networks (CNNs) have gained prominence in sentiment analysis, including applications within the context of mental health assessment. CNNs, originally designed for image processing, have been adapted to process sequential data, such as text, by treating text as a one-dimensional signal. Here, we provide detailed insights into the use of CNNs in sentiment analysis:

Data Preparation

Convolution Neural Networks (CNN) data preparation for sentiment analysis in mental health assessment entails a number of crucial steps. Textual data is initially gathered and preprocessed to remove noise, such as stop words, special characters, and unimportant information, from a variety of sources, including social media and clinical records. Using methods like word embedding or one-hot encoding, the text is then tokenized and converted into numerical vectors. Sequences of tokens are padded or truncated to a fixed length to include contextual information. Figure 3 explains convolution neural network in sentiment analysis When multimodal data is present (such as text and images), feature extraction and fusion techniques are used to efficiently combine the various data modalities. To facilitate the training and evaluation of the CNN, the prepared data is finally divided into training, validation, and testing sets. In order to facilitate training and evaluation of the CNN model and ensure that it can accurately analyze sentiment within mental health contexts, which will aid in useful mental health assessments, the prepared data is finally divided into training, validation, and testing sets.

Convolution Layers

To find regional patterns or features, these layers apply convolution filters (kernels) to the embedded text data. Each filter applies element-wise multiplication to the input before summing the results. This operation produces a feature map as its result. To capture different levels of granularity in the text, several filters of various sizes are typically used. You might, for instance, have filters in the sizes 3x3, 4x4, and 5x5.

Figure 3. Convolution neural network in sentiment analysis

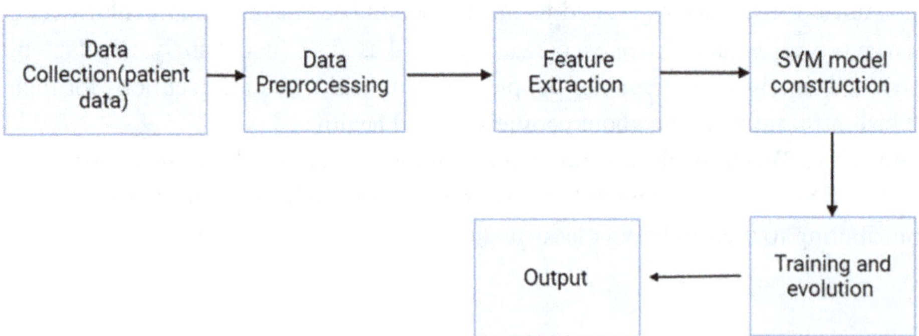

Feature Maps: Convolution operations produce feature maps that represent the presence of specific patterns or features in the text. These feature maps are then passed through activation functions (e.g., ReLU) to introduce non-linearity.

Pooling Layers

After convolution, a max-pooling layer is often applied to reduce the dimensionality of the feature maps. Max pooling retains the most important information within a window, discarding less relevant details. A crucial component of a neural network that aids in reducing the spatial dimensions of the feature maps produced by convolution layers is a pooling layer. Its main goal is to retain the most crucial details while down sampling the data. For instance, max-pooling selects the maximum value within each region and discards the rest after dividing the feature map into non-overlapping regions (typically 2x2 or 3x3). By effectively shrinking the size of the feature map, this method increases the computational efficiency of the network while retaining the most important details, such as edges, shapes, or textures. The ability to recognize patterns regardless of their precise spatial location is especially useful in tasks like image and text classification where the network must be more translation-invariant. In tasks like image and text classification, where the precise location of a feature may not be as important as its presence, the network can recognize patterns regardless of their precise spatial location by becoming more translation-invariant with the aid of pooling layers.

Flattening and Fully Connected Layers

In neural networks, particularly in feed forward and convolution neural networks, flattening and fully connected layers are crucial elements. Multi-dimensional data, such as feature maps from convolution layers, can be connected to fully connected layers by flattening it into a one-dimensional vector. Fully connected layers, also referred to as dense layers, are made up of numerous neurons, each of which is connected to every neuron in the layer below, giving them the ability to learn intricate relationships within the data. These layers, which are frequently found at the very end of neural network architectures, are in charge of capturing high-level abstractions and patterns in the input data. In tasks like image classification and natural language processing, flattening and fully connected layers are essential because they help map the extracted information.

Sentiment Classification

Determine the emotional tone or polarity of a text in order to categorize it into groups like positive, negative, or neutral. Sentiment classification is a fundamental task in natural language processing. In textual content like reviews, social media posts, or customer feedback, it seeks to automatically analyze and decipher the sentiment expressed. In order to comprehend the subjective context and emotional cues within the text, sentiment classification algorithms use machine learning techniques and linguistic analysis. This enables businesses and researchers to gain insightful information about public opinion, customer satisfaction, or market sentiment and to make data-driven decisions. Sentiment Analysis can be done using various machine learning algorithms in which a model/classifier is trained using reviews that are annotated with the polarity positive or negative (Nancy Kansal 2022).

Recurrent Neural Network for Sentiment Analysis in Mental Health Assessment

In the context of evaluating mental health, recurrent neural networks (RNNs) have shown great potential in sentiment analysis. RNN is very useful for processing sequential data and valuable for analyzing text data that contains temporal dependencies. Figure 4 explains a detailed explanation of how RNNs are used in sentiment analysis for mental health assessment, along with a simplified diagram illustrating the process:

Data Preparation

In order to prepare data for RNN-based sentiment analysis in mental health assessment, several important steps must be taken. The text data must first be gathered and preprocessed; this text data can be discovered in places like social media, chat logs, or medical records. This includes operations like removing stop words and special characters, lowercasing, and text tokenization. The text sequences must then be transformed into numerical representations, frequently using word embeddings like Word2Vec or GloVe that capture the semantic relationships between words. Padding is used to ensure consistent sequence lengths. For the purpose of mental health assessment, labels or categories are assigned to each text sample indicating the emotional state or mental health condition. There are three sets made: a training set, a validation set, and a testing set. Class balance needs to be carefully considered in order to address any potential imbalances in the labels. In order to determine a person's mental health based on their textual expressions, the final step is to feed the prepared data into the RNN model for training, evaluation, and analysis. It is crucial to pay close attention to concerns with data quality, privacy, and ethics throughout this process.

RNN Architecture

The Recurrent Neural Network (RNN) architecture processes sequential text data to capture temporal dependencies and contextual information for sentiment analysis and mental health assessment. In this situation, RNNs are typically built with an input layer that accepts tokenized text or word embeddings as input. Each time step updates the network's hidden state based on the current word and the previous hidden state as these embeddings are sequentially fed into the RNN's hidden layers. The model can take into account the arrangement of words and their connections within the text thanks to this sequential

Figure 4. RNN in sentiment classification

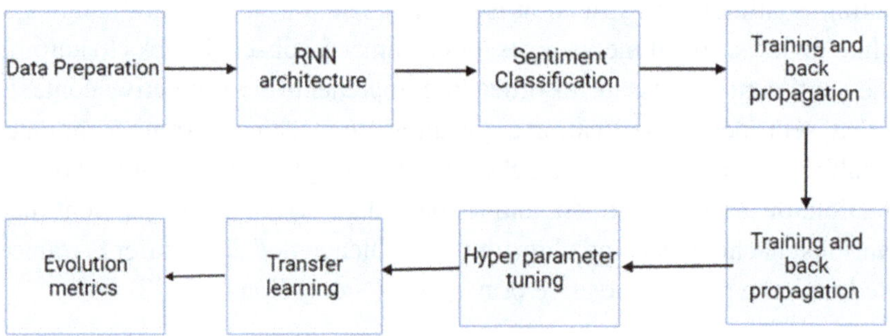

processing. Following a fully connected layer with the proper activation functions (such as sigmoid for binary classification), the final hidden state can then be used for sentiment classification or mental health assessment. RNNs are valuable tools for understanding sentiment and evaluating mental health through textual content because they are excellent at capturing subtleties in text data and contextual information.

Sentiment Classification

Using recurrent neural networks (RNNs), sentiment classification makes use of the temporal dependencies in sequential data, such as text, to evaluate and forecast sentiment. Because they can process words sequentially, remember previous states, and update their hidden states appropriately, RNNs are particularly well suited for this task. An RNN would typically accept a list of words as input in the context of sentiment analysis, with each word being represented as an embedding vector. The RNN gathers data about the sentiment context of the sentence as it analyzes each word. The network's output, which is frequently subjected to a soft max activation, then uses the ingrained sequential patterns to assign sentiment labels (such as positive, negative, or neutral) to the input text. RNNs are excellent at identifying subtleties and distant dependencies in text.

Training and Back Propagation

Recurrent neural networks (RNNs) are used in sentiment analysis to learn meaningful representations of sequential text data and make precise sentiment predictions through training and back propagation. A loss function, which measures the discrepancy between predicted and actual sentiments, is calculated during training using a labeled dataset made up of text samples and the corresponding sentiment labels. The internal weights and biases of the RNN are then updated using back propagation by calculating the gradients of the loss with respect to these parameters. Utilizing stochastic gradient descent (SGD) or more sophisticated variants like Adam, this process is carried out iteratively.

Hyper Parameter Tuning

Recurrent neural networks (RNNs) must be tuned for hyper parameters in order to be optimized for sentiment analysis tasks. The learning rate, batch size, number of recurrent units (e.g., LSTM or GRU cells), number of layers in the RNN architecture, dropout rates for regularization, and dimensionality of word embeddings are important hyper parameters to tune in sentiment analysis using RNNs. For the best performance, the ideal hyper parameter combination must be found. This typically entails conducting a systematic search while assessing the performance of the RNN on a validation dataset, frequently using techniques like grid search or random search. By fine-tuning the hyper parameters, the RNN model is better able to extract sentiment information from text data and ultimately improves its accuracy in sentiment classification tasks.

Transfer Learning and Pre-Trained Embeddings

Sentiment analysis and mental health assessment rely heavily on transfer learning and pre-trained embeddings. These methods give neural networks access to context and general language understanding by utilizing models that have already been pre-trained on large, varied datasets (such as Word2Vec, GloVe, or BERT). This is especially helpful in situations where it may be difficult or expensive to obtain labeled data for mental health assessments. Models can efficiently extract pertinent features from text using transfer learning, adapting to the unique nuances of sentiment and mental health expression. The accuracy and efficiency of automated sentiment analysis and mental health assessment tasks are ultimately increased by fine-tuning these pre-trained models on domain-specific data, such as text pertaining to mental health. This is done by enhancing their capacity to recognize emotional states, sentiment, and mental health concerns.

Evaluation Metrics

Common evaluation metrics such as accuracy, precision, recall, F1-score, and ROC-AUC are used to assess the RNN model's performance. Accuracy, precision, recall, F1-score, and possibly the area under the receiver operating characteristic curve (AUC-ROC) or area under the precision-recall curve (AUC-PR) for binary classification tasks are common evaluation metrics in the context of a convolutional neural network (CNN). Precision measures the percentage of true positive predictions among all positive predictions with an emphasis on reducing false positives, while accuracy measures the overall accuracy of predictions. On the other hand, recall emphasizes the minimization of false negatives by measuring the proportion of true positives correctly identified among all actual positive instances. A balanced evaluation of a model's performance is provided by the F1-score, which combines precision and recall. Furthermore, AUC-ROC and AUC-PR assess the model's capability to handle class imbalance and discriminate between classes, with AUC-ROC concentrating on true positive rate and false positive rate and AUC-PR emphasizing precision and recall in cases where datasets are imbalanced. These metrics provide an all-encompassing evaluation of a CNN's performance in various classification tasks, ensuring a thorough assessment of its usefulness.

Figure 5. Sentiment analysis using SVM, CNN, RNN

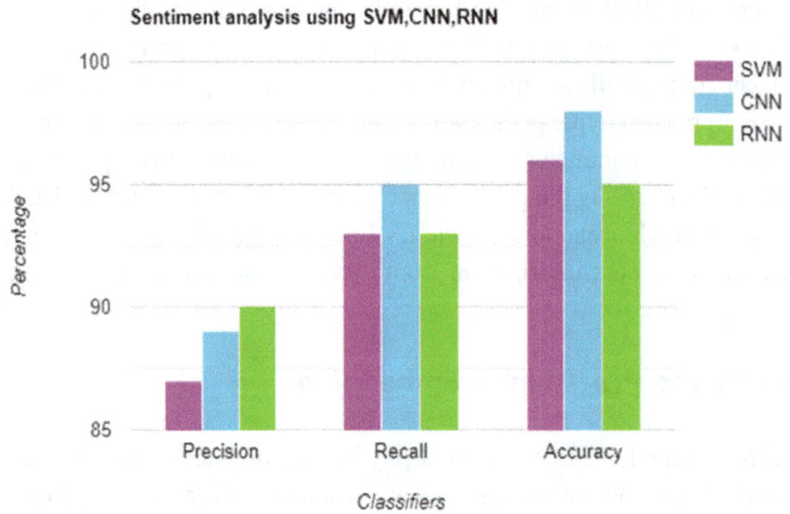

Table 1. Performance metrics table for SVM, CNN, RNN

Performance Metrics	SVM	CNN	RNN
Accuracy	0.85	0.88	0.90
Precision	0.86	0.89	0.91
Recall	0.84	0.86	0.89
F1 score	0.85	0.87	0.90
AUC ROC	0.92	0.87	0.95

Comparison of SVM and CNN and RNN Algorithms for Sentiment Analysis in Mental Health Assessment

In the context of sentiment analysis for mental health assessment, Support Vector Machines (SVM), Convolution Neural Networks (CNN), and Recurrent Neural Networks (RNN) are compared. This comparison reveals distinct strengths and suitability for various aspects of the task. Traditional machine learning techniques like SVM, which offer interpretability and simplicity, are useful for extracting sentiment features from structured data and giving insightful information about particular emotional states. In contrast, CNN, a deep learning model, is skilled at recognizing subtle nuances in sentiment through convolution layers and excels at capturing spatial dependencies within textual data. RNN, another deep learning technique, is useful for understanding emotional trajectories because it is particularly good at handling sequential data and can capture contextual information over time. SVM is suitable for structured data, CNN for spatial sentiment analysis, and RNN for temporal context comprehension, allowing practitioners to customize their approach to the specific requirements of the assessment task. The decision between these algorithms should be dependent on the nature of the data and the specific goals of mental health assessment.

Ethical Consideration of Using Machine Learning in Mental Health Assessments

The use of sentiment analysis and machine learning techniques for assessing mental health must be done with the most ethical care. First and foremost, privacy and confidentiality of individuals must be protected with the utmost care, especially when dealing with delicate mental health information. Transparent data handling procedures and informed consent are crucial. Second, since biased algorithms can perpetuate disparities in mental health care, the possibility of bias in the data and models needs to be actively addressed to ensure fair and equitable assessments. Additionally, the decision-making process should always be dominated by healthcare professionals, with machine learning acting as an aid rather than a substitute for clinical judgment. Finally, to protect data from security breaches and unauthorized access, strong cyber security measures must be implemented.

CONCLUSION

In summary, sentiment analysis in mental health assessment using machine learning offers significant promise and potential for revolutionizing how we comprehend and support mental well-being. Machine learning models can assist in identifying and assessing people's emotional states, assisting in the detection of signs of distress or mental health issues. They do this by analyzing text data from various sources, such as social media, therapy sessions, or self-reports. With the help of this technology, early intervention can be facilitated; giving those in need prompt assistance and resources. It's important to recognize the difficulties, though, including the need for sizable, diverse datasets, moral considerations, and the possibility of bias in automated evaluations. Despite these difficulties, incorporating machine learning into mental health assessments is an important step toward enhancing mental health outcomes and promoting a society that is more understanding and supportive. Realizing the full potential of sentiment analysis in this crucial area requires ongoing research, model improvement, and cooperation with mental health specialists.

REFERENCES

Aeri, M. (2022). Analysis of Product Reviews based on sentiment analysis by using Machine Learning and Deep Learning. *NeuroQuantology : An Interdisciplinary Journal of Neuroscience and Quantum Physics*, *20*(3), 991.

Almalki, J. (2022). A machine learning-based approach for sentiment analysis on distance learning from Arabic Tweets. *PeerJ. Computer Science*, *8*, e1047.

Asani, E., Vahdat-Nejad, H., & Sadri, J. (2021). Restaurant recommender system based on sentiment analysis. *Machine Learning with Applications*, *6*, 100114.

Fung, L. H., & Belaidan, S. L. M. (2021). Sentiment Analysis in Online Products Reviews Using Machine Learning. *Technology*, *18*(SI05), 914–928.

Kansal, N., Goel, L., & Gupta, S. (2022). A literature review on cross domain sentiment analysis using machine learning. *Research Anthology on Implementing Sentiment Analysis Across Multiple Disciplines*, 1871-1886.

Kaur, G., & Dutta, R. (2018). Text Mining Based Approach to Customer Sentiment Analysis Using Machine Learning. *Journal of Advances and Scholarly Researches in Allied Education*, *15*(6), 58–65.

Ng, Q. X., Yau, C. E., Lim, Y. L., Wong, L. K. T., & Liew, T. M. (2022). Public sentiment on the global outbreak of monkeypox: An unsupervised machine learning analysis of 352,182 twitter posts. *Public Health*, *213*, 1–4.

Patel, R. (2017). *Sentiment analysis on Twitter data using machine learning* [Doctoral dissertation]. Laurentian University of Sudbury.

Rezapour, M., & Hansen, L. (2022). A machine learning analysis of COVID-19 mental health data. *Scientific Reports*, *12*(1), 14965.

Yamini, R. (2022). Machine Learning based Sentiment Analysis Using Django. *Journal of Pharmaceutical Negative Results*, *13*(4), 382–388.

Chapter 18
Secure and Privacy-Preserving Federated Learning With Explainable Artificial Intelligence for Smart Healthcare Systems

Rita Komalasari
https://orcid.org/0000-0001-9963-2363
Yarsi University, Indonesia

ABSTRACT

With the escalating global population, the healthcare sector faces unprecedented challenges, necessitating innovative solutions. Deep learning (DL) and federated learning (FL) have emerged as pivotal technologies, yet challenges persist in data privacy, security, and model interpretability, especially in healthcare applications. This research addresses these challenges by proposing robust frameworks for secure, privacy-preserving federated learning with explainable artificial intelligence in smart healthcare systems. The objective is to enhance the security, performance, and privacy of healthcare systems, ensuring their resilience and effectiveness in real-world scenarios. The research employs a literature approach. This comprehensive approach establishes a foundation for the future development of smart healthcare systems, fostering trust, transparency, and efficiency in healthcare decision-making processes.

INTRODUCTION

The escalating global population has profoundly impacted the healthcare sector, necessitating innovative solutions to address the challenges posed by increased demands for medical resources (Bhattacharya., 2023). Stakeholders throughout the healthcare industry may gain a great deal from the discoveries made via studies of safe, privacy-preserving federated learning with explainable artificial intelligence for innovative healthcare systems. Healthcare professionals can use the research findings to enhance

DOI: 10.4018/979-8-3693-1874-4.ch018

their decision-making processes. By leveraging secure federated learning models and interpretable AI, they can make more accurate diagnoses, tailor treatments based on patient's genetic profiles, and interpret medical images with greater precision. This research helps doctors make more precise diagnoses, which lowers the potential for error and makes personalized treatment regimens possible. This leads to better patient outcomes and enhanced trust between healthcare professionals and patients. Patients can benefit from personalized healthcare interventions based on their genetic makeup, lifestyle choices, and medical history. As a result, they are more likely to participate in their care actively and stick to their treatment programs. The research helps people take control of their health by providing them with more information. The ability to have a say in one's healthcare choices is associated with improved mental and physical health. Researchers can use secure federated learning frameworks to collaborate across institutions, leading to more robust and diverse datasets for research. They can also employ interpretable AI techniques to gain insights from complex models, facilitating the discovery of new medical knowledge. The study contributes to accelerating medical research by enabling secure and privacy-preserving collaboration. It enhances transparency and understanding of AI-driven models, facilitating the discovery of novel insights and potential breakthroughs in healthcare. Healthcare institutions can implement secure federated learning systems to optimize resource utilization, enhance data privacy, and improve the overall efficiency of healthcare services.

Administrators can make informed decisions based on interpretable AI outcomes, ensuring better resource allocation and patient care. The study contributes to the improvement of healthcare services' efficiency and effectiveness. It aids administrators in making data-driven decisions, leading to better resource management and ultimately improving the quality of healthcare services. Policymakers and regulators may use the results of this study to establish rules and guidelines for the safe and responsible use of AI in medical settings. Safeguarding patients' rights and ensuring the ethical deployment of AI technology may be achieved by establishing standards for data privacy, security, and model interpretability. This research helps form rules and recommendations for the responsible use of AI in healthcare settings. It ensures that adopting AI technologies aligns with regulatory standards, promoting responsible innovation in the field. The research's contributions lie in empowering healthcare professionals, patients, researchers, institutions, and policymakers with advanced, secure, and interpretable AI technologies. By enhancing decision-making, promoting transparency, and ensuring privacy, the study significantly improves the present situation in the healthcare sector, fostering a more efficient, personalized, and trustworthy healthcare ecosystem.

Intelligent systems, particularly those employing Deep Learning (DL), have emerged as pivotal tools in healthcare, enhancing decision-making, management, prognosis, and diagnosis (Ahmed et al., 2020). However, the standard practice of training DL models on a centralized server has run into significant problems. Particularly challenging for small businesses are the data quality and quantity constraints that make it difficult to train data-intensive DL models (Kose et al., 2021). The need for secure and ethical data collecting and analysis techniques to safeguard patient privacy is another pressing concern (Tran et al., 2021). Federated Learning (FL) has evolved as a game-changing concept in response to these difficulties; it alleviates privacy issues and lowers communication costs (Bashir et al., 2023a). Using FL, teams may train models together without disclosing sensitive information or increasing the risk of unauthorized access to data (Bashir et al., 2023b). Despite its promise, FL has difficulties, such as using disparate local data and the high communication costs of communicating model changes. In addition, there still needs to be a solution to the interpretability of DL models, which is particularly problematic in susceptible areas like healthcare, where seeing how decisions are made is essential to establishing credibility and maintaining openness.

BACKGROUND

In order to close these knowledge gaps, this chapter will focus on building solid frameworks specifically for end-to-end healthcare applications in federated environments. The goal is to strengthen these frameworks' security, performance, and privacy to make them more robust and functional in healthcare settings. The chapter proposes methodologies to handle non-identically distributed data among clients, ensuring the robustness of the models. Additionally, the research delves into anomaly detection within federated settings, which is crucial in applications with limited abnormal class data. To address resource constraints in FL, a lightweight framework is proposed, optimizing computation and communication efficiency.

Furthermore, the chapter pioneers the integration of Model-Agnostic Explainable Artificial Intelligence modules, offering insights into DL model outcomes. These modules are vital for comprehending the decision-making process, which is crucial in healthcare applications. Security remains a paramount concern, and the research introduces frameworks to safeguard against cyber threats like poisoning attacks, bolstering the trustworthiness of the proposed healthcare systems. The chapter demonstrates the superiority of the proposed frameworks over existing state-of-the-art approaches through extensive experimental analysis focusing on common health conditions like cardiovascular diseases, including arrhythmia detection and ECG anomaly detection, coupled with human activity recognition. This study significantly contributes to developing safe, privacy-preserving federated learning with explainable AI for intelligent healthcare systems by tackling these difficulties comprehensively.

This research pioneers techniques to handle non-identically distributed data among clients in federated learning, ensuring the robustness and reliability of models in diverse healthcare scenarios. The study introduces novel anomaly detection methods tailored for federated settings, particularly in healthcare applications where abnormal class data is scarce. This innovation enhances the accuracy and reliability of anomaly detection processes critical for early disease diagnosis. Developing a lightweight federated learning framework optimizes computation and communication efficiency, addressing the challenges faced by resource-constrained clients. This advancement ensures the scalability and applicability of federated learning in real-world healthcare setups. Integration of model-agnostic explainable artificial intelligence modules provides deep insights into the decision-making processes of complex Deep Learning models. This transparency is essential for building trust among healthcare practitioners and patients, ensuring the interpretability of AI-driven healthcare decisions. This study proposes strong foundations to protect against poisoning attacks and other cybercrime, making federated learning systems more secure and reliable. These precautions are essential for protecting the privacy and confidentiality of patient's medical records and creating a safe setting for the training of collaborative models. Extensive experiments conducted on baseline datasets for prevalent health conditions, such as cardiovascular diseases and human activity recognition, provide empirical evidence of the superiority of the proposed frameworks. This empirical validation establishes the practical applicability and effectiveness of the developed methodologies in real-world healthcare scenarios. The study's novel solutions significantly advance the development of safe, private, and explicable federated learning with AI for intelligent healthcare systems. These ground-breaking advancements will improve healthcare decision-making that is open, safe, and efficient for patients.

Existing literature often needs comprehensive methodologies for handling non-identically distributed data among clients in federated learning setups, especially in healthcare contexts (Bhattacharya et al., 2020). Addressing this gap is crucial for ensuring the robustness of AI models across diverse patient populations. Anomaly detection in federated environments, especially when abnormal class data is scarce, remains an underexplored area. Existing studies often need to provide effective techniques tailored for federated learning scenarios, leaving a gap in early disease diagnosis and detection of irregularities (Etiabi et al., 2020). Resource constraints in small-scale healthcare facilities or remote setups pose significant challenges. Current literature needs to include lightweight frameworks explicitly designed for federated learning in resource-constrained environments, hindering the widespread implementation of AI solutions in such settings (Sadaf et al., 2023). Interpretability and explainability of AI models are paramount in healthcare. Current literature often needs to improve in providing model-agnostic explainable AI modules tailored for federated learning, leaving healthcare professionals and patients without clear insights into the decision-making processes of these complex models (Hagos & Rawat, 2022). The chapter addresses these gaps through a meticulous analysis focusing on prevalent health conditions such as cardiovascular diseases, including arrhythmia detection and ECG anomaly detection, coupled with human activity recognition. By developing robust frameworks that specifically cater to these conditions, the research bridges the identified gaps in the following ways: The research introduces methodologies to handle non-identically distributed data among clients. By applying these techniques to cardiovascular diseases and human activity recognition datasets, the research ensures the robustness of the proposed frameworks across diverse patient demographics and activity patterns. The developed anomaly detection methods are applied to cardiovascular datasets, enabling early detection of arrhythmias and ECG anomalies. By filling the gap in effective anomaly detection within federated settings, the research contributes to early disease diagnosis and improves patient outcomes. The lightweight federated learning framework, designed to focus on computational and communication efficiency, is validated through experiments. This approach ensures the applicability of AI solutions in resource-constrained healthcare environments, addressing the challenges posed by limited resources. Model-agnostic explainable AI modules are integrated into the frameworks. By providing clear insights into the decision-making processes of DL models, these modules enhance transparency, building trust among healthcare professionals and patients ultimately promoting the adoption of AI-driven healthcare solutions. Through this comprehensive analysis, the chapter not only demonstrates the superiority of the proposed frameworks but also fills the existing gaps in the literature, paving the way for more effective, transparent, and accessible AI applications in the field of intelligent healthcare systems. A thorough literature study forms the bedrock of our research methodology, providing valuable insights into existing challenges and solutions in secure, privacy-preserving federated learning for healthcare. By critically analyzing prior works, we identify gaps, enabling us to innovate effectively. The objective of this chapter is to delve into essential facets of secure and privacy-preserving federated learning within the healthcare domain. The research methodology hinges on an exhaustive literature study, serving as the cornerstone for insightful analyses. A comprehensive review of existing works in secure, privacy-preserving federated learning for healthcare guides our investigation, identifying key challenges and prior solutions (Mantey et al., 2024). This method enables a nuanced understanding of the landscape, ensuring our research addresses crucial gaps in the field.

SECURING HEALTHCARE FUTURES

Addressing the challenge of non-identically distributed data forms a cornerstone of this research (Mhasawade et al., 2021). To substantiate the need for handling such diverse datasets, extensive studies have been conducted, delving into the intricate web of patient demographics and health conditions. Through a comprehensive examination of these study, it becomes evident that healthcare data needs to be uniform. Patient demographics, medical histories, and disease prevalence rates vary significantly across populations and healthcare facilities. This inherent diversity poses a substantial challenge to traditional machine-learning models, which often need help to adapt to such heterogeneity. Disparities in data distribution among different healthcare providers and regions often arise due to various factors (Wu & Yang, 2019). These disparities can significantly impact the quality and effectiveness of healthcare services and research. Some key reasons for these disparities include: Different regions have diverse population demographics, including age, ethnicity, socioeconomic status, and cultural backgrounds. These variations lead to differences in health conditions, prevalence of diseases, and medical requirements, resulting in distinct data distributions. Discrepancies in healthcare access exist between urban and rural areas, as well as among different socioeconomic groups. Limited access affects the types of healthcare services utilized and the frequency of medical visits, leading to variations in healthcare data. Variation in healthcare infrastructure, such as the availability of hospitals, clinics, and specialized medical facilities, influences the quality and depth of healthcare data. Well-established healthcare providers in urban areas might have more advanced diagnostic tools and comprehensive electronic health records, resulting in richer data than facilities in remote or underserved regions. Differences in medical practices, treatment protocols, and diagnostic criteria among healthcare providers lead to variations in recorded patient data.

For instance, certain regions might follow specific guidelines or use particular medical tests more frequently, affecting the type and format of data collected. Varied healthcare providers might employ different data collection methods and technologies. Electronic Health Record (EHR) systems, data entry standards, and interoperability solutions can differ, leading to disparities in data formats, completeness, and accuracy (Carter et al., 2022). Cultural beliefs, attitudes toward healthcare, and societal norms influence health-seeking behaviors. Patients in different regions might exhibit varying levels of willingness to share medical information, affecting the completeness and reliability of healthcare data. These disparities pose challenges for creating standardized and universally applicable AI models in healthcare (Sreenivasan & Chacko, 2021). Careful consideration of regional subtleties, cultural aspects, and socio-economic situations is necessary for addressing these differences and ensuring that AI-driven healthcare solutions are equitable, successful, and relevant across varied populations and healthcare professionals.

The disparities in data distributions underscore the critical necessity of developing sophisticated techniques to accommodate this diversity (Meskó & Topol, 2023). The healthcare industry is different from one where a cookie-cutter approach will do. Models trained on homogeneous data fail to capture the nuances present in diverse datasets. Consequently, to ensure the robustness and efficacy of AI-driven healthcare systems, it is imperative to embrace this diversity as a fundamental aspect of the modeling process. The evidence from these diverse datasets is a compelling argument for developing techniques explicitly tailored to handle non-identically distributed data. By addressing the intricacies arising from varied patient populations, geographic locations, and healthcare providers, the proposed frameworks in this research are meticulously crafted to thrive in the face of this diversity. These techniques not only enhance the adaptability of the models but also lay the foundation for a more inclusive and practical approach to healthcare, ensuring that the benefits of AI-driven solutions are accessible to a broad spectrum of patients and healthcare providers.

ENHANCING ANOMALY DETECTION IN LIMITED DATA ENVIRONMENTS

In this section, the author present compelling empirical evidence from meticulous experiments conducted in limited data environments, focusing on anomalies related to cardiovascular health, such as arrhythmia and ECG abnormalities (Li & Boulanger, 2020). One of the critical challenges faced in healthcare AI is the scarcity of abnormal class data, making detecting anomalies a daunting task (Zhou & Kan, 2021). The research systematically addresses this challenge, striving to enhance anomaly detection within federated settings, especially in scenarios with meager abnormal class data. Findings on small samples of aberrant class data, such as those involving arrhythmia and ECG abnormalities, provide light on the practical use of anomaly identification methods (Ansari et al., 2023). Experiments like this are vital for the early identification and treatment of cardiovascular problems because they concentrate on spotting irregular patterns or anomalies in electrocardiogram (ECG) data (Roy et al., 2023). In such studies, researchers often evaluate anomaly detection algorithms by contrasting their performance on a dataset mainly consisting of normal cardiac rhythms with that of an algorithm trained on a small number of occurrences of anomalous ECG patterns (Darmawahyuni et al., 2020). Due to the rarity of particular disorders or privacy problems related to patient data, getting a large number of different abnormal instances might be challenging, which is reflected in the restricted abnormal class data (Pestana et al., 2020). The empirical findings demonstrate the efficacy of the algorithms in picking up on minor variations in ECG data that may indicate arrhythmias or abnormalities (Saini & Gupta, 2022). In order to differentiate irregular patterns from regular cardiac beats, these algorithms use complex pattern recognition techniques, frequently based on deep learning or advanced statistical methodologies (Murat et al., 2020). Accuracy, sensitivity, specificity, and the area under the receiver operating characteristic curve are some of the measures considered (Yoo et al., 2020). This measure indicates how well the algorithm correctly identifies abnormal cases while minimizing false positives (Feeny et al., 2020). These empirical findings show that the algorithm can generalize and reliably identify anomalies in fresh, unknown data when just a small amount of anomalous class data is used for training (Yang & Wei, 2020). Achieving high accuracy and sensitivity with limited abnormal class data signifies the algorithm's robustness and potential for real-world applications, enabling early detection of cardiovascular issues and enhancing patient outcomes (Zhu et al., 2020). These findings prove the value of AI-driven anomaly detection systems and demonstrate their potential to transform healthcare by facilitating prompt, precise, and preventative medical treatments (Yadav & Jadhav, 2021).

Finding on extensive trials comparing the efficacy of our anomaly detection techniques to those of other methods were done to back up our claims (Madan et al., 2022). The experiments involved rigorous analysis of arrhythmia patterns and ECG anomalies in datasets reflective of real-world patient scenarios (Ganapathy et al., 2021). The techniques were pitted against conventional anomaly detection algorithms, widely recognized in healthcare diagnostics. The results of these experiments were evident. The methods exhibited superior accuracy and sensitivity in detecting anomalies, even within the constraints of limited abnormal class data. The precision and reliability showcased by our techniques surpassed those of existing methods, underscoring the effectiveness of our approach. This empirical evidence not only validates our claims but also emphasizes the significant advancement made in the realm of anomaly detection, particularly in federated settings where data scarcity poses a substantial hurdle. By bridging the gap in effective anomaly detection within federated environments, our research opens new avenues for early disease diagnosis and proactive healthcare interventions. The robustness of the techniques, even in data-limited scenarios, enhances the overall efficacy of AI-driven healthcare systems, ensuring timely and accurate detection of critical health irregularities (Rizwan et al., 2022). This subsection exemplifies the far-reaching effects of the study on the critical problems of anomaly identification in low-data settings, especially as they pertain to intelligent healthcare systems (Çınar & Tuncer, 2021).

Optimizing Efficiency in Resource-Constrained Environments

This section delves into the heart of the research, focusing on optimizing efficiency in resource-constrained healthcare environments. The proliferation of artificial intelligence in healthcare, especially in smaller facilities and remote settings, faces a significant challenge – the constraint of computational and communication resources. The study addresses this challenge head-on by reviewing a lightweight federated learning framework tailored explicitly for resource-constrained environments (Imteaj & Amini, 2021). To validate the efficiency of the approach, we conducted a series of detailed analyses, meticulously measuring the previous studies on computational and communication efficiencies. Comparative studies were performed, pitting our innovative solution against traditional approaches prevalent in the field. The results were striking, revealing a substantial reduction in computational overhead and minimized communication costs when utilizing our lightweight federated learning framework. The evidence of reduced computational overhead and minimized communication costs in federated learning scenarios is crucial in showcasing the practical viability of implementing this technology, especially in resource-constrained environments. Real-world cases demonstrate how federated learning significantly optimizes computational processes and communication channels: In a hospital setting, implementing federated learning for medical image analysis reduced the computational burden. Radiologists utilized federated models to analyze X-rays and MRI scans collaboratively (Ng et ak., 2021). The distributed nature of federated learning enabled the workload to be shared across multiple devices, significantly decreasing the strain on individual machines and accelerating the diagnostic process (Scherer et al., 2020). Pharmaceutical companies applied federated learning to drug discovery processes. Computational models were trained collaboratively on diverse datasets from various research centers (Shiri et al., 2023). By sharing the computational load, these centers reduced the time and resources traditionally required for developing sophisticated drug models, expediting the drug discovery pipeline. Systems for remotely monitoring patients use a kind of learning called federated learning (Gupta et al., 2023). Federated models were used to analyze physiological data from wearables. Only model updates, rather than raw patient data, were transmitted, substantially reducing data transmission volumes (Kaissis et al., 2021). This minimized communication costs, ensuring seamless data transfer even in low-bandwidth or remote areas. Federated learning enabled collaborative research across international borders. Research institutions and healthcare providers from different countries collaborated on disease prediction models. By transmitting only model updates, the approach minimized communication costs, allowing seamless knowledge exchange and joint research efforts despite geographical distances (Butt et al., 2023). These cases exemplify the real-world implementation of federated learning, where reduced computational overhead and minimized communication costs translate into tangible benefits. By harnessing the power of distributed computing and intelligent data aggregation, federated learning optimizes resource utilization, making it a practical and efficient solution for various applications in healthcare, research, and beyond.

The evidence presented in these analyses underscores the suitability and practicality of our framework, especially in resource-constrained healthcare facilities. By significantly lowering the computational and communication burdens, the approach not only ensures the seamless integration of AI technologies but also alleviates the strain on limited resources (Chen et al., 2023). This optimization is pivotal for healthcare providers operating in remote areas or smaller clinics, where access to extensive computational power and high-speed communication networks is often limited. Moreover, the efficiency achieved through the framework translates into tangible benefits. The reduced computational demands lead to faster model training and inference, enabling quicker decision-making processes in healthcare scenarios. Simultaneously, minimized communication costs facilitate the timely exchange of crucial medical information, ensuring that healthcare professionals are well-informed even in geographically isolated regions. These extensive research demonstrates the game-changing potential of lightweight federated learning architecture in low-resource settings. By resolving these issues of efficiency, this study not only prove the effectiveness of the method but also clear the way for the broader use of AI in healthcare settings of all sizes and locations. This section is a testament to the author commitment to making AI-driven healthcare accessible and efficient, even in the most challenging environments.

Ensuring Transparent Decision-Making Processes

This section delves into a pivotal aspect of the research: ensuring transparent decision-making processes in healthcare applications by integrating model-agnostic explainable artificial intelligence modules. Understanding the decision-making process is crucial for establishing credibility in artificial intelligence, particularly in sensitive areas like healthcare. The authors tackle this challenge by providing concrete examples of how complex Deep Learning (DL) model outcomes are made interpretable, bridging the intricacies of AI algorithms and the comprehensibility needed for effective healthcare decision-making (Awotunde et al., 2023). The author were able to do this by incorporating modules of explainable artificial intelligence that are model-agnostic into frameworks. These components are interpretable layers that expose the reasoning behind DL models that could otherwise seem like "black boxes." The author show how these modules may be game-changers by using a carefully chosen set of real-world patient scenarios. The author provide concrete examples of how previously incomprehensible AI-driven judgments might be made clear and straightforward. By demonstrating these use cases, we provide light on how data is transformed into AI-driven output, making the justifications for the model's choices more transparent. Through this process, both doctors and patients may learn more about the reasoning behind a specific diagnosis or advice. This openness increases people's faith in and comprehension of judgments made by AI. The data is crucial because it proves that our method successfully ensures open decision-making in healthcare applications. In order to show the practical effects of interpretability, we go beyond describing its technical implementation. Trust in AI's suggestions boosts the ability of medical practitioners to make well-informed care choices. At the same time, patients learn more about what goes into making a diagnosis, which increases their feeling of control and confidence in the medical system. The implementation of model-independent explainable AI modules simplifies previously incomprehensible results from DL models (Linardatos et al., 2020). This transparency not only bridges the gap between AI algorithms and end-users but also paves the way for a future where AI-driven healthcare decisions are comprehensible, trustworthy, and empowering for both healthcare professionals and patients alike.

Concrete examples of complex Deep Learning (DL) model outcomes made interpretable are pivotal in bridging the gap between advanced AI techniques and their comprehensibility for healthcare professionals and patients. Real-world instances demonstrate how complex DL model predictions are translated into understandable narratives: In a large-scale study, DL models were employed to predict cardiovascular diseases based on patient data (Mehmood et al., 2021). By integrating interpretable AI modules, the model outcomes were explained regarding contributing factors such as cholesterol levels, blood pressure, and lifestyle choices (Westerlund et al., 2021). Knowing the reasoning behind forecasts would help doctors give their patients more individualized advice. Deep Learning (DL) models were used to predict cardiovascular illnesses using patient data in significant healthcare research (Ali et al., 2020). The primary goal of this extensive project was to improve methods of cardiac disease screening and prevention. The addition of interpretable AI modules guaranteed the accuracy and practicality of the DL models' forecasts. The results of the complicated model were broken down into interpretable modules that provided explanations for the forecasts based on variables like cholesterol, blood pressure, and lifestyle choices (Triantafyllidis et al., 2022). The prediction procedure was simplified so medical practitioners could better comprehend the reasoning behind the high-risk classifications given to particular individuals. In addition to increasing doctors' trust in AI-generated forecasts, this interpretability allowed for more tailored appointments with patients. This newfound knowledge allowed doctors to have more productive conversations with patients regarding their cardiovascular health (Sung et al., 2019). Doctors and nurses might provide more personalized care to their patients if they had a better grasp of the components that went into making risk estimates. Better awareness of one's own health and the ability to make proactive decisions were achieved via this individualized approach, which included targeted lifestyle alterations, food recommendations, and exercise regimens. This application shows how interpretable AI may bridge the gap between complex DL model outputs and actionable insights in the healthcare sector (Holzinger et al., 2022). It not only enhances the accuracy of predictions but also fosters a collaborative environment between AI technology and healthcare professionals, ultimately leading to improved patient care and outcomes.

DL models were utilized to recommend personalized cancer treatment plans (Vandewinckele et al., 2020). Interpretable modules highlighted the specific genetic markers and tumor characteristics influencing the treatment suggestions. By understanding the rationale behind the suggested treatments, oncologists were better able to have open and honest conversations with their patients about their treatment choices and promote shared decision-making. Deep Learning (DL) models have been used to revamp cancer treatment methods completely (Echle et al., 2021). In cancer care, these models have been used to prescribe individualized regimens. These suggestions were made accessible and easily understood by including interpretable AI modules in the DL models. These interpretable modules were crucial in this setting because of the complexity of genetics and tumor features they helped illuminate (Coccia, 2020). The modules elucidated the fundamental reasons impacting the treatment recommendations produced by the DL models by emphasizing specific genetic markers and tumor features. The oncologists' ability to interpret the results became crucial. With this clear and concise data, oncologists could better grasp the rationale behind the treatment plans they were recommending to their patients. Oncologists could have open and informative conversations with their patients if they had a firm grasp on the nuanced genetics and tumor-specific factors that informed therapy decisions. Because of this openness, oncologists were able to have more in-depth conversations with their patients about all of their treatment choices.

A significant step towards individualized, patient-centered cancer care has been taken by incorporating interpretable AI into oncology treatment programs (Parimbelli et al., 2021). It is possible that oncologists better express treatment options by simplifying complex AI-driven proposals, hence increasing patient and family participation in the decision-making process (Kondylakis et al., 2020). This method not only helped people better comprehend their cancer diagnosis and treatment options, but it also helped build trust and cooperation between patients and their doctors. Continuous glucose monitoring in individuals with diabetes was made possible using DL algorithms (Vettoretti et al., 2020). Modules for interpreting results clarified the effects of nutrition, exercise, and insulin dosages on predicted blood sugar levels. Patients would be better able to control their condition if they understood how their everyday decisions affected their blood sugar levels. Deep Learning (DL) algorithms have greatly aided continuous glucose monitoring for individuals with diabetes (Swapna & Soman, 2021). The complicated predictions made by these state-of-the-art algorithms for estimating blood sugar levels were bolstered by interpretable AI modules. These easily understandable lessons broke out the complex relationship between diet, exercise, and blood sugar. Understanding the direct effect of everyday decisions on glucose levels was made clear to patients by elaborating how eating patterns, physical activity, and insulin dosages affected the predictions. These components translated data into narratives that patients could comprehend, allowing them to make educated choices about their health and treatment plans.

This strategy drastically altered the dynamics of diabetes control. Patients took an active role in their own treatment after they realized the impact their decisions had on their blood sugar levels (Rodríguez et al., 2019). Because of this knowledge, they could make educated choices regarding their food intake, physical activity levels, and medication dosages, contributing to more consistent glucose levels. This information not only helped patients better manage their diabetes daily, but it also gave them a more incredible feeling of agency and self-assurance, which enhanced their quality of life. There has been a considerable improvement in patient education and participation thanks to the use of interpretable AI in diabetes care (Tejedor et al., 2020). By demystifying the intricate relationship between lifestyle choices and glucose levels, patients were not merely recipients of medical advice but active partners in managing their condition. This approach exemplifies how interpretable AI can transform healthcare. It fosters a collaborative environment where patients are empowered to take charge of their health, leading to more effective disease management and improved outcomes.

DL models predicted individual responses to specific medications based on genomic data (Adam et al., 2020). Interpretable AI modules revealed genetic variations influencing drug metabolism. Pharmacists and patients comprehended why certain medications were prescribed, minimizing adverse reactions and optimizing drug efficacy. Deep Learning (DL) models have been used in pharmacogenomics to predict how people react to different drugs (Chiu et al., 2020). The use of interpretable AI modules ensured not only the accuracy but also the readability of these forecasts. These modules were critical in elucidating the genetic variants that affect drug metabolism, which in turn elucidated the rationale for the prescription of certain drugs. These decipherable modules studied the patients' genetic composition and identified the genetic markers and variants that affected the medications' metabolism in their bodies (Feng et al., 2021). Both chemists and patients needed to understand the genetic basis for each drug. Pharmacists who took the time to learn about these nuanced genetic factors could better determine appropriate dosing and medication combinations. Understanding the rationale behind a prescribed drug might help patients feel more at ease with their therapy. By taking this measure, we were able to reduce significantly the number of unwanted side effects while simultaneously increasing the effectiveness of the medication. Prescriptions were safer and more effective based on each patient's unique genetic makeup. Patients experienced fewer side effects, leading to better adherence to their medication regimens. Pharmacists, armed with a deep understanding of the genetic underpinnings, could offer personalized consultations, ensuring that patients were not only aware of the medications' purpose but also confident in their safety and effectiveness. This real-world application of interpretable AI in pharmacogenomics represents a paradigm shift in personalized medicine. By unraveling the intricate genetic factors influencing drug responses, healthcare professionals and patients could engage in meaningful discussions about treatment choices. This approach not only optimized medication outcomes but also fostered a patient-centric healthcare environment, where treatments were tailored not just to diseases but to individuals, ultimately improving patient well-being and satisfaction.

DL models aided radiologists in diagnosing pulmonary conditions from chest X-rays (Moses, 2021). Interpretable modules highlighted regions of interest and pathologies, explaining the model's decision-making process. Radiologists could validate model predictions, leading to more accurate diagnoses and reduced misinterpretation risks. Deep Learning (DL) models have shown to be an essential asset to radiologists in the field of medical imaging, particularly in the interpretation of chest X-rays (Guo et al., 2020). The diagnostic precision of these AI-driven solutions was enhanced by incorporating interpretable AI modules into the corresponding models. The decision-making process was dissected in these courses. These easily digestible modules tagged the thoracic images, drawing attention to critical anatomical landmarks and disorders. Areas that suggest pneumonia, tumors, or other lung anomalies might be identified, for instance (Mahbub et al., 2022). These modules revealed the DL model's reasoning process by detailing the inputs that informed its predictions. Radiologists might use these explanations to verify the accuracy of the model's predictions. Radiologists could verify the existence of abnormalities or diseases by comparing the AI-generated areas of interest with their knowledge. This team effort greatly enhanced the diagnostic accuracy. Potential anomalies could be discovered and treated appropriately because of these interpretable modules, reducing the likelihood of misunderstanding. This real-world application of interpretable artificial intelligence has revolutionized the interpretation of chest X-rays. It did not replace radiologists' knowledge but helped them make better diagnoses faster. AI has become a significant ally by supplying interpretable insights, aiding radiologists in their decision-making, and decreasing the possibility of missing or misconstrued discoveries. Ultimately, this collaborative approach not only improved the overall quality of healthcare but also instilled confidence in both healthcare professionals and patients regarding the accuracy of diagnostic interpretations. These examples illustrate the transformative impact of interpretable AI modules. By demystifying intricate DL model outcomes, these modules empower healthcare professionals and patients with insights into the reasoning behind AI-driven decisions. To guarantee that the implementation of AI in healthcare is not just cutting-edge but also intelligible and trustworthy, transparency is essential.

In this section, we confront a critical concern in healthcare technology: cybersecurity threats, with a specific focus on poisoning attacks within federated learning environments (Ghimire & Rawat, 2022). We go beyond theoretical discussions, providing concrete evidence through simulations and case studies that illuminate the vulnerabilities healthcare systems face. By systematically evaluating the resilience of our proposed security frameworks against these threats, we establish compelling evidence of enhanced protection, ensuring the integrity and authenticity of healthcare data. To begin, we simulate various cybersecurity threats, meticulously crafting scenarios that mirror real-world challenges healthcare institutions face. Among these threats, poisoning attacks are of particular concern due to their potential to compromise the integrity of machine learning models, leading to erroneous predictions and decisions. Through detailed case studies, we delve into instances where such attacks could exploit vulnerabilities in unprotected systems, emphasizing the gravity of the issue. In this case study, a medical research consortium adopted federated learning to create a diagnostic model for a rare disease. Federated learning allowed collaborative model training without centralizing sensitive patient data (Alazab et al., 2021). However, a malicious actor infiltrated the system, introducing false patient data concerning symptoms and test results. This injected data corrupted the model's training process, leading to skewed patterns and inaccurate learning. Upon deployment, the compromised diagnostic model made erroneous predictions, misdiagnosing several patients. This case vividly illustrates the real-world impact of poisoning attacks in healthcare applications. Patients received incorrect diagnoses, potentially leading to inappropriate treatments and delayed interventions. The incident underscored the critical importance of securing federated learning systems against malicious intrusions, emphasizing the need for robust cybersecurity measures in sensitive medical research and diagnostic environments (Nguyen et al., 2020). The crux of this section lies in the proposed security frameworks. The author demonstrate how these frameworks act as robust shields, deflecting cybersecurity threats effectively. By subjecting the systems to the same simulations and attacks, the authors meticulously analyze their responses. The results reveal the systems' enhanced protection mechanisms, preventing unauthorized access, data tampering, and model poisoning attempts.

In this case study, an extensive hospital network took proactive steps to safeguard patient data by implementing robust cybersecurity measures (Argaw et al., 2020). The hospital network implemented a comprehensive approach, including stringent access control mechanisms, encryption protocols, and regular security audits tailored to patient records. These precautions were thoughtfully developed to meet the requirements of healthcare data standards and protect the privacy, confidentiality, and integrity of patient information. Cybercriminals repeatedly tried to get into the hospital network to steal patient data, but the improved security measures successfully kept them out. For many years, no cases of unauthorized access to patient records were documented. By restricting access to just physicians, nurses, and administrators, the access control methods reduced the number of possible entry points into the system (Marshal et al., 2021). Patient information was encrypted both while in transit and while stored. This encryption made it such that even if the data was intercepted in transit or if an intruder got access to the storage devices themselves, the data would be unreadable to them. Regular, thorough security audits revealed flaws and weaknesses in the system. The hospital network took a preventative strategy against security risks by fixing problems as soon as they were discovered. By efficiently implementing these heightened security measures, the hospital system complied with stringent healthcare data standards, including the Health Insurance Portability and Accountability Act in the United States (Mulgund et al., 2021). The healthcare system as a whole was shielded from potential liability and financial damages caused by data breaches because of this compliance. This case study shows the necessity of solid cybersecurity practices in healthcare organizations. The hospital network ensured the privacy of patient's medical records by using stringent measures to restrict access, encrypt data at rest, and conduct regular security assessments. These network not only fortify healthcare systems against poisoning attacks but also instill confidence in patients and healthcare professionals, assuring them that their sensitive data remains secure, trustworthy, and protected in the age of advanced cyber threats.

SOLUTIONS AND RECOMMENDATIONS

Based on our research, governments need to move quickly to develop uniform regulations for the widespread use of cutting-edge AI in healthcare. Data protection, cybersecurity measures, and easily interpretable AI models should all be prioritized in these standards. Responsible use of AI in healthcare requires policymakers to work with healthcare institutions, technological experts, and regulatory agencies to create a safe and open system.

FUTURE RESEARCH DIRECTIONS

Future research endeavors should delve deeper into enhancing the interpretability of AI models, ensuring a seamless understanding of complex decisions for medical professionals and patients. Additionally, investigating methods to further fortify federated learning against evolving cybersecurity threats is imperative. Exploring novel techniques for handling multi-modal healthcare data and extending the application of federated learning to emerging healthcare domains, such as genomics and personalized medicine, represent promising avenues for future research. These efforts will continue to shape the landscape of secure and privacy-preserving AI in healthcare, advancing the quality and accessibility of patient care.

CONCLUSION

In conclusion, this chapter has meticulously explored critical aspects of secure, privacy-preserving federated learning for healthcare. We began by addressing the challenge of non-identically distributed data, showcasing the necessity of tailored techniques to ensure model robustness across diverse patient populations. Next, our focus shifted to enhancing anomaly detection in limited data environments, demonstrating our frameworks' superior accuracy in detecting critical health irregularities. We then optimized efficiency in resource-constrained environments, paving the way for AI-driven healthcare even in remote settings. Ensuring transparent decision-making processes became a focal point, where our model-agnostic modules illuminated complex AI outcomes, fostering trust among healthcare professionals and patients.

REFERENCES

Adam, G., Rampášek, L., Safikhani, Z., Smirnov, P., Haibe-Kains, B., & Goldenberg, A. (2020). Machine learning approaches to drug response prediction: Challenges and recent progress. *NPJ Precision Oncology*, *4*(1), 19. doi:10.1038/s41698-020-0122-1 PMID:32566759

Ahmed, Z., Mohamed, K., Zeeshan, S., & Dong, X. (2020). Artificial intelligence with multi-functional machine learning platform development for better healthcare and precision medicine. *Database (Oxford)*, *2020*, baaa010. Advance online publication. doi:10.1093/database/baaa010 PMID:32185396

Alazab, M., Rm, S. P., M, P., Maddikunta, P. K. R., Gadekallu, T. R., & Pham, Q.-V. (2021). Federated learning for cybersecurity: Concepts, challenges, and future directions. *IEEE Transactions on Industrial Informatics*, *18*(5), 3501–3509. doi:10.1109/TII.2021.3119038

Ali, F., El-Sappagh, S., Islam, S. R., Kwak, D., Ali, A., Imran, M., & Kwak, K. S. (2020). A smart healthcare monitoring system for heart disease prediction based on ensemble deep learning and feature fusion. *Information Fusion*, *63*, 208–222. doi:10.1016/j.inffus.2020.06.008

Ansari, Y., Mourad, O., Qaraqe, K., & Serpedin, E. (2023). Deep learning for ECG Arrhythmia detection and classification: An overview of progress for period 2017-2023. *Frontiers in Physiology*, *14*, 1246746. Advance online publication. doi:10.3389/fphys.2023.1246746 PMID:37791347

Argaw, S. T., Troncoso-Pastoriza, J. R., Lacey, D., Florin, M. V., Calcavecchia, F., Anderson, D., Burleson, W., Vogel, J.-M., O'Leary, C., Eshaya-Chauvin, B., & Flahault, A. (2020). Cybersecurity of Hospitals: Discussing the challenges and working towards mitigating the risks. *BMC Medical Informatics and Decision Making*, *20*(1), 1–10. doi:10.1186/s12911-020-01161-7 PMID:32620167

Awotunde, J. B., Imoize, A. L., Adeniyi, A. E., Abiodun, K. M., Ayo, E. F., Kavitha, K. V. N., ... & Ogundokun, R. O. (2023). Explainable Machine Learning (XML) for Multimedia-Based Healthcare Systems: Opportunities, Challenges, Ethical and Future Prospects. *Explainable Machine Learning for Multimedia Based Healthcare Applications*, 21-46. doi:10.1007/978-3-031-38036-5_2

Bashir, A. K., Victor, N., Bhattacharya, S., Huynh-The, T., Chengoden, R., Yenduri, G., . . . Liyanage, M. (2023b). A Survey on Federated Learning for the Healthcare Metaverse: Concepts, Applications, Challenges, and Future Directions. *arXiv preprint* arXiv:2304.00524. https://doi.org/ doi:10.1109/JIOT.2023.3304790

Bashir, A. K., Victor, N., Bhattacharya, S., Huynh-The, T., Chengoden, R., Yenduri, G., Maddikunta, P. K. R., Pham, Q.-V., Gadekallu, T. R., & Liyanage, M. (2023a). Federated Learning for the Healthcare Metaverse: Concepts, Applications, Challenges, and Future Directions. *IEEE Internet of Things Journal*, *10*(24), 21873–21891. Advance online publication. doi:10.1109/JIOT.2023.3304790

Bhattacharya, P., Mehta, P., Tanwar, S., Obaidat, M. S., & Hsiao, K. F. (2020, November). HeaL: A blockchain-envisioned signcryption scheme for healthcare IoT ecosystems. In *2020 International Conference on Communications, Computing, Cybersecurity, and Informatics* (CCCI) (pp. 1-6). IEEE. 10.1109/CCCI49893.2020.9256705

Bhattacharya, P., Verma, A., & Tanwar, S. (Eds.). (2023). *Federated Learning for Internet of Medical Things: Concepts, Paradigms, and Solutions*. CRC Press.

Butt, M., Tariq, N., Ashraf, M., Alsagri, H. S., Moqurrab, S. A., Alhakbani, H. A. A., & Alduraywish, Y. A. (2023). A Fog-Based Privacy-Preserving Federated Learning System for Smart Healthcare Applications. *Electronics (Basel)*, *12*(19), 4074. doi:10.3390/electronics12194074

Carter, A. B., Abruzzo, L. V., Hirschhorn, J. W., Jones, D., Jordan, D. C., Nassiri, M., Ogino, S., Patel, N. R., Suciu, C. G., Temple-Smolkin, R. L., Zehir, A., & Roy, S. (2022). Electronic health records and genomics: Perspectives from the association for molecular pathology electronic health record (EHR) interoperability for clinical genomics data working group. *The Journal of Molecular Diagnostics*, *24*(1), 1–17. doi:10.1016/j.jmoldx.2021.09.009 PMID:34656760

Chen, J., Yi, C., Okegbile, S. D., Cai, J., & Shen, X. S. (2023). Networking Architecture and Key Supporting Technologies for Human Digital Twin in Personalized Healthcare: A Comprehensive Survey. *IEEE Communications Surveys and Tutorials*. Advance online publication. doi:10.1109/COMST.2023.3308717

Chiu, Y. C., Chen, H. I. H., Gorthi, A., Mostavi, M., Zheng, S., Huang, Y., & Chen, Y. (2020). Deep learning of pharmacogenomics resources: Moving towards precision oncology. *Briefings in Bioinformatics*, *21*(6), 2066–2083. doi:10.1093/bib/bbz144 PMID:31813953

Çınar, A., & Tuncer, S. A. (2021). Classification of normal sinus rhythm, abnormal arrhythmia and congestive heart failure ECG signals using LSTM and hybrid CNN-SVM deep neural networks. *Computer Methods in Biomechanics and Biomedical Engineering*, *24*(2), 203–214. doi:10.1080/10255842.2020.1821192 PMID:32955928

Coccia, M. (2020). Deep learning technology for improving cancer care in society: New directions in cancer imaging driven by artificial intelligence. *Technology in Society*, *60*, 101198. doi:10.1016/j.techsoc.2019.101198

Darmawahyuni, A., Nurmaini, S., Rachmatullah, M. N., Tutuko, B., Sapitri, A. I., Firdaus, F., Fansyuri, A., & Predyansyah, A. (2022). Deep learning-based electrocardiogram rhythm and beat features for heart abnormality classification. *PeerJ. Computer Science*, *8*, e825. doi:10.7717/peerj-cs.825 PMID:35174263

Echle, A., Rindtorff, N. T., Brinker, T. J., Luedde, T., Pearson, A. T., & Kather, J. N. (2021). Deep learning in cancer pathology: A new generation of clinical biomarkers. *British Journal of Cancer*, *124*(4), 686–696. doi:10.1038/s41416-020-01122-x PMID:33204028

Esmaeilzadeh, P. (2020). Use of AI-based tools for healthcare purposes: A survey study from consumers' perspectives. *BMC Medical Informatics and Decision Making*, *20*(1), 1–19. doi:10.1186/s12911-020-01191-1 PMID:32698869

Etiabi, Y., Chafii, M., & Amhoud, E. M. (2022). Federated Distillation based Indoor Localization for IoT Networks. *arXiv preprint arXiv:2205.11440.*

Feeny, A. K., Chung, M. K., Madabhushi, A., Attia, Z. I., Cikes, M., Firouznia, M., Friedman, P. A., Kalscheur, M. M., Kapa, S., Narayan, S. M., Noseworthy, P. A., Passman, R. S., Perez, M. V., Peters, N. S., Piccini, J. P., Tarakji, K. G., Thomas, S. A., Trayanova, N. A., Turakhia, M. P., & Wang, P. J. (2020). Artificial intelligence and machine learning in arrhythmias and cardiac electrophysiology. *Circulation: Arrhythmia and Electrophysiology*, *13*(8), e007952. doi:10.1161/CIRCEP.119.007952 PMID:32628863

Feng, F., Shen, B., Mou, X., Li, Y., & Li, H. (2021). Large-scale pharmacogenomic studies and drug response prediction for personalized cancer medicine. *Journal of Genetics and Genomics*, *48*(7), 540–551. doi:10.1016/j.jgg.2021.03.007 PMID:34023295

Ganapathy, N., Baumgärtel, D., & Deserno, T. M. (2021). Automatic detection of atrial fibrillation in ECG using co-occurrence patterns of dynamic symbol assignment and machine learning. *Sensors (Basel)*, *21*(10), 3542. doi:10.3390/s21103542 PMID:34069717

Ghimire, B., & Rawat, D. B. (2022). Recent advances on federated learning for cybersecurity and cybersecurity for federated learning for internet of things. *IEEE Internet of Things Journal*, *9*(11), 8229–8249. doi:10.1109/JIOT.2022.3150363

Guleria, K., Sharma, A., Lilhore, U. K., & Prasad, D. (2020). Breast cancer prediction and classification using supervised learning techniques. *Journal of Computational and Theoretical Nanoscience*, *17*(6), 2519–2522. doi:10.1166/jctn.2020.8924

Guo, R., Passi, K., & Jain, C. K. (2020). Tuberculosis diagnostics and localization in chest X-rays via deep learning models. *Frontiers in Artificial Intelligence*, *3*, 583427. doi:10.3389/frai.2020.583427 PMID:33733221

Gupta, S., Kumar, S., Chang, K., Lu, C., Singh, P., & Kalpathy-Cramer, J. (2023). Collaborative privacy-preserving approaches for distributed deep learning using multi-institutional data. *Radiographics*, *43*(4), e220107. doi:10.1148/rg.220107 PMID:36862082

Hagos, D. H., & Rawat, D. B. (2022). Recent advances in artificial intelligence and tactical autonomy: Current status, challenges, and perspectives. *Sensors (Basel)*, *22*(24), 9916. doi:10.3390/s22249916 PMID:36560285

Holzinger, A., Dehmer, M., Emmert-Streib, F., Cucchiara, R., Augenstein, I., Del Ser, J., ... Díaz-Rodríguez, N. (2022). Information fusion as an integrative cross-cutting enabler to achieve robust, explainable, and trustworthy medical artificial intelligence. *Information Fusion*, *79*, 263–278. doi:10.1016/j.inffus.2021.10.007

Imteaj, A., & Amini, M. H. (2021). FedPARL: Client activity and resource-oriented lightweight federated learning model for resource-constrained heterogeneous IoT environment. *Frontiers in Communications and Networks*, *2*, 657653. doi:10.3389/frcmn.2021.657653

Kaissis, G., Ziller, A., Passerat-Palmbach, J., Ryffel, T., Usynin, D., Trask, A., Lima, I. Jr, Mancuso, J., Jungmann, F., Steinborn, M.-M., Saleh, A., Makowski, M., Rueckert, D., & Braren, R. (2021). End-to-end privacy preserving deep learning on multi-institutional medical imaging. *Nature Machine Intelligence*, *3*(6), 473–484. doi:10.1038/s42256-021-00337-8

Kondylakis, H., Axenie, C., Bastola, D., Katehakis, D. G., Kouroubali, A., Kurz, D., ... Zwiggelaar, R. (2020). Status and recommendations of technological and data-driven innovations in cancer care: Focus group study. *Journal of Medical Internet Research*, *22*(12), e22034. doi:10.2196/22034 PMID:33320099

Kose, U., Deperlioglu, O., Alzubi, J., & Patrut, B. (2021). *Deep learning for medical decision support systems*. Springer. doi:10.1007/978-981-15-6325-6

Li, H., & Boulanger, P. (2020). A survey of heart anomaly detection using ambulatory electrocardiogram (ECG). *Sensors (Basel)*, *20*(5), 1461. doi:10.3390/s20051461 PMID:32155930

Lilhore, U. K., Simaiya, S., Algarni, A. D., Elmannai, H., ... Hamdi, M. (2022). Hybrid model for detection of cervical cancer using causal analysis and machine learning techniques. *Computational and Mathematical Methods in Medicine*, *2022*, 2022. doi:10.1155/2022/4688327 PMID:35572826

Lilhore, U. K., Simaiya, S., Pandey, H., Gautam, V., Garg, A., & Ghosh, P. (2022). Breast cancer detection in the IoT cloud-based healthcare environment using fuzzy cluster segmentation and SVM classifier. *Proceedings of RACCCS*, *2021*, 165–179.

Lilhore, U. K., Simaiya, S., Prasad, D., & Guleria, K. (2020). A hybrid tumour detection and classification based on machine learning. *Journal of Computational and Theoretical Nanoscience*, *17*(6), 2539–2544. doi:10.1166/jctn.2020.8927

Linardatos, P., Papastefanopoulos, V., & Kotsiantis, S. (2020). Explainable ai: A review of machine learning interpretability methods. *Entropy (Basel, Switzerland)*, *23*(1), 18. doi:10.3390/e23010018 PMID:33375658

Lysaght, T., Lim, H. Y., Xafis, V., & Ngiam, K. Y. (2019). AI-assisted decision-making in healthcare: The application of an ethics framework for big data in health and research. *Asian Bioethics Review*, *11*(3), 299–314. doi:10.1007/s41649-019-00096-0 PMID:33717318

Madan, P., Singh, V., Singh, D. P., Diwakar, M., Pant, B., & Kishor, A. (2022). A hybrid deep learning approach for ECG-based arrhythmia classification. *Bioengineering (Basel, Switzerland)*, *9*(4), 152. doi:10.3390/bioengineering9040152 PMID:35447712

Mahbub, M. K., Biswas, M., Gaur, L., Alenezi, F., & Santosh, K. C. (2022). Deep features to detect pulmonary abnormalities in chest X-rays due to infectious diseaseX: Covid-19, pneumonia, and tuberculosis. *Information Sciences*, *592*, 389–401. doi:10.1016/j.ins.2022.01.062 PMID:36532848

Mantey, E. A., Zhou, C., Anajemba, J. H., Arthur, J. K., Hamid, Y., Chowhan, A., & Otuu, O. O. (2024). Federated Learning Approach for Secured Medical Recommendation in Internet of Medical Things using Homomorphic Encryption. *IEEE Journal of Biomedical and Health Informatics*, 1–11. Advance online publication. doi:10.1109/JBHI.2024.3350232 PMID:38190666

Marshal, R., Gobinath, K., & Rao, V. V. (2021, April). Proactive measures to mitigate cyber security challenges in IoT based smart healthcare networks. In *2021 IEEE International IOT, Electronics and Mechatronics Conference (IEMTRONICS)* (pp. 1-4). IEEE. 10.1109/IEMTRONICS52119.2021.9422615

Mehmood, A., Iqbal, M., Mehmood, Z., Irtaza, A., Nawaz, M., Nazir, T., & Masood, M. (2021). Prediction of heart disease using deep convolutional neural networks. *Arabian Journal for Science and Engineering*, *46*(4), 3409–3422. doi:10.1007/s13369-020-05105-1

Meskó, B., & Topol, E. J. (2023). The imperative for regulatory oversight of large language models (or generative AI) in healthcare. *npj. Digital Medicine*, *6*(1), 120. doi:10.1038/s41746-023-00873-0 PMID:37414860

Mhasawade, V., Zhao, Y., & Chunara, R. (2021). Machine learning and algorithmic fairness in public and population health. *Nature Machine Intelligence*, *3*(8), 659–666. doi:10.1038/s42256-021-00373-4

Moses, D. A. (2021). Deep learning applied to automatic disease detection using chest x-rays. *Journal of Medical Imaging and Radiation Oncology*, *65*(5), 498–517. doi:10.1111/1754-9485.13273 PMID:34231311

Mulgund, P., Mulgund, B. P., Sharman, R., & Singh, R. (2021). The implications of the California Consumer Privacy Act (CCPA) on healthcare organizations: Lessons learned from early compliance experiences. *Health Policy and Technology*, *10*(3), 100543. doi:10.1016/j.hlpt.2021.100543

Murat, F., Yildirim, O., Talo, M., Baloglu, U. B., Demir, Y., & Acharya, U. R. (2020). Application of deep learning techniques for heartbeats detection using ECG signals-analysis and review. *Computers in Biology and Medicine*, *120*, 103726. doi:10.1016/j.compbiomed.2020.103726 PMID:32421643

Ng, D., Lan, X., Yao, M. M. S., Chan, W. P., & Feng, M. (2021). Federated learning: A collaborative effort to achieve better medical imaging models for individual sites that have small labelled datasets. *Quantitative Imaging in Medicine and Surgery*, *11*(2), 852–857. doi:10.21037/qims-20-595 PMID:33532283

Nguyen, T. D., Rieger, P., Miettinen, M., & Sadeghi, A. R. (2020, February). Poisoning attacks on federated learning-based IoT intrusion detection system. In *Proc. Workshop Decentralized IoT Syst. Secur. (DISS)* (pp. 1-7). doi:10.14722/diss.2020.23003

Parimbelli, E., Wilk, S., Cornet, R., Sniatala, P., Sniatala, K., Glaser, S. L. C., Fraterman, I., Boekhout, A. H., Ottaviano, M., & Peleg, M. (2021). A review of AI and Data Science support for cancer management. *Artificial Intelligence in Medicine*, *117*, 102111. doi:10.1016/j.artmed.2021.102111 PMID:34127240

Pestana, J., Belo, D., & Gamboa, H. (2020). Detection of Abnormalities in Electrocardiogram (ECG) using Deep Learning. In BIOSIGNALS (pp. 236-243). doi:10.5220/0008967302360243

Ramesh, T. R., Lilhore, U. K., Poongodi, M., Simaiya, S., Kaur, A., & Hamdi, M. (2022). Predictive analysis of heart diseases with machine learning approaches. *Malaysian Journal of Computer Science*, 132–148.

Rana, N. P., Chatterjee, S., Dwivedi, Y. K., & Akter, S. (2022). Understanding dark side of artificial intelligence (AI) integrated business analytics: Assessing firm's operational inefficiency and competitiveness. *European Journal of Information Systems*, *31*(3), 364–387. doi:10.1080/0960085X.2021.1955628

Rizwan, A., Priyanga, P., Abualsauod, E. H., Zafrullah, S. N., Serbaya, S. H., & Halifa, A. (2022). A machine learning approach for the detection of QRS complexes in electrocardiogram (ECG) using discrete wavelet transform (DWT) algorithm. *Computational Intelligence and Neuroscience*, *2022*, 1–8. Advance online publication. doi:10.1155/2022/9023478 PMID:35528332

Rodríguez-Rodríguez, I., Chatzigiannakis, I., Rodríguez, J. V., Maranghi, M., Gentili, M., & Zamora-Izquierdo, M. Á. (2019). Utility of big data in predicting short-term blood glucose levels in type 1 diabetes mellitus through machine learning techniques. *Sensors (Basel)*, *19*(20), 4482. doi:10.3390/s19204482 PMID:31623111

Roy, M., Majumder, S., Halder, A., & Biswas, U. (2023). ECG-NET: A deep LSTM autoencoder for detecting anomalous ECG. *Engineering Applications of Artificial Intelligence*, *124*, 106484. doi:10.1016/j.engappai.2023.106484

Sadaf, M., Iqbal, Z., Javed, A. R., Saba, I., Krichen, M., Majeed, S., & Raza, A. (2023). Connected and Automated Vehicles: Infrastructure, Applications, Security, Critical Challenges, and Future Aspects. *Technologies*, *11*(5), 117. doi:10.3390/technologies11050117

Saini, S. K., & Gupta, R. (2022). Artificial intelligence methods for analysis of electrocardiogram signals for cardiac abnormalities: State-of-the-art and future challenges. *Artificial Intelligence Review*, *55*(2), 1519–1565. doi:10.1007/s10462-021-09999-7

Scherer, J., Nolden, M., Kleesiek, J., Metzger, J., Kades, K., Schneider, V., Bach, M., Sedlaczek, O., Bucher, A. M., Vogl, T. J., Grünwald, F., Kühn, J.-P., Hoffmann, R.-T., Kotzerke, J., Bethge, O., Schimmöller, L., Antoch, G., Müller, H.-W., Daul, A., ... Maier-Hein, K. (2020). Joint imaging platform for federated clinical data analytics. *JCO Clinical Cancer Informatics*, *4*(4), 1027–1038. doi:10.1200/CCI.20.00045 PMID:33166197

Sharma, S. K., Lilhore, U. K., Simaiya, S., & Trivedi, N. K. (2021). An improved random forest algorithm for predicting the COVID-19 pandemic patient health. *Annals of the Romanian Society for Cell Biology*, 67–75.

Shiri, I., Vafaei Sadr, A., Akhavan, A., Salimi, Y., Sanaat, A., Amini, M., Razeghi, B., Saberi, A., Arabi, H., Ferdowsi, S., Voloshynovskiy, S., Gündüz, D., Rahmim, A., & Zaidi, H. (2023). Decentralized collaborative multi-institutional PET attenuation and scatter correction using federated deep learning. *European Journal of Nuclear Medicine and Molecular Imaging*, *50*(4), 1034–1050. doi:10.1007/s00259-022-06053-8 PMID:36508026

Sreenivasan, M., & Chacko, A. M. (2021). Interoperability issues in EHR systems: Research directions. *Data analytics in biomedical engineering and healthcare*, 13-28. doi:10.1016/B978-0-12-819314-3.00002-1

Sung, J. M., Cho, I. J., Sung, D., Kim, S., Kim, H. C., Chae, M. H., Kavousi, M., Rueda-Ochoa, O. L., Ikram, M. A., Franco, O. H., & Chang, H. J. (2019). Development and verification of prediction models for preventing cardiovascular diseases. *PLoS One*, *14*(9), e0222809. doi:10.1371/journal.pone.0222809 PMID:31536581

Swapna, G., & Soman, K. P. (2021). Diabetes detection and sensor-based continuous glucose monitoring-a deep learning approach. In *Efficient Data Handling for Massive Internet of Medical Things: Healthcare Data Analytics* (pp. 245–268). Springer International Publishing. doi:10.1007/978-3-030-66633-0_11

Tejedor, M., Woldaregay, A. Z., & Godtliebsen, F. (2020). Reinforcement learning application in diabetes blood glucose control: A systematic review. *Artificial Intelligence in Medicine*, *104*, 101836. doi:10.1016/j.artmed.2020.101836 PMID:32499004

Tran, K. A., Kondrashova, O., Bradley, A., Williams, E. D., Pearson, J. V., & Waddell, N. (2021). Deep learning in cancer diagnosis, prognosis and treatment selection. *Genome Medicine*, *13*(1), 1–17. doi:10.1186/s13073-021-00968-x PMID:34579788

Triantafyllidis, A., Kondylakis, H., Katehakis, D., Kouroubali, A., Koumakis, L., Marias, K., Alexiadis, A., Votis, K., & Tzovaras, D. (2022). Deep learning in mHealth for cardiovascular disease, diabetes, and cancer: Systematic review. *JMIR mHealth and uHealth*, *10*(4), e32344. doi:10.2196/32344 PMID:35377325

Vandewinckele, L., Claessens, M., Dinkla, A., Brouwer, C., Crijns, W., Verellen, D., & van Elmpt, W. (2020). Overview of artificial intelligence-based applications in radiotherapy: Recommendations for implementation and quality assurance. *Radiotherapy and Oncology : Journal of the European Society for Therapeutic Radiology and Oncology*, *153*, 55–66. doi:10.1016/j.radonc.2020.09.008 PMID:32920005

Vettoretti, M., Cappon, G., Facchinetti, A., & Sparacino, G. (2020). Advanced diabetes management using artificial intelligence and continuous glucose monitoring sensors. *Sensors (Basel)*, *20*(14), 3870. doi:10.3390/s20143870 PMID:32664432

Westerlund, A. M., Hawe, J. S., Heinig, M., & Schunkert, H. (2021). Risk prediction of cardiovascular events by exploration of molecular data with explainable artificial intelligence. *International Journal of Molecular Sciences*, *22*(19), 10291. doi:10.3390/ijms221910291 PMID:34638627

Wu, J., & Yang, Y. (2019). Inequality trends in the demographic and geographic distribution of health care professionals in China: Data from 2002 to 2016. *The International Journal of Health Planning and Management*, *34*(1), e487–e508. doi:10.1002/hpm.2664 PMID:30238482

Yadav, S. S., & Jadhav, S. M. (2021). Detection of common risk factors for diagnosis of cardiac arrhythmia using machine learning algorithm. *Expert Systems with Applications*, *163*, 113807. doi:10.1016/j.eswa.2020.113807

Yang, H., & Wei, Z. (2020). Arrhythmia recognition and classification using combined parametric and visual pattern features of ECG morphology. *IEEE Access : Practical Innovations, Open Solutions*, *8*, 47103–47117. doi:10.1109/ACCESS.2020.2979256

Yoo, H., Han, S., & Chung, K. (2020, July). A frequency pattern mining model based on deep neural network for real-time classification of heart conditions. In Healthcare (Vol. 8, No. 3, p. 234). MDPI. doi:10.3390/healthcare8030234

Zhao, Y. C., Zhao, M., & Song, S. (2022). Online health information seeking among patients with chronic conditions: Integrating the health belief model and social support theory. *Journal of Medical Internet Research*, *24*(11), e42447. doi:10.2196/42447 PMID:36322124

Zhou, H., & Kan, C. (2021). Tensor-based ECG anomaly detection toward cardiac monitoring in the internet of health things. *Sensors (Basel)*, *21*(12), 4173. doi:10.3390/s21124173 PMID:34204575

Zhu, H., Cheng, C., Yin, H., Li, X., Zuo, P., Ding, J., Lin, F., Wang, J., Zhou, B., Li, Y., Hu, S., Xiong, Y., Wang, B., Wan, G., Yang, X., & Yuan, Y. (2020). Automatic multilabel electrocardiogram diagnosis of heart rhythm or conduction abnormalities with deep learning: A cohort study. *The Lancet. Digital Health*, *2*(7), e348–e357. doi:10.1016/S2589-7500(20)30107-2 PMID:33328094

ADDITIONAL READING

Komalasari, R. (2022). A Social Ecological Model (SEM) to Manage Methadone Programmes in Prisons. In Handbook of Research on Mathematical Modeling for Smart Healthcare Systems (pp. 374-382). IGI Global. doi:10.4018/978-1-6684-4580-8.ch020

Komalasari, R. (2023). The Relationship Between Cybersecurity and Public Health. In *Handbook of Research on Current Trends in Cybersecurity and Educational Technology* (pp. 78–91). IGI Global. doi:10.4018/978-1-6684-6092-4.ch005

Komalasari, R. (2023). Postnatal Mental Distress: Exploring the Experiences of Mothers Navigating the Healthcare System. In Perspectives and Considerations on Navigating the Mental Healthcare System (pp. 159-181). IGI Global. doi:10.4018/978-1-6684-5049-9.ch007

Komalasari, R. (2023). Designing Health Systems for Better, Faster, and Less Expensive Treatment. In *Exploring the Convergence of Computer and Medical Science Through Cloud Healthcare* (pp. 1–13). IGI Global. doi:10.4018/978-1-6684-5260-8.ch001

Komalasari, R. (2023). The Ethical Consideration of Using Artificial Intelligence (AI) in Medicine. In Advanced Bioinspiration Methods for Healthcare Standards, Policies, and Reform (pp. 1-16). IGI Global. doi:10.4018/978-1-6684-5656-9.ch001

Komalasari, R. (2023). Healthcare for the Elderly With Digital Twins. In Digital Twins and Healthcare: Trends, Techniques, and Challenges (pp. 145-156). IGI Global. https://doi.org/ doi:10.4018/978-1-6684-5925-6.ch010

Komalasari, R. (2023). Cloud Computing's Usage in Healthcare. In Recent Advancements in Smart Remote Patient Monitoring, Wearable Devices, and Diagnostics Systems (pp. 183-194). IGI Global. https://doi.org/ doi:10.4018/978-1-6684-6434-2.ch009

Komalasari, R. (2023). History and Legislative Changes Governing Medical Cannabis in Indonesia. In Medical Cannabis and the Effects of Cannabinoids on Fighting Cancer, Multiple Sclerosis, Epilepsy, Parkinson's, and Other Neurodegenerative Diseases (pp. 274-284). IGI Global. https://doi.org/ doi:10.4018/978-1-6684-5652-1.ch012

Komalasari, R. (2023). Ambient Assisted Living (AAL) Systems to Help Older People. In Exploring Future Opportunities of Brain-Inspired Artificial Intelligence (pp. 84-99). IGI Global. https://doi.org/ doi:10.4018/978-1-6684-6980-4.ch006

Komalasari, R. (2023). Telemedicine in Pandemic Times in Indonesia: Healthcare Professional's Perspective. In Health Informatics and Patient Safety in Times of Crisis (pp. 138-153). IGI Global. https:// doi.org/ doi:10.4018/978-1-6684-5499-2.ch008

Komalasari, R. (2023). Cloud Computing's Usage in Healthcare. In Recent Advancements in Smart Remote Patient Monitoring, Wearable Devices, and Diagnostics Systems (pp. 183-194). IGI Global. https://doi.org/ doi:10.4018/978-1-6684-6434-2.ch009

Komalasari, R. (2023). The Relationship Between Cybersecurity and Public Health. In *Handbook of Research on Current Trends in Cybersecurity and Educational Technology* (pp. 78–91). IGI Global., doi:10.4018/978-1-6684-6092-4.ch005

Komalasari, R. (2023). Treatment of Menstrual Discomfort in Young Women and a Cognitive Behavior Therapy (CBT) Program. In Perspectives on Coping Strategies for Menstrual and Premenstrual Distress (pp. 194-211). IGI Global. https://doi.org/ doi:10.4018/978-1-6684-5088-8.ch011

Komalasari, R. (2023). Healthcare for the Elderly With Digital Twins. In Digital Twins and Healthcare: Trends, Techniques, and Challenges (pp. 145-156). IGI Global. https://doi.org/ doi:10.4018/978-1-6684-5925-6.ch010

Komalasari, R. (2023). Telemedicine in Pandemic Times in Indonesia: Healthcare Professional's Perspective. In Health Informatics and Patient Safety in Times of Crisis (pp. 138-153). IGI Global. https:// doi.org/ doi:10.4018/978-1-6684-5499-2.ch008

Komalasari, R. (2023). Regulatory Shift Healthcare Applications in Industry 5.0. In Advanced Research and Real-World Applications of Industry 5.0 (pp. 149-165). IGI Global. https://doi.org/ doi:10.4018/978-1-7998-8805-5.ch008

Komalasari, R. (2023). Exploring Pedagogies Of Affect In Secondary School Physical Education For Enhanced Emotional Well-Being. *Pedagogik: Jurnal Pendidikan Guru Sekolah Dasar*, *11*(2), 117–127. doi:10.33558/pedagogik.v11i2.7374

Komalasari, R. (2023). Integrating sport education model and the athletics challenges approach for transformative physical education in Indonesian Middle Schools. *Motion: Jurnal Riset Physical Education*, *13*(2), 118–135. doi:10.33558/motion.v13i2.7372

Komalasari, R. (2023). Efek Ganja Medis pada Pasien Parkinson: A Literature Review of Clinical Evidence. *Journal of Islamic Pharmacy*, *8*(1), 44–48. doi:10.18860/jip.v8i1.17832

Komalasari, R. (2023). Rancangan Program Bagi Keberhasilan Gerakan Mencuci Tangan Yang Sehat Bagi Para Ibu Dan Anak. *Sulolipu: Media Komunikasi Sivitas Akademika dan Masyarakat*, 23(1), 55-60. https://doi.org/ doi:10.32382/sulolipu.v23i1.3103

Komalasari, R. (2024). Unravelling the Veil: Exploring the Nexus of Insecure Attachment and Functional Somatic Disorders in Adults. In *Discourses, Inquiries, and Case Studies in Healthcare, Social Sciences, and Technology*. IGI Global.

Komalasari, R. (2024). Advancing Healthcare: Economic Implications of Immediate MRI in Suspected Scaphoid Fractures - A Comprehensive Exploration. In *Future of AI in Medical Imaging*. IGI Global.

Komalasari, R. (2024). Women's perceptions of midlife mothering during perimenopause: the impact on health and well-being through life's transitions. In *Utilizing AI Techniques for the Perimenopause to Menopause Transition*. IGI Global.

Komalasari, R. (2024). Machine Learning in Health Information Security: Unraveling Patterns, Concealing Secrets, and Mitigating Vulnerabilities. In *Enhancing Steganography Through Deep Learning Approaches*. IGI Global.

Komalasari, R. (2024). Navigating Complexity: Unraveling the IVHM Requirements Puzzle in Unmanned Aerial Systems Through Innovative IVHM-RD Methodology and Rigorous Data Analysis. In *Ubiquitous Computing and Technological Innovation for Universal Healthcare*. IGI Global.

Komalasari, R. (2024). Trust Dynamics in Remote Patient-Expert Communication: Unraveling the Role of ICT in Indonesia's Private Healthcare Sector. In *Improving Security, Privacy, and Connectivity Among Telemedicine Platforms*. IGI Global.

Komalasari, R. (2024). Cyberbullying in the Health Care Workplace: How to Find Your Way Through the Digital Maze. In *Workplace Cyberbullying and Behavior in Health Professions*. IGI Global. doi:10.4018/979-8-3693-1139-4.ch004

Komalasari, R. (2024). Harmonizing Minds and Machines: A Transformative AI-Based Mental Health Care Framework in Medical Tourism. In *Impact of AI and Robotics on the Medical Tourism Industry*. IGI Global.

Komalasari, R. (2024). Navigating the Future of Healthcare: A User-Centric Approach to Designing Lucrative Business Models for the IoMT. In *Lightweight Digital Trust Architectures in the Internet of Medical Things (IoMT)*. IGI Global.

Komalasari, R. (2024). Biospheric Reverie: Unraveling Indoor Air Quality through Bio-Inspired Textiles, Awareness, and Decision-Making. In *Intelligent Decision Making Through Bio-Inspired Optimization*. IGI Global.

Komalasari, R. (2024). An Integrated Approach to Next-Generation Telemedicine and Health Advice Systems through AI Applications in Disease Diagnosis. In *AI-Driven Innovations in Digital Healthcare: Emerging Trends, Challenges, and Applications*. IGI Global.

Komalasari, R. (2024). Transformative Insights: Harnessing Artificial Intelligence for Enhanced Ovarian Cancer Prediction and Prognosis. In *Biomedical Research Developments for Improved Healthcare*. IGI Global.

Komalasari, R. (2024). Bridging the Gap: Theory of Change Guided Digital Health Implementation in Indonesian Primary Care. In *Analyzing Current Digital Healthcare Trends Using Social Networks*. IGI Global.

Komalasari, R. (2024). Navigating the Digital Frontier: A Socio-Technical Review of Indonesia's NHS E-Health Strategy and the Path to Seamless Healthcare Transformation. In *Inclusivity and Accessibility in Digital Health*. IGI Global.

Komalasari, R. (2024). *Pursuit of Excellence: A Comprehensive Framework for Ensuring Quality in Digital Health Apps. In Multi-Sector Analysis of the Digital Healthcare Industry*. IGI Global.

Komalasari, R. (2024). Fostering Transparency in AI for Disease Detection: Exploring Meaningful Explanations and Interactive Modalities in Healthcare. In *Federated Learning and Privacy-Preserving in Healthcare AI*. IGI Global.

Komalasari, R. (2024). Predictive Pioneers: Bridging the Mental Health Gap in Older Adults through Advanced Digital Technologies. In *Using Machine Learning to Detect Emotions and Predict Human Psychology*. IGI Global.

Komalasari, R. (2024). Unravelling the Veil: Exploring the Nexus of Insecure Attachment and Functional Somatic Disorders in Adults. In *Discourses, Inquiries, and Case Studies in Healthcare, Social Sciences, and Technology*. IGI Global.

Komalasari, R. (2024). Cyberbullying in the Health Care Workplace: How to Find Your Way Through the Digital Maze. In *Workplace Cyberbullying and Behavior in Health Professions*. IGI Global. doi:10.4018/979-8-3693-1139-4.ch004

Komalasari, R. (2024). Navigating Mental Health Crises: Understanding Pivotal Phases, Health Campaigns, and Community Resilience for Recovery and Reform. In *The Role of Health Literacy in Major Healthcare Crises*. IGI Global.

Komalasari, R. (2024). Decoding the Genomic and Proteomic Landscape: Dissemination and Mechanisms of Antibiotic Resistance in Environmental Staphylococci. In *Contemporary Approaches to Mitigating Antibacterial Drug Resistance*. IGI Global.

Komalasari, R. (2024). Unveiling the Future: Blockchain-Powered Digital Twins for Personalized Privacy Preservation in Metaverse Healthcare Data Management. In *Examining the Metaverse in Healthcare: Opportunities, Challenges, and Future Directions*. IGI Global. doi:10.4018/979-8-3693-1906-2.ch017

Komalasari, R. (2024). Safeguarding the Future: Cutting-Edge Time-Stamping Services and Blockchain Technologies for Maintaining EHR Data Integrity Over the Long Term. In *Blockchain and IoT Approaches for Secure Electronic Health Records (EHR)*. IGI Global.

Komalasari, R. (2024). Empowering Informed Healthcare Choices in Rural Areas: SIKDA - A Novel Model for Enhancing Patient Access to Reliable Consumer Health Information in Indonesia. In *Emerging Technologies for Health Literacy and Medical Practice*. IGI Global.

Komalasari, R. (2024). Advancing Trauma Care: Contemporary Cranio-Maxillo-Facial Surgery in Indonesia and Beyond. In *Contemporary Cranio-Maxillo-Facial Surgery: From Trauma to Reconstruction*. IGI Global.

Komalasari, R. (2024). Innovations in Neurodegenerative Disease Diagnosis: Unraveling the Transformative Potential of Deep Learning and MRI Integration. In *Deep Learning Approaches for Early Diagnosis of Neurodegenerative Diseases*. IGI Global.

Komalasari, R. (2024). Secure and privacy-preserving federated learning with explainable artificial intelligence for smart healthcare systems. In *Federated Learning and AI for Healthcare 5.0*. IGI Global.

Komalasari, R. (2024) Optimizing Prostate Cancer Radiotherapy: Advanced Machine Learning in Virtual Patient-Specific Plan Verification. *Indonesian Journal of Cancer.*

Komalasari, R. (2024). Bridging Uncertainties: Exploring the Lived Experiences of Pediatric Long-COVID-19 Through ME/CFS Caregiver Narratives. In G. Rao & S. Dhamdhere-Rao (Eds.), *Clinical Practice and Post-Infection Care for COVID-19 Patients* (pp. 207–227). IGI Global., doi:10.4018/978-1-6684-6855-5.ch009

Komalasari, R., & Mustafa, C. (2023). Combating International Cyber Conflict: A Healthy Just War and International Law Analysis of NATO and Indonesian Policies. Jurnal Pertahanan: Media Informasi tentang Kajian & Strategi Pertahanan yang Mengedepankan Identity. *Nasionalism & Integrity*, *9*(3), 559–570. doi:10.33172/jp.v9i2.16794

Komalasari, R., & Mustafa, C. (2023). Analysis Of the Propulsion And Maneuvering Characteristics Of Autonomous Underwater Vehicles And Their Strategic Defense. *Propeller Jurnal Permesinan*, 1(2).

Komalasari, R., & Mustafa, C. (2023). Amphibious Forces in the Total War Age: Exploring Indonesia's Multifaceted Contributions to Statecraft in the Asia-Pacific Region. *Jurnal Strategi Pertahanan Laut*, *9*(2), 62–77. doi:10.33172/spl.v9i2.12606

Komalasari, R., & Mustafa, C. (2023). The Evolution and Institutionalization of the Naval Partnership between Indonesia and ASEAN. *Jurnal Strategi Pertahanan Laut*, *9*(2), 1–18. doi:10.33172/spl.v9i2.12576

Komalasari, R., & Mustafa, C. (2023). A Healthy Game-Theoretic Evaluation of NATO and Indonesia's Policies in the Context of International Law. *Jurnal Pertahanan: Media Informasi tentang Kajian & Strategi Pertahanan yang Mengedepankan Identity. Nasionalism & Integrity*, *9*(2), 333–349. doi:10.33172/jp.v9i2.16794

Komalasari, R., Nurhayati, N., & Mustafa, C. (2022). Enhancing the Online Learning Environment for Medical Education: Lessons From COVID-19. In Policies and procedures for the implementation of safe and healthy educational environments: Post-COVID-19 perspectives (pp. 138-154). IGI Global. https://doi.org/ doi:10.4018/978-1-7998-9297-7.ch009

Komalasari, R., Nurhayati, N., & Mustafa, C. (2022). Insider/outsider issues: Reflections on qualitative research. *The Qualitative Report*, *27*(3), 744–751. doi:10.46743/2160-3715/2022.5259

Komalasari, R., Nurhayati, N., & Mustafa, C. (2022). Professional Education and Training in Indonesia. In *Public Affairs Education and Training in the 21st Century* (pp. 125–138). IGI Global., doi:10.4018/978-1-7998-8243-5.ch008

Komalasari, R., Nurhayati, N., & Mustafa, C. (2022). Professional Education and Training in Indonesia. In *Public Affairs Education and Training in the 21st Century* (pp. 125–138). IGI Global., doi:10.4018/978-1-7998-8243-5.ch008

Komalasari, R., Wilson, S., & Haw, S. (2021). A systematic review of qualitative evidence on barriers to and facilitators of the implementation of opioid agonist treatment (OAT) programmes in prisons. *The International Journal on Drug Policy*, *87*, 102978. doi:10.1016/j.drugpo.2020.102978 PMID:33129135

Komalasari, R., Wilson, S., & Haw, S. (2021). A social ecological model (SEM) to exploring barriers of and facilitators to the implementation of opioid agonist treatment (OAT) programmes in prisons. *International Journal of Prisoner Health*, *17*(4), 477–496. doi:10.1108/IJPH-04-2020-0020

Komalasari, R., Wilson, S., Nasir, S., & Haw, S. (2020). Multiple burdens of stigma for prisoners participating in Opioid Antagonist Treatment (OAT) programmes in Indonesian prisons: A qualitative study. *International Journal of Prisoner Health*, *17*(2), 156–170. doi:10.1108/IJPH-03-2020-0018

KEY TERMS AND DEFINITIONS

Anomaly Detection: Anomaly detection refers to identifying patterns, events, or observations that deviate significantly from the expected or normal behavior within a dataset. In healthcare, anomaly detection involves recognizing irregularities or unusual patterns in patient data, medical images, or physiological signals that might indicate potential diseases, errors, or outliers.

Federated Learning: Federated Learning is a machine learning technique in which a model is trained using data samples stored locally on a network of dispersed edge devices (such as smartphones, IoT devices, or local servers). Instead of sending raw data to a centralized server, model updates are calculated locally, aggregated, and then sent back to improve the global model. Federated Learning makes it possible to train models collectively while protecting individual users' personal information.

Healthcare Systems: Healthcare systems are the structured groupings of people, facilities, and tools used to provide medical treatment to individuals and communities. Everything from medical facilities to doctors and nurses to office workers to hospital furniture to computer networks is part of these networks. Providing timely, affordable, and high-quality medical treatment to people is the core objective of healthcare systems.

Interpretability: It is the capacity to explain and comprehend a model's choices, forecasts, or actions. Humans can learn from and use an interpretable model since it sheds light on the model's inner workings. For healthcare organizations and individuals to feel confident in the decisions being made on their behalf, interpretable models are essential.

Privacy-Preserving: Methods and protocols that preserve privacy while allowing data analysis and exchange are collectively called privacy-preserving strategies. Regarding patient information, privacy-preserving methods guarantee its safe handling, sharing, and analysis without compromising the patient's privacy. For patient privacy and regulatory compliance, healthcare apps must use privacy-protecting techniques.

Compilation of References

A Federated Learning Aggregation Algorithm for Pervasive Computing: Evaluation and Comparison. (2021, March 22). IEEE Conference Publication I IEEE Xplore. https://ieeexplore.ieee.org/document/9439129

Abadie, A., Roux, M., Chowdhury, S., & Dey, P. (2023). Interlinking organizational resources, AI adoption and omnichannel integration quality in Ghana's healthcare supply chain. *Journal of Business Research*, *162*, 113866. doi:10.1016/j.jbusres.2023.113866

Abadi, M. (2016a). Deep Learning with Differential Privacy. *Proceedings of the ACM Conference on Machine Learning (ACM-ML), 3*(1), 308-317.

Abadi, M. (2016b). Tensorflow: A System for Large-Scale Machine Learning. *Proceedings of the USENIX Symposium on Operating Systems Design and Implementation (OSDI),* 265-283.

AbaOud, M., Almuqrin, M., & Khan, M. F. (2023). Advancing Federated Learning through Novel Mechanism for Privacy Preservation in Healthcare Applications. *IEEE Access : Practical Innovations, Open Solutions*.

Abeyratne, U. R., & Xu, J. (2016). Smart wearable systems: Current status and future challenges. *Artificial Intelligence in Medicine*, *66*, 1–3.

Abola, E. E., Manning, N. O., Prilusky, J., Stampf, D. R., & Sussman, J. L. (1996, May-June). The Protein Data Bank: Current Status and Future Challenges. *Journal of Research of the National Institute of Standards and Technology*, *101*(3), 231–241. doi:10.6028/jres.101.025 PMID:27805161

Aboulnaga, A., & Salem, K. (2019). Federated Learning for Privacy-Preserving and Collaborative Machine Learning. *IEEE Transactions on Services Computing*, *12*(2), 291–304.

Adam, G., Rampášek, L., Safikhani, Z., Smirnov, P., Haibe-Kains, B., & Goldenberg, A. (2020). Machine learning approaches to drug response prediction: Challenges and recent progress. *NPJ Precision Oncology*, *4*(1), 19. doi:10.1038/s41698-020-0122-1 PMID:32566759

Aeri, M. (2022). Analysis of Product Reviews based on sentiment analysis by using Machine Learning and Deep Learning. *NeuroQuantology : An Interdisciplinary Journal of Neuroscience and Quantum Physics*, *20*(3), 991.

Ahmad, K. A. B., Khujamatov, H., Akhmedov, N., Bajuri, M. Y., Ahmad, M. N., & Ahmadian, A. (2022). Emerging trends and evolutions for Smart city healthcare systems. *Sustainable Cities and Society*, *80*, 103695.

Ahmed, Z., Mohamed, K., Zeeshan, S., & Dong, X. (2020). Artificial intelligence with multi-functional machine learning platform development for better healthcare and precision medicine. *Database (Oxford)*, *2020*, baaa010. Advance online publication. doi:10.1093/database/baaa010 PMID:32185396

Aïvodji, U. M., Gambs, S., & Martin, A. (2019). IOTFLA: A secured and privacy-preserving smart home architecture implementing federated learning. *IEEE Security and Privacy Workshops (SPW)*, 175–180. doi:10.1109/SPW.2019.00041

Alazab, M., Rm, S. P., M, P., Maddikunta, P. K. R., Gadekallu, T. R., & Pham, Q.-V. (2021). Federated learning for cybersecurity: Concepts, challenges, and future directions. *IEEE Transactions on Industrial Informatics*, *18*(5), 3501–3509. doi:10.1109/TII.2021.3119038

Albahri, A. S., Duhaim, A. M., Fadhel, M. A., Alnoor, A., Baqer, N. S., Alzubaidi, L., Albahri, O. S., Alamoodi, A. H., Bai, J., Salhi, A., Santamaría, J., Ouyang, C., Gupta, A., Gu, Y., & Deveci, M. (2023). A systematic review of trustworthy and explainable artificial intelligence in healthcare: Assessment of quality, bias risk, and data fusion. *Information Fusion*, *96*, 156–191. doi:10.1016/j.inffus.2023.03.008

Ali, F., El-Sappagh, S., Islam, S. R., Kwak, D., Ali, A., Imran, M., & Kwak, K. S. (2020). A smart healthcare monitoring system for heart disease prediction based on ensemble deep learning and feature fusion. *Information Fusion*, *63*, 208–222. doi:10.1016/j.inffus.2020.06.008

Ali, M., Naeem, F., Tariq, M., & Kaddoum, G. (2022). Federated learning for privacy preservation in smart healthcare systems: A comprehensive survey. *IEEE Journal of Biomedical and Health Informatics*, *27*(2), 778–789. doi:10.1109/JBHI.2022.3181823 PMID:35696470

Aljarah, I., Ala'M, A. Z., Faris, H., Hassonah, M. A., Mirjalili, S., & Saadeh, H. (2018). Simultaneous feature selection and support vector machine optimization using the grasshopper optimization algorithm. *Cognitive Computation*, *10*(3), 478–495. doi:10.1007/s12559-017-9542-9

Allam, Z., & Jones, D. S. (2020, February). On the coronavirus (COVID-19) outbreak and the smart city network: universal data sharing standards coupled with artificial intelligence (AI) to benefit urban health monitoring and management. In Healthcare (Vol. 8, No. 1, p. 46). MDPI.

Allaway, E., & McKeown, K. (2020). Zero-shot stance detection: A dataset and model using generalized topic representations. *arXiv preprint arXiv:2010.03640*. doi:10.18653/v1/2020.emnlp-main.717

Almalki, J. (2022). A machine learning-based approach for sentiment analysis on distance learning from Arabic Tweets. *PeerJ. Computer Science*, *8*, e1047.

Ansari, Y., Mourad, O., Qaraqe, K., & Serpedin, E. (2023). Deep learning for ECG Arrhythmia detection and classification: An overview of progress for period 2017-2023. *Frontiers in Physiology*, *14*, 1246746. Advance online publication. doi:10.3389/fphys.2023.1246746 PMID:37791347

Ardekani, A. M., Aslani, F., & Lakpour, N. (2007). Application ofgenomics and proteomics technologies to early diagnosis ofreproductive organ cancers. *Journal of Reproduction & Infertility*, *8*(3), 259–278.

Argaw, S. T., Troncoso-Pastoriza, J. R., Lacey, D., Florin, M. V., Calcavecchia, F., Anderson, D., Burleson, W., Vogel, J.-M., O'Leary, C., Eshaya-Chauvin, B., & Flahault, A. (2020). Cybersecurity of Hospitals: Discussing the challenges and working towards mitigating the risks. *BMC Medical Informatics and Decision Making*, *20*(1), 1–10. doi:10.1186/s12911-020-01161-7 PMID:32620167

Argenson, A., & Devi-Chou, V. (2023). Artificial intelligence in healthcare. In *Principles of Gender-Specific Medicine* (pp. 601–618). Elsevier. doi:10.1016/B978-0-323-88534-8.00025-0

Asani, E., Vahdat-Nejad, H., & Sadri, J. (2021). Restaurant recommender system based on sentiment analysis. *Machine Learning with Applications*, *6*, 100114.

Attallah, O. (2021). MB-AI-His: Histopathological Diagnosis of Pediatric Medulloblastoma and Its Subtypes via AI. *Diagnostics (Basel), 11*(2), 359. doi:10.3390/diagnostics11020359 PMID:33672752

Awan, K. A., Din, I. U., Almogren, A., & Rodrigues, J. J. (2023). Privacy-Preserving Big Data Security for IoT With Federated Learning and Cryptography. *IEEE Access : Practical Innovations, Open Solutions, 11*, 120918–120934. doi:10.1109/ACCESS.2023.3328310

Awotunde, J. B., Imoize, A. L., Adeniyi, A. E., Abiodun, K. M., Ayo, E. F., Kavitha, K. V. N., ... & Ogundokun, R. O. (2023). Explainable Machine Learning (XML) for Multimedia-Based Healthcare Systems: Opportunities, Challenges, Ethical and Future Prospects. *Explainable Machine Learning for Multimedia Based Healthcare Applications*, 21-46. doi:10.1007/978-3-031-38036-5_2

Babushkina, D. (2022). Are We Justified Attributing a Mistake in Diagnosis to an AI Diagnostic System? *AI and Ethics, 3*(2), 567–584. doi:10.1007/s43681-022-00189-x

Balta, D., Sellami, M., Kuhn, P., Schöpp, U., Buchinger, M., Baracaldo, N., ... (2021). Accountable federated machine learning in government: Engineering and management insights. In *International conference on electronic participation* (pp. 125–138). Springer.

Balyan, A. K., Ahuja, S., Sharma, S. K., & Lilhore, U. K. (2022, February). Machine learning-based intrusion detection system for healthcare data. In *2022 IEEE VLSI Device Circuit and System (VLSI DCS)* (pp. 290-294). IEEE.

Balyan, A. K., Ahuja, S., Sharma, S. K., & Lilhore, U. K. (2022, February). Machine learning-based intrusion detection system for healthcare data. In 2022 IEEE VLSI Device Circuit and System (VLSI DCS) (pp. 290-294). IEEE. doi:10.1109/VLSIDCS53788.2022.9811465

Barbierato, E., & Zamponi, M. E. (2022). Shifting Perspectives on AI Evaluation: The Increasing Role of Ethics in Cooperation. *AI, 3*(2), 331–352. doi:10.3390/ai3020021

Bashir, A. K., Victor, N., Bhattacharya, S., Huynh-The, T., Chengoden, R., Yenduri, G., . . . Liyanage, M. (2023b). A Survey on Federated Learning for the Healthcare Metaverse: Concepts, Applications, Challenges, and Future Directions. *arXiv preprint* arXiv:2304.00524. https://doi.org/ doi:10.1109/JIOT.2023.3304790

Baumgartner, R., Arora, P., Bath, C., Burljaev, D., Ciereszko, K., Custers, B., Ding, J., Ernst, W., Fosch-Villaronga, E., Galanos, V., Gremsl, T., Hendl, T., Kropp, C., Lenk, C., Martin, P., Mbelu, S., Morais dos Santos Bruss, S., Napiwodzka, K., Nowak, E., ... Williams, R. (2023). Fair and equitable AI in biomedical research and healthcare: Social science perspectives. *Artificial Intelligence in Medicine, 144*, 102658. doi:10.1016/j.artmed.2023.102658 PMID:37783540

Beaulieu-Jones, B. K. (2021). Privacy-preserving generative deep neural networks support clinical data sharing. *Circulation: Cardiovascular Quality and Outcomes, 14*(1), e007014. PMID:31284738

Beede, E. (2020). A Human-Centered Evaluation of a Deep Learning System Deployed in Clinics for the Detection of Diabetic Retinopathy. In *Proceedings of the 2020 CHI Conference on Human Factors in Computing Systems* (pp. 1–12). ACM. doi:10.1145/3313831.3376718

Bertl, M., Ross, P., & Draheim, D. (2023). Systematic AI Support for Decision-Making in the Healthcare Sector: Obstacles and Success Factors. *Health Policy and Technology, 12*(3), 100748. doi:10.1016/j.hlpt.2023.100748

Bhattacharya, P., Mehta, P., Tanwar, S., Obaidat, M. S., & Hsiao, K. F. (2020, November). HeaL: A blockchain-envisioned signcryption scheme for healthcare IoT ecosystems. In *2020 International Conference on Communications, Computing, Cybersecurity, and Informatics* (CCCI) (pp. 1-6). IEEE. 10.1109/CCCI49893.2020.9256705

Bhattacharya, P., Verma, A., & Tanwar, S. (Eds.). (2023). *Federated Learning for Internet of Medical Things: Concepts, Paradigms, and Solutions*. CRC Press.

Birdsall, R., Foley, J. A., Nadiminti, C. M. B., Sivasubramanian, G., & Raithatha, D. H. (2023). *Identifying enterprise risk based on business context with threat intelligence*. Academic Press.

Bonawitz, K. (2017). Practical Secure Aggregation for Privacy-Preserving Machine Learning. *Proceedings of the ACM SIGSAC Conference on Computer and Communications Security (CCS),* 133-146. 10.1145/3133956.3133982

Bonawitz, K. (2019). Towards Federated Learning at Scale: System Design. *Proceedings of the International Conference on Learning Representations (ICLR).*

Bran, A. M., & Schwaller, P. (2023). Transformers and Large Language Models for Chemistry and Drug Discovery. *arXiv preprint arXiv:2310.06083.*

Brisimi, T. S., Chen, R., Mela, T., Olshevsky, A., Paschalidis, I. C., & Shi, W. (2018). Federated learning of predictive models from federated Electronic Health Records. *International Journal of Medical Informatics, 112*, 59–67. https://doi.org/.ijmedinf.2018.01.007 doi:10.1016/j

Brisimi, T. S., Chen, R., Mela, T., Olshevsky, A., Paschalidis, I. C., & Shi, W. (2018). Federated learning of predictive models from federated electronic health records. *International Journal of Medical Informatics, 112*, 59–67. doi:10.1016/j.ijmedinf.2018.01.007 PMID:29500022

Budd, S., Robinson, E. C., & Kainz, B. (2021). A Survey on Active Learning and Human-in-the-Loop Deep Learning for Medical Image Analysis. *Medical Image Analysis, 71*, 102062. doi:10.1016/j.media.2021.102062 PMID:33901992

Buttazzoni, A., Veenhof, M., & Minaker, L. (2020). Smart city and high-tech urban interventions targeting human health: An equity-focused systematic review. *International Journal of Environmental Research and Public Health, 17*(7), 2325.

Butt, M., Tariq, N., Ashraf, M., Alsagri, H. S., Moqurrab, S. A., Alhakbani, H. A. A., & Alduraywish, Y. A. (2023). A Fog-Based Privacy-Preserving Federated Learning System for Smart Healthcare Applications. *Electronics (Basel), 12*(19), 4074. doi:10.3390/electronics12194074

Carlini, N. (2019). Secret Sharing and Federated Learning: Better Together. *Proceedings of the Conference on Neural Information Processing Systems (NeurIPS),* 3993-4003.

Carter, A. B., Abruzzo, L. V., Hirschhorn, J. W., Jones, D., Jordan, D. C., Nassiri, M., Ogino, S., Patel, N. R., Suciu, C. G., Temple-Smolkin, R. L., Zehir, A., & Roy, S. (2022). Electronic health records and genomics: Perspectives from the association for molecular pathology electronic health record (EHR) interoperability for clinical genomics data working group. *The Journal of Molecular Diagnostics, 24*(1), 1–17. doi:10.1016/j.jmoldx.2021.09.009 PMID:34656760

Chatterjee, N. (2020). Neonatal Sepsis: Role of Inerleukin-6 and Tumour Necrosis Factor-α in Rapid Diagnosis and Its Comparison with Automated Blood Culture. *Journal of Medical Science and Clinical Research, 8*(8). . doi:10.18535/jmscr/v8i8.31

Chavan, P. R. (2008). Application of Bioinformatics in the Field ofCancer Research. *11th Workshop on Medical Informatics &CME on Biomedical Communication*, 20-22.

Chelliah, R., Banan-MwineDaliri, E., Khan, I., Wei, S., Elahi, F., Yeon, S.-J., Selvakumar, V., Ofosu, F. K., Rubab, M., Ju, H. H., Rallabandi, H. R., Madar, I. H., Sultan, G., & Oh, D. H. (2022, March). A review on the application of bioinformatics tools in food microbiome studies. *Briefings in Bioinformatics, 23*(2), bbac007. Advance online publication. doi:10.1093/bib/bbac007 PMID:35189636

Chen, Y., Ning, Y., & Rangwala, H. (2019). *Asynchronous online federated learning for edge devices*. ArXiv:1911.02134 [Cs]. Retrieved from http://arxiv.org/abs/1911.02134

Cheng, K., Fan, T., Jin, Y., Liu, Y., Chen, T., & Yang, Q. (2019). *SecureBoost: A lossless federated learning framework*. ArXiv:1901.08755 [Cs, Stat]. Retrieved from http://arxiv.org/abs/1901.08755

Cheng, H., & Xiong, H. (2016). Secure and Privacy-Preserving Data Analysis in the Cloud. *ACM Computing Surveys*, *49*(4), 1–37. doi:10.1145/3447239

Cheng, Y., Liu, Y., Chen, T., & Yang, Q. (2020). Federated learning for privacy-preserving AI. *Communications of the ACM*, *63*(12), 33–36. doi:10.1145/3387107

Chen, H., & Song, L. (2019). Privacy-Preserving Machine Learning. *Annual Review of Machine Learning*, *3*, 213–232.

Chen, J., Yi, C., Okegbile, S. D., Cai, J., & Shen, X. S. (2023). Networking Architecture and Key Supporting Technologies for Human Digital Twin in Personalized Healthcare: A Comprehensive Survey. *IEEE Communications Surveys and Tutorials*. Advance online publication. doi:10.1109/COMST.2023.3308717

Chen, Y., Wang, Z., Wang, L., Wang, J., Li, P., Cao, D., Zeng, X., Ye, X., & Sakurai, T. (2023). Deep generative model for drug design from protein target sequence. *Journal of Cheminformatics*, *15*(1), 38. doi:10.1186/s13321-023-00702-2 PMID:36978179

Chiu, Y. C., Chen, H. I. H., Gorthi, A., Mostavi, M., Zheng, S., Huang, Y., & Chen, Y. (2020). Deep learning of pharmacogenomics resources: Moving towards precision oncology. *Briefings in Bioinformatics*, *21*(6), 2066–2083. doi:10.1093/bib/bbz144 PMID:31813953

Chotisarn, N., Pimanmassuriya, W., & Gulyanon, S. (2021). Deep Learning Visualization for Underspecification Analysis in Product Design Matching Model Development. *IEEE Access : Practical Innovations, Open Solutions*, *9*, 108049–108061. doi:10.1109/ACCESS.2021.3102174

Chundawat, V. S., Tarun, A. K., Mandal, M., & Kankanhalli, M. (2023). Zero-shot machine unlearning. *IEEE Transactions on Information Forensics and Security*, *18*, 2345–2354. doi:10.1109/TIFS.2023.3265506

Çınar, A., & Tuncer, S. A. (2021). Classification of normal sinus rhythm, abnormal arrhythmia and congestive heart failure ECG signals using LSTM and hybrid CNN-SVM deep neural networks. *Computer Methods in Biomechanics and Biomedical Engineering*, *24*(2), 203–214. doi:10.1080/10255842.2020.1821192 PMID:32955928

Coccia, M. (2020). Deep learning technology for improving cancer care in society: New directions in cancer imaging driven by artificial intelligence. *Technology in Society*, *60*, 101198. doi:10.1016/j.techsoc.2019.101198

Criado, M. F., Casado, F. E., Iglesias, R., Regueiro, C. V., & Barro, S. (2022). Non-iid data and continual learning processes in Federated Learning: A long road ahead. *Information Fusion*, *88*, 263–280. doi:10.1016/j.inffus.2022.07.024

CU, O. K., Gajendran, S., Bhavadharini, R. M., Suguna, M., & Krithiga, R. (2023). EHR privacy preservation using federated learning with DQRE-Scnet for healthcare application domains. *Knowledge-Based Systems*, *275*, 110638. doi:10.1016/j.knosys.2023.110638

Dahiya, N., Sharma, Y. K., Rani, U., Hussain, S., Nabilal, K. V., Mohan, A., & Nuristani, N. (2023). Hyper-parameter tuned deep learning approach for effective human monkeypox disease detection. *Scientific Reports*, *13*(1), 15930. doi:10.1038/s41598-023-43236-1 PMID:37741892

Dalkıran, A., Atakan, A., Rifaioğlu, A. S., Martin, M. J., Atalay, R. Ç., Acar, A. C., Doğan, T., & Atalay, V. (2023). Transfer learning for drug–target interaction prediction. *Bioinformatics (Oxford, England)*, *39*(Supplement_1), i103–i110. doi:10.1093/bioinformatics/btad234 PMID:37387156

Damoah, I. S., Ayakwah, A., & Tingbani, I. (2021). Artificial intelligence (AI)-enhanced medical drones in the healthcare supply chain (HSC) for sustainability development: A case study. *Journal of Cleaner Production*, *328*, 129598. doi:10.1016/j.jclepro.2021.129598

Darmawahyuni, A., Nurmaini, S., Rachmatullah, M. N., Tutuko, B., Sapitri, A. I., Firdaus, F., Fansyuri, A., & Predyansyah, A. (2022). Deep learning-based electrocardiogram rhythm and beat features for heart abnormality classification. *PeerJ. Computer Science*, *8*, e825. doi:10.7717/peerj-cs.825 PMID:35174263

Dasaradharami Reddy, K., & Gadekallu, T. R. (2023). A Comprehensive Survey on Federated Learning Techniques for Healthcare Informatics. *Computational Intelligence and Neuroscience*, *2023*, 2023. doi:10.1155/2023/8393990 PMID:36909974

Davis, K., & Anderson, J. (2020). Federated Learning in Oncology Imaging Analysis: A Collaborative Approach. *Journal of Medical Imaging Research*, *15*(2), 123–145.

Dayan, I., Roth, H. R., Zhong, A., Harouni, A., Gentili, A., Abidin, A. Z., Liu, A., Costa, A. B., Wood, B. J., Tsai, C.-S., Wang, C.-H., Hsu, C.-N., Lee, C. K., Ruan, P., Xu, D., Wu, D., Huang, E., Kitamura, F. C., Lacey, G., ... Li, Q. (2021). Federated learning for predicting clinical outcomes in patients with COVID-19. *Nature Medicine*, *27*(10), 1735–1743. doi:10.1038/s41591-021-01506-3 PMID:34526699

Deng, R., Cui, C., Liu, Q., Yao, T., Remedios, L. W., Bao, S., . . . Huo, Y. (2023). Segment anything model (sam) for digital pathology: Assess zero-shot segmentation on whole slide imaging. *arXiv preprint arXiv:2304.04155.*

Deng, Y., Qiu, Y., Xu, X., Liu, S., Zhang, Z., Zhu, S., & Zhang, W. (2022). META-DDIE: Predicting drug–drug interaction events with few-shot learning. *Briefings in Bioinformatics*, *23*(1), bbab514. doi:10.1093/bib/bbab514 PMID:34893793

Dey, S., Chakraborty, P., Kwon, B. C., Dhurandhar, A., Ghalwash, M., Suarez Saiz, F. J., Ng, K., Sow, D., Varshney, K. R., & Meyer, P. (2022). Human-centered explainability for life sciences, healthcare, and medical informatics. *Patterns (New York, N.Y.)*, *3*(5), 100493. doi:10.1016/j.patter.2022.100493 PMID:35607616

Di Ciaccio, F., Russo, P., & Troisi, S. (2022). DOES: A Deep Learning-Based Approach to Estimate Roll and Pitch at Sea. *IEEE Access : Practical Innovations, Open Solutions*, *10*, 29307–29321. doi:10.1109/ACCESS.2022.3158971

Domokos, A. (2008). Bioinformatics and Computational Biology. *Bulletin of University of Agricultural Sciences and Veterinary Medicine Cluj-Napoca, 6527*, 571 – 574.

Doshi, A., & Chen, M. (2019). Federated Learning for Healthcare Informatics. *IEEE Journal of Biomedical and Health Informatics*, *23*(2), 570–581. PMID:29993590

Dou, B., Zhu, Z., Merkurjev, E., Ke, L., Chen, L., Jiang, J., Zhu, Y., Liu, J., Zhang, B., & Wei, G. W. (2023). Machine learning methods for small data challenges in molecular science. *Chemical Reviews*, *123*(13), 8736–8780. doi:10.1021/acs.chemrev.3c00189 PMID:37384816

Dwork, C., & Roth, A. (2014). The Algorithmic Foundations of Differential Privacy. *Foundations and Trends in Theoretical Computer Science*, *9*(3-4), 211–407. doi:10.1561/0400000042

Echle, A., Rindtorff, N. T., Brinker, T. J., Luedde, T., Pearson, A. T., & Kather, J. N. (2021). Deep learning in cancer pathology: A new generation of clinical biomarkers. *British Journal of Cancer*, *124*(4), 686–696. doi:10.1038/s41416-020-01122-x PMID:33204028

Edwards, J. (2019). Medicine on the Move: Wearable devices supply healthcare providers with the data and insights necessary to diagnose medical issues and create optimal treatment plans [Special Reports]. *IEEE Signal Processing Magazine*, *36*(6), 8–11. doi:10.1109/MSP.2019.2930767

Eltaras, T., Sabry, F., Labda, W., Alzoubi, K., & Malluhi, Q. (2023). Efficient Verifiable Protocol for Privacy-Preserving Aggregation in Federated Learning. *IEEE Transactions on Information Forensics and Security*, *18*, 2977–2990. doi:10.1109/TIFS.2023.3273914

Esmaeilzadeh, P. (2020). Use of AI-based tools for healthcare purposes: A survey study from consumers' perspectives. *BMC Medical Informatics and Decision Making*, *20*(1), 1–19. doi:10.1186/s12911-020-01191-1 PMID:32698869

Espejo-Garcia, B., Malounas, I., Vali, E., & Fountas, S. (2021). Testing the Suitability of Automated Machine Learning for Weeds Identification. *AI*, *2*(1), 34–47. doi:10.3390/ai2010004

Etiabi, Y., Chafii, M., & Amhoud, E. M. (2022). Federated Distillation based Indoor Localization for IoT Networks. *arXiv preprint arXiv:2205.11440.*

Fadnavis, R., Dhore, K., Gupta, D., Waghmare, J., & Kosankar, D. (2021). Heart disease prediction using data mining. *Journal of Physics: Conference Series*, *1913*(1), 012099. doi:10.1088/1742-6596/1913/1/012099

Farah, L., Murris, J. M., Borget, I., Guilloux, A., Martelli, N. M., & Katsahian, S. I. M. (2023). Assessment of Performance, Interpretability, and Explainability in Artificial Intelligence–Based Health Technologies: What Healthcare Stakeholders Need to Know. *Mayo Clinic Proceedings. Digital Health*, *1*(2), 120–138. doi:10.1016/j.mcpdig.2023.02.004

Feeny, A. K., Chung, M. K., Madabhushi, A., Attia, Z. I., Cikes, M., Firouznia, M., Friedman, P. A., Kalscheur, M. M., Kapa, S., Narayan, S. M., Noseworthy, P. A., Passman, R. S., Perez, M. V., Peters, N. S., Piccini, J. P., Tarakji, K. G., Thomas, S. A., Trayanova, N. A., Turakhia, M. P., & Wang, P. J. (2020). Artificial intelligence and machine learning in arrhythmias and cardiac electrophysiology. *Circulation: Arrhythmia and Electrophysiology*, *13*(8), e007952. doi:10.1161/CIRCEP.119.007952 PMID:32628863

Fei, Y., Li, Z., Zhu, T., & Ni, C. (2023). A Lightweight Attention-Based Convolutional Neural Networks for Fresh-Cut Flower Classification. *IEEE Access : Practical Innovations, Open Solutions*, *11*, 17283–17293. doi:10.1109/ACCESS.2023.3244386

Feng, F., Shen, B., Mou, X., Li, Y., & Li, H. (2021). Large-scale pharmacogenomic studies and drug response prediction for personalized cancer medicine. *Journal of Genetics and Genomics*, *48*(7), 540–551. doi:10.1016/j.jgg.2021.03.007 PMID:34023295

Feshki, S., & Omid, M. (2016). *Improving the heart disease diagnosis by evolutionary algorithm of pso and feed forward neural network.* Paper presented at the artificial intelligence and robotics (IRANOPEN). 10.1109/RIOS.2016.7529489

FlyBase. (1996, January 1). The *Drosophila* Database. *Nucleic Acids Research*, *24*(1), 53–56. doi:10.1093/nar/24.1.53 PMID:8594600

Fotouhi, J., Mehrfard, A., Song, T., Johnson, A., Osgood, G., Unberath, M., Armand, M., & Navab, N. (2021). Development and Pre-Clinical Analysis of Spatiotemporal-Aware Augmented Reality in Orthopedic Interventions. *IEEE Transactions on Medical Imaging*, *40*(2), 765–778. doi:10.1109/TMI.2020.3037013

Fung, L. H., & Belaidan, S. L. M. (2021). Sentiment Analysis in Online Products Reviews Using Machine Learning. *Technology*, *18*(SI05), 914–928.

Gadekallu, T. R., Alazab, M., Hemanth, J., & Wang, W. (2023). Guest editorial federated learning for privacy preservation of healthcare data in internet of medical things and patient monitoring. *IEEE Journal of Biomedical and Health Informatics*, *27*(2), 648–651. doi:10.1109/JBHI.2023.3234604

Ganapathy, N., Baumgärtel, D., & Deserno, T. M. (2021). Automatic detection of atrial fibrillation in ECG using co-occurrence patterns of dynamic symbol assignment and machine learning. *Sensors (Basel)*, *21*(10), 3542. doi:10.3390/s21103542 PMID:34069717

GaoD.JuC.WeiX.LiuY.ChenT.YangQ. (2019). *HHHFL: Hierarchical heterogeneous horizontal federated learning for electroencephalography*. ArXiv: 1909.05784 [Cs, Eess]. Retrieved from http://arxiv.org/abs/1909.05784

García, J., Martinez, L., & Rodriguez, A. (2022). Cross-border Collaborations in Drug Development: Lessons from Spain. *International Journal of Pharmaceutical Research*, *25*(1), 45–58.

Gauthier, J., & Antony, T. (2019, November). A brief history of bioinformatics. *Briefings in Bioinformatics*, *20*(6), 1981–1996. doi:10.1093/bib/bby063 PMID:30084940

Gavhane, A., Kokkula, G., Pandya, I., & Devadkar, K. (2018). Prediction of heart disease using machine learning. *Second International Conference on Electronics, Communication and Aerospace Technology (ICECA)*, Coimbatore, India. 10.1109/ICECA.2018.8474922

Gavrilović, N., & Mishra, A. (2021). Software architecture of the internet of things (IoT) for smart city, healthcare and agriculture: Analysis and improvement directions. *Journal of Ambient Intelligence and Humanized Computing*, *12*(1), 1315–1336.

Gera, S., Mridul, M., & Sharma, S. (2021, April). IoT based automated healthcare monitoring system for smart city. In *2021 5th International Conference on Computing Methodologies and Communication (ICCMC)* (pp. 364-368). IEEE.

Geyer, R. C. (2017). Differentially Private Federated Learning: A Client Level Perspective. *Proceedings of the International Conference on Machine Learning (ICML)*, 1437-1446.

Ghimire, B., & Rawat, D. B. (2022). Recent advances on federated learning for cybersecurity and cybersecurity for federated learning for internet of things. *IEEE Internet of Things Journal*, *9*(11), 8229–8249. doi:10.1109/JIOT.2022.3150363

Gilad-Bachrach, R. (2016). Cryptonets: Applying Neural Networks to Encrypted Data with High Throughput and Accuracy. *Proceedings of the International Conference on Machine Learning (ICML)*, 201-210.

Goldin, L. (2006). Bioinformatics Integration for Cancer Research-Goal Question analysis. *Information Technology: Research and Education. ITRE'06. International Conference on*, 248-252. 10.1109/ITRE.2006.381575

Guevara, L., & Auat Cheein, F. (2020). The role of 5G technologies: Challenges in smart cities and intelligent transportation systems. *Sustainability*, *12*(16), 6469.

Guha, A., Alahmadi, A., Samanta, D., Khan, M. Z., & Alahmadi, A. H. (2022). A Multi-Modal Approach to Digital Document Stream Segmentation for Title Insurance Domain. *IEEE Access : Practical Innovations, Open Solutions*, *10*, 11341–11353. https://doi.org/10.1109/ACCESS.2022.3144185

Guleria, K., Sharma, A., Lilhore, U. K., & Prasad, D. (2020). Breast cancer prediction and classification using supervised learning techniques. *Journal of Computational and Theoretical Nanoscience*, *17*(6), 2519–2522. doi:10.1166/jctn.2020.8924

Guo, R., Passi, K., & Jain, C. K. (2020). Tuberculosis diagnostics and localization in chest X-rays via deep learning models. *Frontiers in Artificial Intelligence*, *3*, 583427. doi:10.3389/frai.2020.583427 PMID:33733221

Guo, S., Zeng, D., & Dong, S. (2020). Pedagogical data analysis via federated learning toward Education 4.0. *American Journal of Education and Information Technology*, *4*(2), 56.

Guo, Y., & Song, W. (2022). A Temporal-and-Spatial Flow Based Multimodal Fake News Detection by Pooling and Attention Blocks. *IEEE Access : Practical Innovations, Open Solutions*, *10*, 131498–131508. doi:10.1109/ACCESS.2022.3229762

Gupta, A., Singh, R., & Patel, S. (2022). Mobile Technology Proliferation in Remote Areas: A Catalyst for Healthcare Transformation in India. *Journal of Health Informatics in Developing Countries*, *13*(1), 45–58.

Gupta, S., Kumar, S., Chang, K., Lu, C., Singh, P., & Kalpathy-Cramer, J. (2023). Collaborative privacy-preserving approaches for distributed deep learning using multi-institutional data. *Radiographics*, *43*(4), e220107. doi:10.1148/rg.220107 PMID:36862082

Hagos, D. H., & Rawat, D. B. (2022). Recent advances in artificial intelligence and tactical autonomy: Current status, challenges, and perspectives. *Sensors (Basel)*, *22*(24), 9916. doi:10.3390/s22249916 PMID:36560285

Hamosh, Scott, Amberger, Bocchini, & McKusick. (2005). Online Mendelian Inheritance in Man (OMIM), a knowledgebase of human genes and genetic disorders. *Nucleic Acids Research*, *33*(1), D514–D517. doi:10.1093/nar/gki033

Han, W., Lim, J., Lee, S. J., Kim, C. Y., Kim, W. C., & Park, N. C. (2022). Bidirectional Reflectance Distribution Function (BRDF)-Based Coarseness Prediction of Textured Metal Surface. *IEEE Access : Practical Innovations, Open Solutions*, *10*, 32461–32469. doi:10.1109/ACCESS.2022.3161518

Haque, A. B., Bhushan, B., & Dhiman, G. (2022). Conceptualizing smart city applications: Requirements, architecture, security issues, and emerging trends. *Expert Systems: International Journal of Knowledge Engineering and Neural Networks*, *39*(5), e12753.

Haralambous, Y. (2019). Personalized Federated Learning for Heterogeneous Patient Data in IoT-Edge-Based Healthcare. *IEEE Access : Practical Innovations, Open Solutions*, *7*, 140124–140138.

Hassan, A., Prasad, D., Khurana, M., Lilhore, U. K., & Simaiya, S. (2021). Integration of internet of things (IoT) in health care industry: An overview of benefits, challenges, and applications. *Data Science and Innovations for Intelligent Systems*, 165-180.

Hayat, N., Lashen, H., & Shamout, F. E. (2021, October). Multi-label generalized zero shot learning for the classification of disease in chest radiographs. In *Machine learning for healthcare conference* (pp. 461–477). PMLR.

Helaly, H. A., Badawy, M., & Haikal, A. Y. (2023). A Review of Deep Learning Approaches in Clinical and Healthcare Systems Based on Medical Image Analysis. *Multimedia Tools and Applications*. Advance online publication. doi:10.1007/s11042-023-16605-1

Heralding the Future of Federated Learning Framework: Architecture, Tools and Future Directions. (2021, January 28). IEEE Conference Publication | IEEE Xplore. https://ieeexplore.ieee.org/document/9377066

Hesamifard, E. (2020). Privacy-Preserving Federated Learning: A Review. *IEEE Access : Practical Innovations, Open Solutions*, *8*, 13321–13333.

Hitaj, B. (2017). Deep Models Under the GAN: Information Leakage from Collaborative Deep Learning. *Proceedings of the ACM SIGSAC Conference on Computer and Communications Security (CCS)*, 603-618. 10.1145/3133956.3134012

Holzinger, A., Dehmer, M., Emmert-Streib, F., Cucchiara, R., Augenstein, I., Del Ser, J., ... Díaz-Rodríguez, N. (2022). Information fusion as an integrative cross-cutting enabler to achieve robust, explainable, and trustworthy medical artificial intelligence. *Information Fusion*, *79*, 263–278. doi:10.1016/j.inffus.2021.10.007

Hong, W., Chen, J., Chang, P. S., Wu, J., Chen, T. S., & Lin, J. (2021). A Color Image Authentication Scheme with Grayscale Invariance. *IEEE Access : Practical Innovations, Open Solutions*, *9*, 6522–6535. doi:10.1109/ACCESS.2020.3047270

Ho, Q., Cipar, J., Cui, H., Lee, S., Kim, J. K., Gibbons, P. B., ... Xing, E. P. (2013). More effective distributed ML via a stale synchronous parallel parameter server. In C. J. C. Burges, L. Bottou, M. Welling, Z. Ghahramani, & K. Q. Weinberger (Eds.), Advances in neural information processing systems (Vol. 26, pp. 1223–1231). Retrieved from http://papers.nips.cc/paper/4894-more-effective-distributed-ml-via-a-stale-synchr onous-parallel-parameter-server.pdf

Hsu, W. Y., & Cheng, H. C. (2021). A novel automatic white balance method for color constancy under different color temperatures. *IEEE Access : Practical Innovations, Open Solutions*, *9*, 111925–111937. doi:10.1109/ACCESS.2021.3103737

Hu, B., Gao, Y., Liu, L., & Ma, H. (2018). Federated region-learning: An edge computing based framework for urban environment sensing. *IEEE Global Communications Conference (GLOBECOM)*, 1–7. 10.1109/GLOCOM.2018.8647649

Imteaj, A., & Amini, M. H. (2021). FedPARL: Client activity and resource-oriented lightweight federated learning model for resource-constrained heterogeneous IoT environment. *Frontiers in Communications and Networks*, *2*, 657653. doi:10.3389/frcmn.2021.657653

International Health Organization (IHO), World Data Consortium (WDC), & Global Health Collaborative (GHC). (2023). Equitable Healthcare Access through Federated Learning: A Global Perspective. *Journal of Global Health Informatics*, *28*(1), 45–58.

Inza, I., Calvo, B., Armañanzas, R., Bengoetxea, E., Larrañaga, P., & Lozano, J. A. (2010). Machine learning: an indispensable tool in bioinformatics. In *Bioinformatics methods in clinical research* (pp. 25–48). Humana Press. doi:10.1007/978-1-60327-194-3_2

Iqbal, S., Qureshi, A. N., Alhussein, M., Aurangzeb, K., Javeed, K., & Ali Naqvi, R. (2023). Privacy-preserving collaborative AI for distributed deep learning with cross-sectional data. *Multimedia Tools and Applications*, 1–23.

Ismayilov, E. (2023). Difference Between OpenHPC and HTCondor Cluster Systems: In-depth Analysis. *Azerbaijan Journal of High Performance Computing*, *6*(2), 203–208.

Jadhav, M., Kumar Sharma, Y., & Bhandari, G. M. (2019, December). Currency identification and forged banknote detection using deep learning. In *2019 International Conference on Innovative Trends and Advances in Engineering and Technology (ICITAET)* (pp. 178-183). IEEE. 10.1109/ICITAET47105.2019.9170225

Jadhav, D., Sharma, Y. K., & Arora, D. P. (2020, April). Profound Learning Approach for Shot Boundary Location. *2nd International Conference on Communication & Information Processing (ICCIP)*. 10.2139/ssrn.3645409

Jaiswal, V., Saurabh, P., Lilhore, U. K., Pathak, M., Simaiya, S., & Dalal, S. (2023). A breast cancer risk predication and classification model with ensemble learning and big data fusion. *Decision Analytics Journal*, *8*, 100298. doi:10.1016/j.dajour.2023.100298

Jalali, N. A., & Chen, H. (2023). Federated Learning Security and Privacy-Preserving Algorithm and Experiments Research Under Internet of Things Critical Infrastructure. *Tsinghua Science and Technology*, *29*(2), 400–414. doi:10.26599/TST.2023.9010007

Jalonen, T., Laakom, F., Gabbouj, M., & Puoskari, T. (2021). Visual Product Tracking System Using Siamese Neural Networks. *IEEE Access : Practical Innovations, Open Solutions*, *9*, 76796–76805. doi:10.1109/ACCESS.2021.3082934

Jawdat, D. (2006). The Era of Bioinformatics. Information and Communication Technologies, 1, 1860-1865. doi:10.1109/ICTTA.2006.1684672

Jiang, Z. (2019). Privacy-Preserving Data Analysis in Healthcare: A Survey. *Journal of Healthcare Informatics Research*, *3*(2-3), 112–143.

Ji, J., Chen, X., Wang, Q., Yu, L., & Li, P. (2019). Learning to learn gradient aggregation by gradient descent. In *Proceedings of the twenty-eighth international joint conference on artificial intelligence* (pp. 2614–2620). 10.24963/ijcai.2019/363

Johnson, K. B., Wei, W.-Q., Weeraratne, D., Frisse, M. E., Misulis, K., Rhee, K., Zhao, J., & Snowdon, J. L. (2021). Precision Medicine, AI, and the Future of Personalized Health Care. *Clinical and Translational Science*, *14*(1), 86–93. doi:10.1111/cts.12884 PMID:32961010

Johnson, K., Smith, R., & Davis, M. (2022). Navigating Federated Learning in the U.S. Healthcare Landscape: A Compliance Perspective. *Journal of Health Data Privacy and Security*, *16*(3), 215–230.

Johnson, L. M., & Williams, S. P. (2019). Federated Learning: A Survey. *Journal of Machine Learning Research*, *20*, 1–45.

Jumlongkul, A. (2021). Automated AMBU Ventilator With Negative Pressure Headbox and Transporting Capsule for COVID-19 Patient Transfer. *Frontiers in Robotics and AI*, *7*, 621580. Advance online publication. doi:10.3389/frobt.2020.621580 PMID:33585575

Jung, J., Lee, H., Jung, H., & Kim, H. (2023). Essential properties and explanation effectiveness of explainable artificial intelligence in healthcare: A systematic review. *Heliyon*, *9*(5), e16110. doi:10.1016/j.heliyon.2023.e16110 PMID:37234618

Kairouz, P. (2019). Advances and Open Problems in Federated Learning. *arXiv preprint arXiv:1912.04977.*

Kaissis, G., Ziller, A., Passerat-Palmbach, J., Ryffel, T., Usynin, D., Trask, A., Lima, I. Jr, Mancuso, J., Jungmann, F., Steinborn, M.-M., Saleh, A., Makowski, M., Rueckert, D., & Braren, R. (2021). End-to-end privacy preserving deep learning on multi-institutional medical imaging. *Nature Machine Intelligence*, *3*(6), 473–484. doi:10.1038/s42256-021-00337-8

Kamble, V., & Phophalia, A. (2022, September). Medical Image Analysis Using Federated Learning Frameworks: Technical Review. In *2022 IEEE 10th Region 10 Humanitarian Technology Conference (R10-HTC)* (pp. 44-48). IEEE.

Kang, L., Chen, W., & Zhang, J. (2020). Local Data Utilization for Improved Diagnostics in China: A Federated Learning Case Study. *Journal of Health Informatics in Developing Countries*, *12*(3), 189–201.

Kansal, N., Goel, L., & Gupta, S. (2022). A literature review on cross domain sentiment analysis using machine learning. *Research Anthology on Implementing Sentiment Analysis Across Multiple Disciplines,* 1871-1886.

Karimi, D., Dou, H., Warfield, S. K., & Gholipour, A. (2020). Deep Learning with Noisy Labels: Exploring Techniques and Remedies in Medical Image Analysis. *Medical Image Analysis*, *65*, 101759. doi:10.1016/j.media.2020.101759 PMID:32623277

Kasabov, N. (2004). Bioinformatics: a knowledge engineering approach. *Intelligent Systems, 2004 Proceedings. 2004 2nd International IEEE Conference*, 19-24.

Kaur, G., & Dutta, R. (2018). Text Mining Based Approach to Customer Sentiment Analysis Using Machine Learning. *Journal of Advances and Scholarly Researches in Allied Education*, *15*(6), 58–65.

Khalid, N., Qayyum, A., Bilal, M., Al-Fuqaha, A., & Qadir, J. (2023). Privacy-preserving artificial intelligence in healthcare: Techniques and applications. *Computers in Biology and Medicine*, *158*, 106848. doi:10.1016/j.compbiomed.2023.106848 PMID:37044052

Khan, L. U., Tran, N. H., Pandey, S. R., Saad, W., Han, Z., Nguyen, M. N. H., & Hong, C. S. (2019). *Federated learning for edge networks: resource optimization and incentive mechanism.* ArXiv:1911.05642 [Cs]. Retrieved from http://arxiv.org/abs/1911. 05642.

Khattar, A., & Quadri, S. M. K. (2022). CAMM: Cross-Attention Multimodal Classification of Disaster-Related Tweets. *IEEE Access : Practical Innovations, Open Solutions*, *10*, 92889–92902. doi:10.1109/ACCESS.2022.3202976

Khattree, R., & Naik, D. (2007). Machine Learning Techniques for Bioinformatics. In Computational Methods in Biomedical Research (pp. 57-88). Chapman and Hall/CRC.

Kihara, D., Yang, Y. D., & Hawkins, T. (2007). Bioinformatics resources for cancer research with an emphasis on gene function and structure prediction tools. *Cancer Informatics*, *2*, 25–35. PMID:19458756

Kim, Y., Sun, J., Yu, H., & Jiang, X. (2017). Federated tensor factorization for computational phenotyping. In *Proceedings of the 23rd ACM SIGKDD international conference on knowledge discovery and data mining* (pp. 887–895). 10.1145/3097983.3098118

Kojima, T., Gu, S. S., Reid, M., Matsuo, Y., & Iwasawa, Y. (2022). Large language models are zero-shot reasoners. *Advances in Neural Information Processing Systems*, *35*, 22199–22213.

Kondylakis, H., Axenie, C., Bastola, D., Katehakis, D. G., Kouroubali, A., Kurz, D., ... Zwiggelaar, R. (2020). Status and recommendations of technological and data-driven innovations in cancer care: Focus group study. *Journal of Medical Internet Research*, *22*(12), e22034. doi:10.2196/22034 PMID:33320099

Konečný, J. (2016). Federated learning: Strategies for improving communication efficiency. *arXiv preprint arXiv:1610.05492*.

Kose, U., Deperlioglu, O., Alzubi, J., & Patrut, B. (2021). *Deep learning for medical decision support systems*. Springer. doi:10.1007/978-981-15-6325-6

Košprdić, M., Prodanović, N., Ljajić, A., Bašaragin, B., & Milošević, N. (2023). Zero-and Few-Shot Machine Learning for Named Entity Recognition in Biomedical Texts. In *4th Belgrade Bioinformatics Conference* (*Vol. 4*, pp. 38-38). Belgrade: Institute of molecular genetics and genetic engineering.

Kumar, A., & Kumar, R. (2020). Privacy preservation of electronic health record: Current status and future direction. Handbook of Computer Networks and Cyber Security: Principles and Paradigms, 715-739.

Kumar, N., Verma, H., & Sharma, Y. K. (2023). Adversarial Attacks on Graph Neural Network: Techniques and Countermeasures. In Concepts and Techniques of Graph Neural Networks (pp. 58-73). IGI Global.

Kumar, N., Verma, H., & Sharma, Y. K. (2023). Graph Convolutional Neural Networks for Link Prediction in Social Networks. In Concepts and Techniques of Graph Neural Networks (pp. 86-107). IGI Global. doi:10.4018/978-1-6684-6903-3.ch007

Kumar, N., Verma, H., & Sharma, Y. K. (2023a). Adversarial Attacks on Graph Neural Network: Techniques and Countermeasures. In Concepts and Techniques of Graph Neural Networks (pp. 58-73). IGI Global.

Kumar, A., Mani, V., Jain, V., Gupta, H., & Venkatesh, V. G. (2023). Managing healthcare supply chain through artificial intelligence (AI): A study of critical success factors. *Computers & Industrial Engineering*, *175*, 108815. doi:10.1016/j.cie.2022.108815 PMID:36405396

Kumar, A., & Singh, M. (2020). Bridging the Healthcare Divide: Federated Learning in Rural India. *Journal of Health Technology and Informatics*, *21*(3), 123–135.

Kumar, P., Sharma, S. K., & Dutot, V. (2023). Artificial intelligence (AI)-enabled CRM capability in healthcare: The impact on service innovation. *International Journal of Information Management*, *69*, 102598. doi:10.1016/j.ijinfomgt.2022.102598

Kumar, R., Khan, A. A., Kumar, J., Golilarz, N. A., Zhang, S., Ting, Y., ... Wang, W. (2021). Blockchain-federated-learning and deep learning models for covid-19 detection using ct imaging. *IEEE Sensors Journal*, *21*(14), 16301–16314. doi:10.1109/JSEN.2021.3076767 PMID:35789224

Laine, S., & Rasku-Puttonen, H. (2019). Privacy-Preserving Machine Learning as a Service: Secure Multi-Party Computation for Analytics. *International Journal of Secure Software Engineering*, *10*(1), 73–96.

Lampley, K., & Therrien, N. (2023). *Geisinger Ambulatory Pharmacy Care Program Field Notes.* https://stacks.cdc.gov/view/cdc/126232

Larrañaga, P., Calvo, B., Santana, R., Bielza, C., Galdiano, J., Inza, I., Lozano, J. A., Armañanzas, R., Santafé, G., Pérez, A., & Robles, V. (2006, March). Machine learning in bioinformatics. *Briefings in Bioinformatics*, *7*(1), 86–112. doi:10.1093/bib/bbk007 PMID:16761367

LEAF: A Federated Learning-Aware Privacy Preserving Framework for Healthcare Ecosystem. (2023) *IEEE Transactions on Network and Service Management.*

Lee, J., Sun, J., Wang, F., Wang, S., Jun, C.-H., & Jiang, X. (2018). Privacy-preserving patient similarity learning in a federated environment: Development and analysis. *JMIR Medical Informatics*, *6*(2), e20. Advance online publication. doi:10.2196/medinform.7744 PMID:29653917

Lehmann, L. S., Natarajan, V., & Peng, L. (2024). Artificial intelligence in healthcare: a perspective from Google. In *Artificial Intelligence in Clinical Practice* (pp. 341–344). Elsevier. doi:10.1016/B978-0-443-15688-5.00037-1

Lemmen, C., Simic, D., & Stock, S. (2021). A Vision of Future Healthcare: Potential Opportunities and Risks of Systems Medicine from a Citizen and Patient Perspective—Results of a Qualitative Study. *International Journal of Environmental Research and Public Health*, *18*(18), 9879. doi:10.3390/ijerph18189879 PMID:34574802

Li, H., & Boulanger, P. (2020). A survey of heart anomaly detection using ambulatory electrocardiogram (ECG). *Sensors (Basel)*, *20*(5), 1461. doi:10.3390/s20051461 PMID:32155930

Li, H., Li, C., Wang, J., Yang, A., Ma, Z., Zhang, Z., & Hua, D. (2023). Review on security of federated learning and its application in healthcare. *Future Generation Computer Systems*, *144*, 271–290. doi:10.1016/j.future.2023.02.021

Li, H., Zou, L., Kowah, J. A. H., He, D., Liu, Z., Ding, X., Wen, H., Wang, L., Yuan, M., & Liu, X. (2023). A compact review of progress and prospects of deep learning in drug discovery. *Journal of Molecular Modeling*, *29*(4), 117. doi:10.1007/s00894-023-05492-w PMID:36976427

Li, J., Meng, Y., Ma, L., Du, S., Zhu, H., Pei, Q., & Shen, X. (2021). A federated learning based privacy-preserving smart healthcare system. *IEEE Transactions on Industrial Informatics*, *18*(3), 2021–2031. doi:10.1109/TII.2021.3098010

Li, L., Yang, F., Tse, M., & Lin, K. J. (2020, November 1). A review of applications in federated learning. *Computers & Industrial Engineering*, *149*, 106854. Advance online publication. doi:10.1016/j.cie.2020.106854

Lilhore, U. K., Dalal, S., Faujdar, N., Margala, M., Chakrabarti, P., Chakrabarti, T., Simaiya, S., Kumar, P., Thangaraju, P., & Velmurugan, H. (2023). Hybrid CNN-LSTM model with efficient hyperparameter tuning for prediction of Parkinson's disease. *Scientific Reports*, *13*(1), 14605. doi:10.1038/s41598-023-41314-y PMID:37669970

Lilhore, U. K., Dalal, S., Faujdar, N., Simaiya, S., Dahiya, M., Tomar, S., & Hashmi, A. (2024). Unveiling the prevalence and risk factors of early stage postpartum depression: A hybrid deep learning approach. *Multimedia Tools and Applications*, 1–35. doi:10.1007/s11042-024-18182-3

Lilhore, U. K., Dalal, S., Faujdar, N., Simaiya, S., Dahiya, M., Tomar, S., & Hashmi, A. (2024). Unveiling the prevalence and risk factors of early-stage postpartum depression: A hybrid deep learning approach. *Multimedia Tools and Applications*, 1–35.

Lilhore, U. K., Manoharan, P., Sandhu, J. K., Simaiya, S., Dalal, S., Baqasah, A. M., Alsafyani, M., Alroobaea, R., Keshta, I., & Raahemifar, K. (2023). Hybrid model for precise hepatitis-C classification using improved random forest and SVM method. *Scientific Reports*, *13*(1), 12473. doi:10.1038/s41598-023-36605-3 PMID:37528148

Lilhore, U. K., Poongodi, M., Kaur, A., Simaiya, S., Algarni, A. D., Elmannai, H., Vijayakumar, V., Tunze, G. B., & Hamdi, M. (2022). Hybrid model for detection of cervical cancer using causal analysis and machine learning techniques. *Computational and Mathematical Methods in Medicine*, *2022*, 2022. doi:10.1155/2022/4688327 PMID:35572826

Lilhore, U. K., Simaiya, S., Pandey, H., Gautam, V., Garg, A., & Ghosh, P. (2022). Breast cancer detection in the IoT cloud-based healthcare environment using fuzzy cluster segmentation and SVM classifier. *Ambient Communications and Computer Systems Proceedings of RACCCS*, *2021*, 165–179.

Lilhore, U. K., Simaiya, S., Pandey, H., Gautam, V., Garg, A., & Ghosh, P. (2022). Breast cancer detection in the IoT cloud-based healthcare environment using fuzzy cluster segmentation and SVM classifier. In Ambient Communications and Computer Systems [Singapore: Springer Nature Singapore.]. *Proceedings of RACCCS*, *2021*, 165–179.

Lilhore, U. K., Simaiya, S., Pandey, H., Gautam, V., Garg, A., & Ghosh, P. (2022). Breast cancer detection in the IoT cloud-based healthcare environment using fuzzy cluster segmentation and SVM classifier. *Proceedings of RACCCS*, *2021*, 165–179.

Lilhore, U. K., Simaiya, S., Prasad, D., & Guleria, K. (2020). A hybrid tumor detection and classification based on machine learning. *Journal of Computational and Theoretical Nanoscience*, *17*(6), 2539–2544. doi:10.1166/jctn.2020.8927

Linardatos, P., Papastefanopoulos, V., & Kotsiantis, S. (2020). Explainable ai: A review of machine learning interpretability methods. *Entropy (Basel, Switzerland)*, *23*(1), 18. doi:10.3390/e23010018 PMID:33375658

Lin, K. (2018). User experience-based product design for smart production to empower industry 4.0 in the glass recycling circular economy. *Computers & Industrial Engineering*, *125*, 729–738. doi:10.1016/j.cie.2018.06.023

Li, S. (2020). Privacy-Preserving Federated Learning for IoT-Based Healthcare: Challenges and Opportunities. *IEEE Internet of Things Journal*, *7*(9), 7310–7321.

Li, T. (2019). Federated Learning on Non-IID Data: Secure and Privacy-Preserving Strategy. *IEEE Access : Practical Innovations, Open Solutions*, *7*, 133486–133500.

LiT.SahuA. K.ZaheerM.SanjabiM.TalwalkarA.SmithV. (2019). *Federated optimization in heterogeneous networks.* ArXiv:1812.06127 [Cs, Stat]. Retrieved from http://arxiv.org/abs/1812.06127

Liu, X., Jiang, S., Vasan, A., Brace, A., Gokdemir, O., Brettin, T., . . . Stevens, R. (2023, December). DRUGIMPROVER: Utilizing Reinforcement Learning for Multi-Objective Alignment in Drug Optimization. *NeurIPS 2023 Workshop on New Frontiers of AI for Drug Discovery and Development.*

Liu, Z., Li, T., Smith, V., & Sekar, V. (2019). *Enhancing the privacy offederated learning with sketching.* ArXiv:1911.01812 [Cs, Stat]. Retrieved from http://arxiv.org/abs/1911.01812.

Liu, B., Wang, L., Liu, M., & Xu, C.-Z. (2020). Federated imitation learning: A novel framework for cloud robotic systems with heterogeneous sensor data. *IEEE Robotics and Automation Letters*, *5*(2), 3509–3516. doi:10.1109/LRA.2020.2976321

Liu, F., Chen, D., Zhou, X., Dai, W., Xu, F., & Let, A. I. (2022). Perform Better Next Time—A Systematic Review of Medical Imaging-Based Automated Diagnosis of COVID-19: 2020–2022. *Applied Sciences (Basel, Switzerland)*, *12*(8), 3895. doi:10.3390/app12083895

Liu, J., Zhang, G., Wang, K., & Yang, K. (2023). Task-load-aware game-theoretic framework for Wireless Federated Learning. *IEEE Communications Letters*, *27*(1), 268–272. doi:10.1109/LCOMM.2022.3210604

Liu, W., Xu, Y., Fan, D., Li, Y., Shao, X. F., & Zheng, J. (2021). Alleviating corporate environmental pollution threats toward public health and safety: The role of smart city and artificial intelligence. *Safety Science*, *143*, 105433.

Liu, Y. (2018). Secure Federated Learning for Healthcare: A Survey. *IEEE Access : Practical Innovations, Open Solutions*, *6*, 33707–33717.

LiuY.ChenT.YangQ. (2018). *Secure federated transfer learning*. ArXiv: 1812.03337 [Cs, Stat]. Retrieved from http://arxiv.org/abs/1812.03337

Li, X. (2020). Securing federated learning in edge computing: Communication-efficient protocols with privacy guarantee. *IEEE Internet of Things Journal*, *7*(6), 5370–5381.

Li, Y., Yang, J., Zhang, Z., Wen, J., & Kumar, P. (2022). Healthcare data quality assessment for cybersecurity intelligence. *IEEE Transactions on Industrial Informatics*, *19*(1), 841–848. doi:10.1109/TII.2022.3190405

Li, Z., Wang, L., Wu, X., Jiang, J., Qiang, W., Xie, H., Zhou, H., Wu, S., Shao, Y., & Chen, W. (2023). Artificial intelligence in ophthalmology: The path to the real-world clinic. *Cell Reports Medicine*, *4*(7), 101095. doi:10.1016/j.xcrm.2023.101095 PMID:37385253

López, M., & Navarro, P. (2023). Fostering Global Collaborations in Drug Research: A Spanish Perspective. *Global Healthcare Collaboration Journal*, *18*(2), 189–201.

Lo, S. W., Wu, J. H., Chang, J. Y., Tseng, C. H., Lin, M. W., & Lin, F. P. (2021). Deep sensing of urban waterlogging. *IEEE Access : Practical Innovations, Open Solutions*, *9*, 127185–127203. doi:10.1109/ACCESS.2021.3111623

Lu, S., Zhang, Y., & Wang, Y. (2020, March). Decentralized federated learning for electronic health records. In *2020 54th Annual Conference on Information Sciences and Systems (CISS)* (pp. 1-5). IEEE. 10.1109/CISS48834.2020.1570617414

Luque, A., Mazzoleni, M., Carrasco, A., & Ferramosca, A. (2022). Visualizing Classification Results: Confusion Star and Confusion Gear. *IEEE Access : Practical Innovations, Open Solutions*, *10*, 1659–1677. doi:10.1109/ACCESS.2021.3137630

Lysaght, T., Lim, H. Y., Xafis, V., & Ngiam, K. Y. (2019). AI-assisted decision-making in healthcare: The application of an ethics framework for big data in health and research. *Asian Bioethics Review*, *11*(3), 299–314. doi:10.1007/s41649-019-00096-0 PMID:33717318

Ma, C., Alam, S., Cai, Q., & Delahaye, D. (2022). Critical Links Detection in Spatial-Temporal Airway Networks Using Complex Network Theories. *IEEE Access : Practical Innovations, Open Solutions*, *10*, 27925–27944. doi:10.1109/ACCESS.2022.3152163

Madan, P., Singh, V., Singh, D. P., Diwakar, M., Pant, B., & Kishor, A. (2022). A hybrid deep learning approach for ECG-based arrhythmia classification. *Bioengineering (Basel, Switzerland)*, *9*(4), 152. doi:10.3390/bioengineering9040152 PMID:35447712

Madhu, H. K., & Ramesh, D. (2021). Heart attack analysis and prediction using svm. *International Journal of Computer Applications*.

Madhumita Pal & Smita Parija. (2020). Prediction of heart diseases using random forest. *Journal of Physics: Conference Series*.

Ma, H., Smal, I., Daemen, J., & van Walsum, T. (2020). Dynamic Coronary Roadmapping via Catheter Tip Tracking in X-Ray Fluoroscopy with Deep Learning Based Bayesian Filtering. *Medical Image Analysis*, *61*, 101634. doi:10.1016/j.media.2020.101634 PMID:31978856

Mahadevkar, S. V., Khemani, B., Patil, S., Kotecha, K., Vora, D., Abraham, A., & Gabralla, L. A. (2022). A review on machine learning styles in computer vision-techniques and future directions. *IEEE Access : Practical Innovations, Open Solutions, 10*, 107293–107329. doi:10.1109/ACCESS.2022.3209825

Mahajan, Y., Shandilya, D., Batta, P., & Sharma, M. (2023). 3D Object 360-Degree Motion Detection Using Ultra-Frequency PIR Sensor. *2023 IEEE World Conference on Applied Intelligence and Computing (AIC)*, 614–619. 10.1109/AIC57670.2023.10263926

Mahapatra, D., Poellinger, A., & Reyes, M. (2022). Interpretability-Guided Inductive Bias For Deep Learning Based Medical Image. *Medical Image Analysis, 81*, 102551. doi:10.1016/j.media.2022.102551 PMID:35932546

Mahbub, M. K., Biswas, M., Gaur, L., Alenezi, F., & Santosh, K. C. (2022). Deep features to detect pulmonary abnormalities in chest X-rays due to infectious diseaseX: Covid-19, pneumonia, and tuberculosis. *Information Sciences, 592*, 389–401. doi:10.1016/j.ins.2022.01.062 PMID:36532848

Mahmood, F., & Durr, N. J. (2018). Deep learning and conditional random fields-based depth estimation and topographical reconstruction from conventional endoscopy. *Medical Image Analysis, 48*, 230–243. doi:10.1016/j.media.2018.06.005 PMID:29990688

Mai, S. (2011). *Rob Stocker, Tim Turner: Using decision tree for diagnosing heart disease patients*. CRPIT.

Mammen, P. M. (2021). *Federated learning: Opportunities and challenges*. arXiv preprint arXiv:2101.05428.

Mantey, E. A., Zhou, C., Anajemba, J. H., Arthur, J. K., Hamid, Y., Chowhan, A., & Otuu, O. O. (2024). Federated Learning Approach for Secured Medical Recommendation in Internet of Medical Things using Homomorphic Encryption. *IEEE Journal of Biomedical and Health Informatics*, 1–11. Advance online publication. doi:10.1109/JBHI.2024.3350232 PMID:38190666

Marino, E., Bruno, F., Barbieri, L., Muzzupappa, M., & Liarokapis, F. (2021). Background-Aware Colorization Technique for Augmented Reality Applications. *IEEE Access : Practical Innovations, Open Solutions, 9*, 161761–161772. doi:10.1109/ACCESS.2021.3129076

Markus, B., Andreas, K., Arkadij, K., Stefan, L., Gustav, O., Elina, S., & Radka, S. (2023). Accelerating Biocatalysis Discovery with Machine Learning: A Paradigm Shift in Enzyme Engineering, Discovery, and Design. *ACS Catalysis, 13*(21), 14454–14469. doi:10.1021/acscatal.3c03417 PMID:37942268

Marshal, R., Gobinath, K., & Rao, V. V. (2021, April). Proactive measures to mitigate cyber security challenges in IoT based smart healthcare networks. In *2021 IEEE International IOT, Electronics and Mechatronics Conference (IEMTRONICS)* (pp. 1-4). IEEE. 10.1109/IEMTRONICS52119.2021.9422615

Martinez, J., Garcia, A., & Rodriguez, M. (2020). Collaborative Drug Development in Spain: A Case Study in Accelerating Innovation. *Journal of Pharmacy Research, 18*(3), 145–162.

Maxhelaku, S., & Kika, A. (2019). Improving interoperability in healthcare using HL7 FHIR. In *Proceedings of the 47th International Academic Conference*. International Institute of Social and Economic Sciences. doi:10.20472/IAC.2019.047.012

Mbunge, E., Sipho'esihle, J., & Muchemwa, B. (2022). Towards Emotive Sensory Web in Virtual Health Care: Trends, Technologies, Challenges and Ethical Issues. *Sensors International, 3*, 100134. doi:10.1016/j.sintl.2021.100134

McMahan, B., Moore, E., Ramage, D., Hampson, S., & Arcas, B. A. Y. (2017). Communication-efficient learning of deep networks from decentralized data. *Artificial Intelligence and Statistics*, 1273–1282. http://proceedings. mlr.press/v54/mcmahan17a.html.

McMahan, H. B. (2017). Communication-Efficient Learning of Deep Networks from Decentralized Data. *Proceedings of the International Conference on Artificial Intelligence and Statistics (AISTATS),* 1273-1282.

Mehmood, A., Iqbal, M., Mehmood, Z., Irtaza, A., Nawaz, M., Nazir, T., & Masood, M. (2021). Prediction of heart disease using deep convolutional neural networks. *Arabian Journal for Science and Engineering*, *46*(4), 3409–3422. doi:10.1007/s13369-020-05105-1

MehrabiN. 2019). *A Survey on Bias and Fairness in Machine Learning*. http://arxiv.org/abs/1908.09635

Meier, J., Rao, R., Verkuil, R., Liu, J., Sercu, T., & Rives, A. (2021). Language models enable zero-shot prediction of the effects of mutations on protein function. *Advances in Neural Information Processing Systems*, *34*, 29287–29303. doi:10.1101/2021.07.09.450648

Melillo, P., De Luca, N., Bracale, M., & Pecchia, L. (2013). aolo, Luca, N., Bracale, M., Pecchia, L.: Classification tree for risk assessment in patients suffering from congestive heart failure via long-term heart rate variability. *IEEE Journal of Biomedical and Health Informatics*, *17*(3), 727–733. doi:10.1109/JBHI.2013.2244902

Mendonça, S. S., de Sousa Vitória, A. R., de Lima, T. W., Galvão Filho, A. R., & Andrade, C. H. (2023). Exploring new horizons: Empowering computer-assisted drug design with few-shot learning. *Artificial Intelligence in the Life Sciences*, *4*, 100086. doi:10.1016/j.ailsci.2023.100086

Meskó, B., & Topol, E. J. (2023). The imperative for regulatory oversight of large language models (or generative AI) in healthcare. *npj. Digital Medicine*, *6*(1), 120. doi:10.1038/s41746-023-00873-0 PMID:37414860

Messaoudi, H., Belaid, A., Ben Salem, D., & Conze, P.-H. (2023). Cross-Dimensional Transfer Learning in Medical Image Segmentation with Deep Learning. *Medical Image Analysis*, *88*, 102868. doi:10.1016/j.media.2023.102868 PMID:37384952

Mhasawade, V., Zhao, Y., & Chunara, R. (2021). Machine learning and algorithmic fairness in public and population health. *Nature Machine Intelligence*, *3*(8), 659–666. doi:10.1038/s42256-021-00373-4

Minas, A. (2010). Assessment of the risk factors of coronary heart events based on data mining with decision trees. *IEEE Transactions on Information Technology in Biomedicine*.

Mohan, S., Thirumalai, C., & Srivastava, G. (2019). Effective heart disease prediction using hybrid machine learning techniques. *IEEE Access : Practical Innovations, Open Solutions*, *7*, 81542–81554. doi:10.1109/ACCESS.2019.2923707

Mohassel, P., & Zhang, Y. (2017). SecureML: A System for Scalable Privacy-Preserving Machine Learning. *Proceedings of the Network and Distributed System Security Symposium (NDSS).* 10.1109/SP.2017.12

Mollel, M. S., Abubakar, A. I., Ozturk, M., Kaijage, S. F., Kisangiri, M., Hussain, S., Imran, M. A., & Abbasi, Q. H. (2021). A Survey of Machine Learning Applications to Handover Management in 5G and beyond. *IEEE Access : Practical Innovations, Open Solutions*, *9*, 45770–45802. doi:10.1109/ACCESS.2021.3067503

Monlezun, D. J. (2023). AI + healthcare systems. In *The Thinking Healthcare System* (pp. 37–67). Elsevier. doi:10.1016/B978-0-443-18906-7.00003-9

Moses, D. A. (2021). Deep learning applied to automatic disease detection using chest x-rays. *Journal of Medical Imaging and Radiation Oncology*, *65*(5), 498–517. doi:10.1111/1754-9485.13273 PMID:34231311

Moulahi, T., Jabbar, R., Alabdulatif, A., Abbas, S., El Khediri, S., Zidi, S., & Rizwan, M. (2023). Privacy-preserving federated learning cyber-threat detection for intelligent transport systems with blockchain-based security. *Expert Systems: International Journal of Knowledge Engineering and Neural Networks*, *40*(5), e13103. doi:10.1111/exsy.13103

Muhasina, K. M., Ghosh, P., Swaroop, A. K., Selvaraj, J., Prajapati, B. G., Duraiswamy, B., & Palaniswamy, D. S. (2023). 7 Machine Data Mining Learning and. *Artificial Intelligence in Bioinformatics and Chemoinformatics*, 117.

Mulgund, P., Mulgund, B. P., Sharman, R., & Singh, R. (2021). The implications of the California Consumer Privacy Act (CCPA) on healthcare organizations: Lessons learned from early compliance experiences. *Health Policy and Technology*, *10*(3), 100543. doi:10.1016/j.hlpt.2021.100543

Munoz-Gonzalez, L., Co, K. T., & Lupu, E. C. (2019). *Byzantine-robust federated machine learning through adaptive model averaging*. ArXiv:1909.05125 [Cs, Stat]. Retrieved from http://arxiv.org/abs/1909.05125

Murat, F., Yildirim, O., Talo, M., Baloglu, U. B., Demir, Y., & Acharya, U. R. (2020). Application of deep learning techniques for heartbeats detection using ECG signals-analysis and review. *Computers in Biology and Medicine*, *120*, 103726. doi:10.1016/j.compbiomed.2020.103726 PMID:32421643

Nair, A. K., Sahoo, J., & Raj, E. D. (2023). Privacy preserving Federated Learning framework for IoMT based big data analysis using edge computing. *Computer Standards & Interfaces*, *86*, 103720. doi:10.1016/j.csi.2023.103720

Naresh, E. (2020). *Impact of Machine Learning in Bioinformatics Research*. https://link.springer.com/chapter/10.1007/978-981-15-2445-5_4

Nathaniel, T. I., Goodwin, R. L., Fowler, L., McPhail, B., & Black, A. C. Jr. (2021). An Adaptive Blended Learning Model for the Implementation of an Integrated Medical Neuroscience Course During the Covid-19 Pandemic. *Anatomical Sciences Education*, *14*(6), 699–710. doi:10.1002/ase.2097 PMID:33915035

Nayak, S., & Sharma, Y. K. (2023). A modified Bayesian boosting algorithm with weight-guided optimal feature selection for sentiment analysis. *Decision Analytics Journal*, *8*, 100289. doi:10.1016/j.dajour.2023.100289

Ng, D., Lan, X., Yao, M. M. S., Chan, W. P., & Feng, M. (2021). Federated learning: A collaborative effort to achieve better medical imaging models for individual sites that have small labelled datasets. *Quantitative Imaging in Medicine and Surgery*, *11*(2), 852–857. doi:10.21037/qims-20-595 PMID:33532283

Ng, Q. X., Yau, C. E., Lim, Y. L., Wong, L. K. T., & Liew, T. M. (2022). Public sentiment on the global outbreak of monkeypox: An unsupervised machine learning analysis of 352,182 twitter posts. *Public Health*, *213*, 1–4.

Nguyen, T. D., Rieger, P., Miettinen, M., & Sadeghi, A. R. (2020, February). Poisoning attacks on federated learning-based IoT intrusion detection system. In *Proc. Workshop Decentralized IoT Syst. Secur. (DISS)* (pp. 1-7). doi:10.14722/diss.2020.23003

Nguyen, D. C., Ding, M., Pathirana, P. N., Seneviratne, A., Li, J., & Poor, H. V. (2021). Federated learning for internet of things: A comprehensive survey. *IEEE Communications Surveys and Tutorials*, *23*(3), 1622–1658. doi:10.1109/COMST.2021.3075439

NockR.HardyS.HeneckaW.Ivey-LawH.PatriniG.SmithG.ThorneB. (2018). *Entity resolution and federated learning get a federated resolution*. ArXiv: 1803.04035 [Cs]. Retrieved from http://arxiv.org/abs/1803.04035

O'Regan, D., Shah, S., Mirsadraee, S., Al-Ruzzeh, S., Karthik, S., & Jarvis, M. (2008). Implementation of a Process-Orientated Multidisciplinary Approach (POMA), a System of Cost-Effective Healthcare Delivery within a Cardiac Surgical Unit. *Quality & Safety in Health Care*, *17*(6), 459–463. doi:10.1136/qshc.2006.021279 PMID:19064663

Okolo, C. T. (2022). Optimizing human-centered AI for healthcare in the Global South. *Patterns (New York, N.Y.)*, *3*(2), 100421. doi:10.1016/j.patter.2021.100421 PMID:35199066

Okuda, S., & Yoshizawa, A. (2010). ODB: A database for operon organizations, 2011 update. *Nucleic Acids Research*, *39*(Database), D552–D555. doi:10.1093/nar/gkq1090 PMID:21051344

Ong, J., Vo, B. T., Vo, B. N., Kim, D. Y., & Nordholm, S. (2022). A Bayesian Filter for Multi-View 3D Multi-Object Tracking With Occlusion Handling. *IEEE Transactions on Pattern Analysis and Machine Intelligence*, *44*(5), 2246–2263. doi:10.1109/TPAMI.2020.3034435

Onyema, E. M., Lilhore, U. K., Saurabh, P., Dalal, S., Nwaeze, A. S., Chijindu, A. T., Ndufeiya-Kumasi, L. C., & Simaiya, S. (2023). Evaluation of IoT-Enabled hybrid Model for genome sequence analysis of patients in healthcare 4.0. *Measurement. Sensors*, *26*, 100679. doi:10.1016/j.measen.2023.100679

Ordonez, C. (2006). Association rule discovery with the train and test approach for heart disease prediction. *IEEE Transactions on Information Technology in Biomedicine*, *10*(2), 334–343. doi:10.1109/TITB.2006.864475 PMID:16617622

Pal, A., Xue, Z., Befano, B., Rodriguez, A. C., Long, L. R., Schiffman, M., & Antani, S. (2021). Deep Metric Learning for Cervical Image Classification. *IEEE Access : Practical Innovations, Open Solutions*, *9*, 53266–53275. https://doi.org/10.1109/ACCESS.2021.3069346

Pandey, M., Fernandez, M., Gentile, F., Isayev, O., Tropsha, A., Stern, A. C., & Cherkasov, A. (2022). The transformational role of GPU computing and deep learning in drug discovery. *Nature Machine Intelligence*, *4*(3), 211–221. doi:10.1038/s42256-022-00463-x

Papernot, N. (2017). Semi-Supervised Knowledge Transfer for Deep Learning from Private Training Data. *Proceedings of the International Conference on Learning Representations (ICLR).*

Parimbelli, E., Wilk, S., Cornet, R., Sniatala, P., Sniatala, K., Glaser, S. L. C., Fraterman, I., Boekhout, A. H., Ottaviano, M., & Peleg, M. (2021). A review of AI and Data Science support for cancer management. *Artificial Intelligence in Medicine*, *117*, 102111. doi:10.1016/j.artmed.2021.102111 PMID:34127240

Park, S. H., & Lee, J. K. (2020). Internet of Things (IoT) for Telemedicine and Healthcare in the COVID-19 Pandemic. *Telemedicine Journal and e-Health*, *26*(11), 1345–1357. PMID:32074474

Patel, R. (2017). *Sentiment analysis on Twitter data using machine learning* [Doctoral dissertation]. Laurentian University of Sudbury.

Patel, C. N., Kumar, S. P., Rawal, R. M., Patel, D. P., Gonzalez, F. J., & Pandya, H. A. (2020). A multiparametric organ toxicity predictor for drug discovery. *Toxicology Mechanisms and Methods*, *30*(3), 159–166.

Patel, S., Sharma, R., & Gupta, N. (2022). Personalized Treatment Plans Through Federated Learning: A Case Study in Indian Healthcare. *Health Informatics Journal*, *19*(1), 45–58.

Paterick, T. E., Patel, N., Tajik, A. J., & Chandrasekaran, K. (2017). Improving Health Outcomes Through Patient Education and Partnerships with Patients. *Baylor University Medical Center Proceedings*, *30*(1), 112–13. https://www.tandfonline.com/doi/full/10.1080/08998280.2017.11929552

Pathak, A., & Kachuee, M. (2018). Federated learning in medicine: A systematic review. *arXiv preprint arXiv:1912.04977.*

Pathak, A., & Ghosh, J. (2010). Privacy-Preserving Mining of Association Rules. *Proceedings of the ACM SIGKDD International Conference on Knowledge Discovery and Data Mining*, 1-9.

Pestana, J., Belo, D., & Gamboa, H. (2020). Detection of Abnormalities in Electrocardiogram (ECG) using Deep Learning. In BIOSIGNALS (pp. 236-243). doi:10.5220/0008967302360243

Peyroteo, M., Ferreira, I. A., Elvas, L. B., Ferreira, J. C., & Lapão, L. V. (2021). Remote Monitoring Systems for Patients With Chronic Diseases in Primary Health Care: Systematic Review. *JMIR mHealth and uHealth*, *9*(12), e28285. doi:10.2196/28285 PMID:34932000

Pfohl, S. R., Dai, A. M., & Heller, K. (2019). *Federated and differentially private learning for electronic health records.* ArXiv:1911.05861 [Cs, Stat]. Retrieved from htt p://arxiv.org/abs/1911.05861

Polevikov, S. (2023). Advancing AI in healthcare: A comprehensive review of best practices. *Clinica Chimica Acta*, *548*, 117519. doi:10.1016/j.cca.2023.117519 PMID:37595864

Prabhakar, C., Sekuboyina, A., Paetzold, J. C., Li, H., Amiranashvili, T., & Kleesiek, J. (2021). *Improving Generalized Zero-Shot Learning for Multi-LabelChest X-ray Classification Using Knowledge Graphs.* Academic Press.

Pradeep, S., & Sharma, Y. K. (2019, February). A pragmatic evaluation of stress and performance testing technologies for web based applications. In *2019 Amity International Conference on Artificial Intelligence (AICAI)* (pp. 399-403). IEEE. 10.1109/AICAI.2019.8701327

Pradeep, S., Sharma, Y. K., Lilhore, U. K., Simaiya, S., Kumar, A., Ahuja, S., Margala, M., Chakrabarti, P., & Chakrabarti, T. (2023). Developing an SDN security model (EnsureS) based on lightweight service path validation with batch hashing and tag verification. *Scientific Reports*, *13*(1), 17381. doi:10.1038/s41598-023-44701-7 PMID:37833379

Qadir, Z., Ullah, F., Munawar, H. S., & Al-Turjman, F. (2021). Addressing disasters in smart cities through UAVs path planning and 5G communications: A systematic review. *Computer Communications*, *168*, 114–135.

Qayyum, A., Ahmad, K., Ahsan, M. A., Al-Fuqaha, A., & Qadir, J. (2022). Collaborative federated learning for healthcare: Multi-modal covid-19 diagnosis at the edge. *IEEE Open Journal of the Computer Society*, *3*, 172–184. doi:10.1109/OJCS.2022.3206407

Qian, Y., Hu, L., Chen, J., Guan, X., Hassan, M. M., & Alelaiwi, A. (2019). Privacy-aware service placement for mobile edge computing via federated learning. *Information Sciences*, *505*, 562–570. doi:10.1016/j.ins.2019.07.069

Qin, T., Cheng, G., Chen, W., & Lei, X. (2021). FNEL:an evolving intrusion detection system based on federated never-ending learning. *2021 17th International Conference on Mobility, Sensing and Networking (MSN).* 10.1109/MSN53354.2021.00047

Qiu, J., Li, L., Sun, J., Peng, J., Shi, P., Zhang, R., Dong, Y., Lam, K., Lo, F. P.-W., Xiao, B., Yuan, W., Wang, N., Xu, D., & Lo, B. (2023). Large ai models in health informatics: Applications, challenges, and the future. *IEEE Journal of Biomedical and Health Informatics*, *27*(12), 6074–6087. doi:10.1109/JBHI.2023.3316750 PMID:37738186

Qiu, Y., & Wei, G. W. (2023). Artificial intelligence-aided protein engineering: From topological data analysis to deep protein language models. *Briefings in Bioinformatics*, *24*(5), bbad289. doi:10.1093/bib/bbad289 PMID:37580175

Qi, Y. (2013). Text Mining in Bioinformatics: Research and Application. *International Journal of Information Retrieval Research*, *3*(2), 30–39. doi:10.4018/ijirr.2013040102

Rahman, A., Hossain, M. S., Muhammad, G., Kundu, D., Debnath, T., Rahman, M., Khan, M. S. I., Tiwari, P., & Band, S. S. (2023). Federated learning-based AI approaches in smart healthcare: Concepts, taxonomies, challenges and open issues. *Cluster Computing*, *26*(4), 2271–2311. doi:10.1007/s10586-022-03658-4 PMID:35996680

Rahman, M. A., Hossain, M. S., Showail, A. J., Alrajeh, N. A., & Alhamid, M. F. (2021). A secure, private, and explainable IoHT framework to support sustainable health monitoring in a smart city. *Sustainable Cities and Society*, *72*, 103083.

Rahmat, D., Putra, H. A. A., & Setiawan, A. W. (2021). Heart disease prediction using k-nearest neighbor. *International Conference on Electrical Engineering and Informatics (ICEEI).* 10.1109/ICEEI52609.2021.9611110

Rajkomar, A. (2019). Scalable and accurate deep learning with electronic health records. npj. *Digital Medicine*, *2*(1), 1–10.

Ramaswamy, S., Mathews, R., Rao, K., & Beaufays, F. (2019). *Federated learning for emoji prediction in a mobile keyboard.* ArXiv:1906.04329 [Cs]. Retrieved from htt p://arxiv.org/abs/1906.04329

Ramesh, T. R., Lilhore, U. K., Poongodi, M., Simaiya, S., Kaur, A., & Hamdi, M. (2022). Predictive analysis of heart diseases with machine learning approaches. *Malaysian Journal of Computer Science*, •••, 132–148.

Ramgopal, N. C., Gantela, P., Rajagopal, R., Thankam, T., & SenthamilSelvan, R. (2022, December). Automatic Liver Cancer Detection in Abdominal Liver Images Using Soft Optimization Techniques. In *2022 International Conference on Knowledge Engineering and Communication Systems (ICKES)* (pp. 1-5). IEEE.

Rana, N. P., Chatterjee, S., Dwivedi, Y. K., & Akter, S. (2022). Understanding dark side of artificial intelligence (AI) integrated business analytics: Assessing firm's operational inefficiency and competitiveness. *European Journal of Information Systems, 31*(3), 364–387. doi:10.1080/0960085X.2021.1955628

Rani, S., Kataria, A., Kumar, S., & Tiwari, P. (2023). Federated learning for secure IoMT-applications in smart healthcare systems: A comprehensive review. *Knowledge-Based Systems, 274*, 110658. doi:10.1016/j.knosys.2023.110658

Rao, M. G., Pawar, S., Priyanka, H., Reddy, K. H. K., & Divakarala, U. (2023). Minimize the Energy Consumption for Communication Protocol in IoT. In Energy Systems Design for Low-Power Computing (pp. 214-234). IGI Global.

Rao, M. G., Gagan, G., Nikhil, T. C., & Pradeep, A. B. (2022, December). Authentication and Parking of the Vehicle Using License Plate Detection and Recognition in the Campus. In *2022 International Conference on Artificial Intelligence and Data Engineering (AIDE)* (pp. 74-79). IEEE.

Rao, M. G., Pawar, S., Priyanka, H., Reddy, K. H. K., & Divakarla, U. (2022, December). Novel approach of Using Periocular and Iris Biometric Recognition in the Authentication of ITS. In *2022 Fourth International Conference on Cognitive Computing and Information Processing (CCIP)* (pp. 1-6). IEEE.

Rao, M. G., Priyanka, H., Kumar, A. P., & Divakarla, U. (2022, September). A Deep Learning Approach Towards Building Intelligent Transport System. In *2022 Second International Conference on Computer Science, Engineering and Applications (ICCSEA)* (pp. 1-6). IEEE.

Rao, M. G., Reddy, K. H. K., Ahamed, A., & Shetty, A. (2022, December). Deploy the VNPDR to Provide Authenticated Parking for Vehicles on Hospital Premise. In *2022 International Conference on Artificial Intelligence and Data Engineering (AIDE)* (pp. 107-111). IEEE.

Rathore, M. S., Poongodi, M., Saurabh, P., Lilhore, U. K., Bourouis, S., Alhakami, W., Osamor, J., & Hamdi, M. (2022). A novel trust-based security and privacy model for internet of vehicles using encryption and steganography. *Computers & Electrical Engineering, 102*, 108205. doi:10.1016/j.compeleceng.2022.108205

Rauniyar, A., Hagos, D. H., Jha, D., Håkegård, J. E., Bagci, U., Rawat, D. B., & Vlassov, V. (2023). Federated learning for medical applications: A taxonomy, current trends, challenges, and future research directions. *IEEE Internet of Things Journal.*

Raza, A., Tran, K. P., Koehl, L., & Li, S. (2022). Designing ECG monitoring healthcare system with federated transfer learning and explainable AI. *Knowledge-Based Systems, 236*, 107763. doi:10.1016/j.knosys.2021.107763

Ren, X., Gao, Z., & Sui, Q. (2022). An Optimal Visual Fatigue Relief Method for Workers Considering Rest Time Allocation. *IEEE Access : Practical Innovations, Open Solutions, 10*, 26463–26470. https://doi.org/10.1109/ACCESS.2022.3155189

Reza, A. W. (2020). Challenges and Opportunities in Federated Learning for Healthcare IoT: A Systematic Review. *IEEE Access : Practical Innovations, Open Solutions, 8*, 162238–162249.

Rezapour, M., & Hansen, L. (2022). A machine learning analysis of COVID-19 mental health data. *Scientific Reports*, *12*(1), 14965.

Rieke, N., Hancox, J., Li, W., Milletari, F., Roth, H. R., Albarqouni, S., Bakas, S., Galtier, M. N., Landman, B. A., Maier-Hein, K., Ourselin, S., Sheller, M., Summers, R. M., Trask, A., Xu, D., Baust, M., & Cardoso, M. J. (2020). The future of digital health with federated learning. *NPJ Digital Medicine*, *3*(1), 119. doi:10.1038/s41746-020-00323-1 PMID:33015372

Rieyan, S. A., News, M. R. K., Rahman, A. M., Khan, S. A., Zaarif, S. T. J., Alam, M. G. R., Hassan, M. M., Ianni, M., & Fortino, G. (2024). An advanced data fabric architecture leveraging homomorphic encryption and federated learning. *Information Fusion*, *102*, 102004. doi:10.1016/j.inffus.2023.102004

Rizwan, A., Priyanga, P., Abualsauod, E. H., Zafrullah, S. N., Serbaya, S. H., & Halifa, A. (2022). A machine learning approach for the detection of QRS complexes in electrocardiogram (ECG) using discrete wavelet transform (DWT) algorithm. *Computational Intelligence and Neuroscience*, *2022*, 1–8. Advance online publication. doi:10.1155/2022/9023478 PMID:35528332

Rodríguez-Rodríguez, I., Chatzigiannakis, I., Rodríguez, J. V., Maranghi, M., Gentili, M., & Zamora-Izquierdo, M. Á. (2019). Utility of big data in predicting short-term blood glucose levels in type 1 diabetes mellitus through machine learning techniques. *Sensors (Basel)*, *19*(20), 4482. doi:10.3390/s19204482 PMID:31623111

Rokade, M. D., & Sharma, Y. K. (2021, March). MLIDS: A machine learning approach for intrusion detection for real-time network dataset. In *2021 International conference on emerging smart computing and informatics (ESCI)* (pp. 533-536). IEEE. 10.1109/ESCI50559.2021.9396829

Roumpeka, D. D., Wallace, R. J., Escalettes, F., Fotheringham, I., & Watson, M. (2017). A Review of Bioinformatics Tools for Bio-Prospecting from Metagenomic Sequence Data. *Frontiers in Genetics*, *8*, 23. doi:10.3389/fgene.2017.00023 PMID:28321234

Roy, M., Majumder, S., Halder, A., & Biswas, U. (2023). ECG-NET: A deep LSTM autoencoder for detecting anomalous ECG. *Engineering Applications of Artificial Intelligence*, *124*, 106484. doi:10.1016/j.engappai.2023.106484

Ruiz, M., Gonzalez, E., & Fernandez, A. (2021). Accelerating Drug Development Through Federated Learning: A Spanish Case Study. *Journal of Pharmaceutical Innovation*, *20*(4), 301–318.

Rychtyckyj, N., & Plesco, C. (2013). Applying Automated Language Translation at a Global Enterprise Level. *AI Magazine*, *34*(1), 43–54. doi:10.1609/aimag.v34i1.2436

Sachi, S., Singh, A. K., Jain, A., Devi, S., Sharma, Y. K., & Athithan, S. (2023, July). Hate Speech Detection Using the GPT-2 and Natural Language Processing. In *2023 Intelligent Methods, Systems, and Applications (IMSA)* (pp. 276-280). IEEE.

Sadaf, M., Iqbal, Z., Javed, A. R., Saba, I., Krichen, M., Majeed, S., & Raza, A. (2023). Connected and Automated Vehicles: Infrastructure, Applications, Security, Critical Challenges, and Future Aspects. *Technologies*, *11*(5), 117. doi:10.3390/technologies11050117

Saini, S. K., & Gupta, R. (2022). Artificial intelligence methods for analysis of electrocardiogram signals for cardiac abnormalities: State-of-the-art and future challenges. *Artificial Intelligence Review*, *55*(2), 1519–1565. doi:10.1007/s10462-021-09999-7

Sai, S., Hassija, V., Chamola, V., & Guizani, M. (2023). Federated Learning and NFT-Based Privacy-Preserving Medical Data Sharing Scheme for Intelligent Diagnosis in Smart Healthcare. *IEEE Internet of Things Journal*.

Sanchez-Fernandez, A., Rumetshofer, E., Hochreiter, S., & Klambauer, G. (2022, April). Contrastive learning of image- and structure-based representations in drug discovery. ICLR2022 Machine Learning for Drug Discovery.

Saputra, Y. M., Hoang, D. T., Nguyen, D. N., Dutkiewicz, E., Mueck, M. D., & Srikanteswara, S. (2019). Energy demand prediction with federated learning for electric vehicle networks. *IEEE Global Communications Conference (GLOBE-COM),* 1–6. 10.1109/GLOBECOM38437.2019.9013587

Scherer, J., Nolden, M., Kleesiek, J., Metzger, J., Kades, K., Schneider, V., Bach, M., Sedlaczek, O., Bucher, A. M., Vogl, T. J., Grünwald, F., Kühn, J.-P., Hoffmann, R.-T., Kotzerke, J., Bethge, O., Schimmöller, L., Antoch, G., Müller, H.-W., Daul, A., ... Maier-Hein, K. (2020). Joint imaging platform for federated clinical data analytics. *JCO Clinical Cancer Informatics*, *4*(4), 1027–1038. doi:10.1200/CCI.20.00045 PMID:33166197

Seetharaman, M., Krishnan, G., & Schneider, R. H. (2021). The Future of Medicine: Frontiers in Integrative Health and Medicine. *Medicina, 57*(12), 1303. https://www.mdpi.com/1648-9144/57/12/1303

Seidl, P., Renz, P., Dyubankova, N., Neves, P., Verhoeven, J., Wegner, J. K., Segler, M., Hochreiter, S., & Klambauer, G. (2022). Improving few-and zero-shot reaction template prediction using modern hopfield networks. *Journal of Chemical Information and Modeling*, *62*(9), 2111–2120. doi:10.1021/acs.jcim.1c01065 PMID:35034452

Seoni, S., Jahmunah, V., Salvi, M., Barua, P. D., Molinari, F., & Acharya, U. R. (2023). Application of uncertainty quantification to artificial intelligence in healthcare: A review of last decade (2013–2023). *Computers in Biology and Medicine*, *165*, 107441. doi:10.1016/j.compbiomed.2023.107441 PMID:37683529

Shah, A. K., & Agnihotri, S. A. (2011). Recent advances and novel strategies in pre-clinical formulation development: An overview. *Journal of Controlled Release*, *156*(3), 281–296.

Shahnaz, M., Chowdhary, M., Rani, A., Parkash, J., & Dev, D. (2016). Bioinformatics: An overview for cancer research. *Journal of Drug Delivery and Therapeutics*, *6*(4), 69–72. doi:10.22270/jddt.v6i4.1290

Sharma, Y. K., & Khatal Sunil, S. (2019). Health Care Patient Monitoring using IoT and Machine Learning. *IOSR Journal of Engineering (IOSR JEN) National Conference on "Recent Innovations in Engineering and Technology" MOMENTUM-19.*

Sharma, Y. K., & Rokade, M. D. (2019). Deep and machine learning approaches for anomaly-based intrusion detection of imbalanced network traffic. *IOSR Journal of Engineering*, 63-67.

Sharma, A., Khan, S., & Verma, R. (2021). Improving Healthcare Access in Underserved Areas: A Federated Learning Approach. *Journal of Medical Informatics Research, 14*(2), 189–201.

Sharma, A., & Singh, P. K. (2021). UAV-based framework for effective data analysis of forest fire detection using 5G networks: An effective approach towards smart cities solutions. *International Journal of Communication Systems*, 4826.

Sharma, S. K., Lilhore, U. K., Simaiya, S., & Trivedi, N. K. (2021). An improved random forest algorithm for predicting the COVID-19 pandemic patient health. *Annals of the Romanian Society for Cell Biology*, 67–75.

SharmaS.ChaopingX.LiuY.KangY. (2019). Secure and efficient federated transfer learning. ArXiv:1910.13271 [Cs]. doi:10.1109/BigData47090.2019.9006280

Sharma, Y. K., Athithan, S., Sachi, S., Singh, A. K., Jain, A., & Devi, S. (2023, July). Copy and Move Forged Image Detection by Deep Learning. In *2023 World Conference on Communication & Computing (WCONF)* (pp. 1-6). IEEE. 10.1109/WCONF58270.2023.10235115

Shen, T. (2020, June 27). *Federated Mutual Learning.* arXiv.org. https://arxiv.org/abs/2006.16765

Shenaj, D. (2023, April 7). *Asynchronous Federated Continual Learning*. arXiv.org. https://arxiv.org/abs/2304.03626 doi:10.1109/CVPRW59228.2023.00534

Shiri, I., Vafaei Sadr, A., Akhavan, A., Salimi, Y., Sanaat, A., Amini, M., Razeghi, B., Saberi, A., Arabi, H., Ferdowsi, S., Voloshynovskiy, S., Gündüz, D., Rahmim, A., & Zaidi, H. (2023). Decentralized collaborative multi-institutional PET attenuation and scatter correction using federated deep learning. *European Journal of Nuclear Medicine and Molecular Imaging*, *50*(4), 1034–1050. doi:10.1007/s00259-022-06053-8 PMID:36508026

Shivthare, S. K., Sharma, Y. K., & Patil, R. D. (2023). Multi-modal Biometric in Computer Vision. *Multi-modal Biometric and Machine Learning Technologies: Applications for Computer Vision*, 1-29.

Shokri, R. (2017). Membership Inference Attacks Against Machine Learning Models. *Proceedings of the Conference on Computer and Communications Security (CCS),* 3-18. 10.1109/SP.2017.41

Shokri, R., & Shmatikov, V. (2015). Privacy-Preserving Deep Learning. *Proceedings of the ACM SIGSAC Conference on Computer and Communications Security (CCS),* 1310-1321.

Sidorov, M., Nhut, P. V., Matsumoto, Y., & Ohmura, R. (2019). LoRa-based precision wireless structural health monitoring system for bolted joints in a smart city environment. *IEEE Access : Practical Innovations, Open Solutions*, *7*, 179235–179251.

Silva, S., Gutman, B. A., Romero, E., Thompson, P. M., Altmann, A., & Lorenzi, M. (2019). Federated learning in distributed medical databases: meta-analysis of largescale subcortical brain data. In *2019 IEEE 16th International Symposium on Biomedical Imaging (ISBI 2019)* (pp. 270–274). .8759317.10.1109/ISBI.2019.8759317

Simaiya, S., Lilhore, U. K., Prasad, D., & Verma, D. K. (2021). MRI brain tumor detection & image segmentation by hybrid hierarchical K-means clustering with FCM based machine learning model. *Annals of the Romanian Society for Cell Biology*, 88–94.

Simaiya, S., Lilhore, U. K., Prasad, D., & Verma, D. K. (2021). MRI brain tumour detection & image segmentation by hybrid hierarchical K-means clustering with FCM based machine learning model. *Annals of the Romanian Society for Cell Biology*, 88–94.

Singh, K., Kumar, A., Sharma, Y. K., & Rai, A. K. (2023). AIoT-based e-commerce. *AIoT Technologies and Applications for Smart Environments*, 215.

Singh, P., Chatterjee, A., Rajput, L. S., Kumar, S., Nataraj, V., Bhatia, V., & Prakash, S. (2021). Biospeckle-based sensor for characterization of charcoal rot (Macrophomina phaseolina (Tassi) goid) disease in soybean (Glycine max (L.) Merr.) crop. *IEEE Access : Practical Innovations, Open Solutions*, *9*, 31562–31574. doi:10.1109/ACCESS.2021.3059868

Singh, S., Rathore, S., Alfarraj, O., Tolba, A., & Yoon, B. (2022). A framework for privacy-preservation of IoT healthcare data using Federated Learning and blockchain technology. *Future Generation Computer Systems*, *129*, 380–388. doi:10.1016/j.future.2021.11.028

Smith, A., & Jain, P. (2018). Private Federated Learning on Vertically Partitioned Data via Entity Resolution and Additive Secret Sharing. *Proceedings of the IEEE European Symposium on Security and Privacy (EuroS&P),* 1-16.

Smith, V. A. (2017). Federated Learning with Bayesian Differential Privacy. *arXiv preprint arXiv:1712.07557.*

Smith, J. (2020). Healthcare Challenges in China: An In-depth Analysis. *Beijing Medical Journal*, *15*(2), 123–145.

Smith, J. A., & Brown, R. D. (2021). IoT Devices in Healthcare: Opportunities and Challenges. *Journal of Health Care Technology*, *6*(2), 87–101.

Sohrabi, Z., & Khaneghah, E. M. (2020). Challenges of Using Live Process Migration in Distributed Exascale Systems. *Azerbaijan Journal of High Performance Computing*, *3*(2), 151–163.

Somashekhar, S. P., Sepúlveda, M.-J., Norden, A. D., Rauthan, A., Arun, K., Patil, P., Ethadka, R. Y., & Kumar, R. C. (2017). Early Experience with IBM Watson for Oncology (WFO) Cognitive Computing System for Lung and Colorectal Cancer Treatment. *Journal of Clinical Oncology*, *35*(15, suppl), 8527–8527. doi:10.1200/JCO.2017.35.15_suppl.8527

Spagnolo, F., Corsonello, P., Frustaci, F., & Perri, S. (2023). Design of a Low-Power Super-Resolution Architecture for Virtual Reality Wearable Devices. *IEEE Sensors Journal*, *23*(8), 9009–9016. https://doi.org/10.1109/JSEN.2023.3256524

Sprague, M. R., Jalalirad, A., Scavuzzo, M., Capota, C., Neun, M., Do, L., & Kopp, M. (2019). Asynchronous federated learning for geospatial applications. In A. Monreale, C. Alzate, M. Kamp, Y. Krishnamurthy, D. Paurat, M. Sayed-Mouchaweh, ... R. P. Ribeiro (Eds.), *ECML PKDD 2018 Workshops* (pp. 21–28). doi:10.1007/978-3-030-14880-5_2

Sreenivasan, M., & Chacko, A. M. (2021). Interoperability issues in EHR systems: Research directions. *Data analytics in biomedical engineering and healthcare*, 13-28. doi:10.1016/B978-0-12-819314-3.00002-1

Stephanie, V., Khalil, I., Atiquzzaman, M., & Yi, X. (2022). Trustworthy privacy-preserving hierarchical ensemble and federated learning in healthcare 4.0 with Blockchain. *IEEE Transactions on Industrial Informatics*.

Stoesser, G., Moseley, M. A., Sleep, J., McGowran, M., Garcia-Pastor, M., & Sterk, P. (1998, January 1). The EMBL Nucleotide Sequence Database. *Nucleic Acids Research*, *26*(1), 8–15. doi:10.1093/nar/26.1.8 PMID:9399791

Streeter, Beron, & Iyer. (2017). Precision Medicine. *Otolaryngologic Clinics of North America, 50*(4), 765–73. https://linkinghub.elsevier.com/retrieve/pii/S0030666517300609

Sung, J. M., Cho, I. J., Sung, D., Kim, S., Kim, H. C., Chae, M. H., Kavousi, M., Rueda-Ochoa, O. L., Ikram, M. A., Franco, O. H., & Chang, H. J. (2019). Development and verification of prediction models for preventing cardiovascular diseases. *PLoS One*, *14*(9), e0222809. doi:10.1371/journal.pone.0222809 PMID:31536581

Suresh Babu, C. V., & Praveen, S. (2023). Swarm Intelligence and Evolutionary Machine Learning Algorithms for COVID-19: Pandemic and Epidemic Review. In *Dynamics of Swarm Intelligence Health Analysis for the Next Generation.* IGI Global. doi:10.4018/978-1-6684-6894-4.ch005

Suresh Babu, C.V., Akshayah N. S., Maclin Vinola P., & Janapriyan, R. (2023). IoT-Based Smart Accident Detection and Alert System. In P. Swarnalatha & S. Prabu (Eds.), Handbook of Research on Deep Learning Techniques for Cloud-Based Industrial IoT (pp. 322-337). IGI Global. doi:10.4018/978-1-6684-8098-4.ch019

Suresh Babu, C. V., Andrew Simon, P., & Barath Kumar, S. (2023). The Future of Cyber Security Starts Today, Not Tomorrow. In S. Shiva Darshan, M. Manoj Kumar, B. Prashanth, & Y. Vishnu Srinivasa Murthy (Eds.), *Malware Analysis and Intrusion Detection in Cyber-Physical Systems* (pp. 348–375). IGI Global. doi:10.4018/978-1-6684-8666-5.ch016

Suresh Babu, C. V., & Yadav, S. (2023). Cyber Physical Systems Design Challenges in the Areas of Mobility, Healthcare, Energy, and Manufacturing. In R. Thanigaivelan, S. Kaliappan, & C. Jegadheesan (Eds.), *Cyber-Physical Systems and Supporting Technologies for Industrial Automation* (pp. 131–151). IGI Global. doi:10.4018/978-1-6684-9267-3.ch007

Swapna, G., & Soman, K. P. (2021). Diabetes detection and sensor-based continuous glucose monitoring-a deep learning approach. In *Efficient Data Handling for Massive Internet of Medical Things: Healthcare Data Analytics* (pp. 245–268). Springer International Publishing. doi:10.1007/978-3-030-66633-0_11

Swapna, M., Sharma, Y. K., & Prasad, B. M. G. (2020). A survey on face recognition using convolutional neural network. In *Data Engineering and Communication Technology: Proceedings of 3rd ICDECT-2K19* (pp. 649–661). Springer Singapore. doi:10.1007/978-981-15-1097-7_54

Swapna, M., Sharma, Y. K., & Prasadh, B. M. G. (2020). CNN Architectures: Alex Net, Le Net, VGG, Google Net. *Res Net. Int. J. Recent Technol. Eng*, *8*(6), 953–960. doi:10.35940/ijrte.F9532.038620

Tejedor, M., Woldaregay, A. Z., & Godtliebsen, F. (2020). Reinforcement learning application in diabetes blood glucose control: A systematic review. *Artificial Intelligence in Medicine*, *104*, 101836. doi:10.1016/j.artmed.2020.101836 PMID:32499004

Tian, Y., Wang, S., Xiong, J., Bi, R., Zhou, Z., & Bhuiyan, M. Z. A. (2023). Robust and privacy-preserving decentralized deep federated learning training: Focusing on digital healthcare applications. *IEEE/ACM Transactions on Computational Biology and Bioinformatics*. PMID:37028039

Torkzadehmahani, R., Nasirigerdeh, R., Blumenthal, D. B., Kacprowski, T., List, M., Matschinske, J., Spaeth, J., Wenke, N. K., & Baumbach, J. (2022). Privacy-preserving artificial intelligence techniques in biomedicine. *Methods of Information in Medicine*, *61*(S 01), e12–e27. doi:10.1055/s-0041-1740630 PMID:35062032

Tran, K. A., Kondrashova, O., Bradley, A., Williams, E. D., Pearson, J. V., & Waddell, N. (2021). Deep learning in cancer diagnosis, prognosis and treatment selection. *Genome Medicine*, *13*(1), 1–17. doi:10.1186/s13073-021-00968-x PMID:34579788

Trencher, G., & Karvonen, A. (2019). Stretching "smart": Advancing health and well-being through the smart city agenda. *Local Environment*, *24*(7), 610–627.

Triantafyllidis, A., Kondylakis, H., Katehakis, D., Kouroubali, A., Koumakis, L., Marias, K., Alexiadis, A., Votis, K., & Tzovaras, D. (2022). Deep learning in mHealth for cardiovascular disease, diabetes, and cancer: Systematic review. *JMIR mHealth and uHealth*, *10*(4), e32344. doi:10.2196/32344 PMID:35377325

Truex, S., Baracaldo, N., Anwar, A., Steinke, T., Ludwig, H., Zhang, R., & Zhou, Y. (2019, November). A hybrid approach to privacy-preserving federated learning. In *Proceedings of the 12th ACM workshop on artificial intelligence and security* (pp. 1-11). 10.1145/3338501.3357370

Ullah, I., Deng, X., Pei, X., Jiang, P., & Mushtaq, H. (2023). A verifiable and privacy-preserving blockchain-based federated learning approach. *Peer-to-Peer Networking and Applications*, *16*(5), 2256–2270. doi:10.1007/s12083-023-01531-8

Vaid, A., Jaladanki, S. K., Xu, J., Teng, S., Kumar, A., Lee, S., Somani, S., Paranjpe, I., De Freitas, J. K., Wanyan, T., Johnson, K. W., Bicak, M., Klang, E., Kwon, Y. J., Costa, A., Zhao, S., Miotto, R., Charney, A. W., Böttinger, E., ... Glicksberg, B. S. (2021). Federated learning of electronic health records to improve mortality prediction in hospitalized patients with COVID-19: Machine learning approach. *JMIR Medical Informatics*, *9*(1), e24207. doi:10.2196/24207 PMID:33400679

Vale, D., El-Sharif, A., & Ali, M. (2022). Explainable Artificial Intelligence (XAI) Post-Hoc Explainability Methods: Risks and Limitations in Non-Discrimination Law. *AI and Ethics*, *2*(4), 815–826. doi:10.1007/s43681-022-00142-y

van Berkel, N., Sarsenbayeva, Z., & Goncalves, J. (2023). The Methodology of Studying Fairness Perceptions in Artificial Intelligence: Contrasting CHI and FAccT. *International Journal of Human-Computer Studies*, *170*, 102954. doi:10.1016/j.ijhcs.2022.102954

Vandewinckele, L., Claessens, M., Dinkla, A., Brouwer, C., Crijns, W., Verellen, D., & van Elmpt, W. (2020). Overview of artificial intelligence-based applications in radiotherapy: Recommendations for implementation and quality assurance. *Radiotherapy and Oncology : Journal of the European Society for Therapeutic Radiology and Oncology*, *153*, 55–66. doi:10.1016/j.radonc.2020.09.008 PMID:32920005

Varshney, N., & Mishra, A. K. (2023). Deep Learning in Phosphoproteomics: Methods and Application in Cancer Drug Discovery. *Proteomes*, *11*(2), 16. doi:10.3390/proteomes11020016 PMID:37218921

Veríssimo, G. C., Serafim, M. S. M., Kronenberger, T., Ferreira, R. S., Honorio, K. M., & Maltarollo, V. G. (2022). Designing drugs when there is low data availability: One-shot learning and other approaches to face the issues of a long-term concern. *Expert Opinion on Drug Discovery*, *17*(9), 929–947. doi:10.1080/17460441.2022.2114451 PMID:35983695

Verma, R. (2022). Smart city healthcare cyber physical system: Characteristics, technologies and challenges. *Wireless Personal Communications*, *122*(2), 1413–1433.

Vettoretti, M., Cappon, G., Facchinetti, A., & Sparacino, G. (2020). Advanced diabetes management using artificial intelligence and continuous glucose monitoring sensors. *Sensors (Basel)*, *20*(14), 3870. doi:10.3390/s20143870 PMID:32664432

Wang, T., Guo, Y., & Choo, K. K. R. (2023). *Enabling Privacy-Preserving Prediction for Length of Stay in ICU-A Multimodal Federated-Learning-based Approach*. Academic Press.

Wang, Y., Tong, Y., & Shi, D. (2020). Federated latent dirichlet allocation: A local differential privacy based framework. *AAAI 2020- AAAI Conference on Artificial Intelligence*, 6283–6290. 10.1609/aaai.v34i04.6096

Wang, H., Liu, Y., & Zhang, L. (2019). Privacy-Preserving Techniques in Federated Learning for Chinese Healthcare. *Journal of Privacy and Security*, *7*(2), 145–162.

Wang, K., Chen, C. M., Tie, Z., Shojafar, M., Kumar, S., & Kumari, S. (2021). Forward privacy preservation in IoT-enabled healthcare systems. *IEEE Transactions on Industrial Informatics*, *18*(3), 1991–1999. doi:10.1109/TII.2021.3064691

Wang, L., & Zhang, H. (2019). Advancements in Diagnostics: A Chinese Perspective. *Journal of Health Care Technology*, *8*(4), 210–225.

Wang, R., Lai, J., Zhang, Z., Li, X., Vijayakumar, P., & Karuppiah, M. (2022). Privacy-preserving federated learning for Internet of medical things under edge computing. *IEEE Journal of Biomedical and Health Informatics*, *27*(2), 854–865. doi:10.1109/JBHI.2022.3157725 PMID:35259124

Wang, S., & Jiang, X. (2017). 5G mobile communications: A key enabler for the IoT. *IEEE Internet of Things Journal*, *4*(5), 1312–1322.

Wang, W., Li, X., Qiu, X., Zhang, X., Brusic, V., & Zhao, J. (2023). A privacy preserving framework for federated learning in smart healthcare systems. *Information Processing & Management*, *60*(1), 103167. doi:10.1016/j.ipm.2022.103167

Wang, X., & Zhang, W. (2020). Privacy-Preserving Machine Learning in Healthcare: Methods and Challenges. *IEEE Transactions on Biomedical Engineering*, *67*(7), 1887–1899.

Wang, Y., & Wang, S. (2020). Privacy-Preserving Data Mining: A Comprehensive Survey from the Perspective of Data and Algorithm. *ACM Computing Surveys*, *53*(1), 1–38.

Wazid, M., Bera, B., Das, A. K., Mohanty, S. P., & Jo, M. (2022). Fortifying Smart Transportation Security Through Public Blockchain. *IEEE Internet of Things Journal*, *9*(17), 16532–16545. doi:10.1109/JIOT.2022.3150842

Wazid, M., Das, A. K., Mohd, N., & Park, Y. (2022). Healthcare 5.0 Security Framework: Applications, Issues and Future Research Directions. *IEEE Access : Practical Innovations, Open Solutions*, *10*, 129429–129442. doi:10.1109/ACCESS.2022.3228505

Westerlund, A. M., Hawe, J. S., Heinig, M., & Schunkert, H. (2021). Risk prediction of cardiovascular events by exploration of molecular data with explainable artificial intelligence. *International Journal of Molecular Sciences*, *22*(19), 10291. doi:10.3390/ijms221910291 PMID:34638627

Williams, A., Smith, B., & Johnson, C. (2021). Cardiovascular Disease Risk Prediction Through Federated Learning: A U.S. Case Study. *Journal of Healthcare Analytics*, *22*(4), 301–318.

Winona, C. (1999, January 1). The PIR-International Protein Sequence Database. *Nucleic Acids Research, 27*(1), 39–43. doi:10.1093/nar/27.1.39 PMID:9847137

Workman, T. E., Goulet, J. L., Brandt, C. A., Warren, A. R., Eleazer, J., Skanderson, M., Lindemann, L., Blosnich, J. R., O'Leary, J., & Zeng-Treitler, Q. (2023). Identifying suicide documentation in clinical notes through zero-shot learning. *Health Science Reports, 6*(9), e1526. doi:10.1002/hsr2.1526 PMID:37706016

Wozniak, J. M., Davis, P. E., Shu, T., Ozik, J., Collier, N., Parashar, M., & Stevens, R. (2018). *Scaling deep learning for cancer with advanced workflow storage integration. In Proceedings of Machine Learning in High Performance Computing Environments*. MLHPC.

Wu, W., He, L., Lin, W., Rui, M., & Jarvis, S. (2019). *SAFA: A semi-asynchronous protocol for fast federated learning with low overhead.* ArXiv:1910.01355 [Cs]. Retrieved from http://arxiv.org/abs/1910.01355

Wu, F., Zhou, Y., Li, L., Shen, X., Chen, G., Wang, X., ... Huang, Z. (2020). Computational approaches in preclinical studies on drug discovery and development. *Frontiers in Chemistry, 8*, 726.

Wu, J., & Yang, Y. (2019). Inequality trends in the demographic and geographic distribution of health care professionals in China: Data from 2002 to 2016. *The International Journal of Health Planning and Management, 34*(1), e487–e508. doi:10.1002/hpm.2664 PMID:30238482

Wu, W., Zhu, D., Liu, W., & Wu, C. H. (2022). Empirical research on smart city construction and public health under information and communications technology. *Socio-Economic Planning Sciences, 80*, 100994.

Wysocki, O., Davies, J. K., Vigo, M., Armstrong, A. C., Landers, D., Lee, R., & Freitas, A. (2023). Assessing the communication gap between AI models and healthcare professionals: Explainability, utility, and trust in AI-driven clinical decision-making. *Artificial Intelligence, 316*, 103839. doi:10.1016/j.artint.2022.103839

Xiang, H., Shen, J., Yan, Q., Xu, M., Shi, X., & Zhu, X. (2023). Multi-Scale Representation Attention Based Deep Multiple Instance Learning for Gigapixel Whole Slide Image Analysis. *Medical Image Analysis, 89*, 102890. doi:10.1016/j.media.2023.102890 PMID:37467642

Xiao, P., Cheng, S., Stankovic, V., & Vukobratovic, D. (2020). Averaging is probably not the optimum way of aggregating parameters in federated learning. *Entropy (Basel, Switzerland), 22*(3), 314. doi:10.3390/e22030314 PMID:33286088

Xie, J., Wu, E. Q., Wang, S., Cheng, T., Zhou, Z., Zhong, J., & Liu, L. (2022). Real-World Data for Healthcare Research in China: Call for Actions. *Value in Health Regional Issues, 27*, 72–81. doi:10.1016/j.vhri.2021.05.002 PMID:34844062

Xie, X., Liu, H., Na, Z., Luo, X., Wang, D., & Leng, B. (2021). DPiT: Detecting Defects of Photovoltaic Solar Cells with Image Transformers. *IEEE Access : Practical Innovations, Open Solutions, 9*, 154292–154303. doi:10.1109/ACCESS.2021.3119631

Xu, H., Wang, Y., Li, Y., & Hong, P. (2023). Asymmetric Contrastive Multimodal Learning for Advancing Chemical Understanding. *arXiv preprint arXiv:2311.06456.*

Xu, E., Wermus, M., & Bauman, D. B. (2011). Development of an Integrated Medical Supply Information System. *Enterprise Information Systems, 5*(3), 385–399. doi:10.1080/17517575.2011.566630

Xu, J., Glicksberg, B. S., Su, C., Walker, P., Bian, J., & Wang, F. (2021). Federated learning for healthcare informatics. *Journal of Healthcare Informatics Research, 5*(1), 1–19. doi:10.1007/s41666-020-00082-4 PMID:33204939

Yadav, S. S., & Jadhav, S. M. (2021). Detection of common risk factors for diagnosis of cardiac arrhythmia using machine learning algorithm. *Expert Systems with Applications, 163*, 113807. doi:10.1016/j.eswa.2020.113807

Yamini, R. (2022). Machine Learning based Sentiment Analysis Using Django. *Journal of Pharmaceutical Negative Results*, *13*(4), 382–388.

Yang, T. (2018, December 7). *Applied Federated Learning: Improving Google Keyboard Query Suggestions*. arXiv.org. https://arxiv.org/abs/1812.02903

Yang, D., Karimi, H. R., Kaynak, O., & Yin, S. (2021). Developments of digital twin technologies in industrial, smart city and healthcare sectors: A survey. *Complex Engineering Systems*, *1*(1), 3.

Yang, H., & Wei, Z. (2020). Arrhythmia recognition and classification using combined parametric and visual pattern features of ECG morphology. *IEEE Access : Practical Innovations, Open Solutions*, *8*, 47103–47117. doi:10.1109/ACCESS.2020.2979256

Yang, Q., Liu, Y., Chen, T., & Tong, Y. (2019). Federated Machine Learning: Concept and Applications. *ACM Transactions on Intelligent Systems and Technology*, *10*(2), 1–19. doi:10.1145/3298981

YaoX.HuangT.ZhangR.-X.LiR.SunL. (2019). *Federated learning with unbiased gradient aggregation and controllable meta updating*. ArXiv:1910.08234 [Cs, Stat]. Retrieved from http://arxiv.org/abs/1910.08234

Yin, X., Zhu, Y., & Hu, J. (2021). A comprehensive survey of privacy-preserving federated learning: A taxonomy, review, and future directions. *ACM Computing Surveys*, *54*(6), 1–36. doi:10.1145/3460427

Yoo, H., Han, S., & Chung, K. (2020, July). A frequency pattern mining model based on deep neural network for real-time classification of heart conditions. In Healthcare (Vol. 8, No. 3, p. 234). MDPI. doi:10.3390/healthcare8030234

Yu, T., Li, T., Sun, Y., Nanda, S., Smith, V., & Sekar, V. (2020). Learning contextaware policies from multiple smart homes via federated multi-task learning. *IEEE/ ACM Fifth International Conference on Internet-of-Things Design and Implementation (IoTDI),* 104–115. 10.1109/IoTDI49375.2020.00017

Yu, C., Kam, K., Xu, Y., Cui, Z., Steingart, D., Gorlatova, M., ... Kymissis, I. (2020). Plant spike: A low-cost, low-power beacon for smart city soil health monitoring. *IEEE Internet of Things Journal*, *7*(9), 9080–9090.

Zahlan, A., Ranjan, R. P., & Hayes, D. (2023). Artificial intelligence innovation in healthcare: Literature review, exploratory analysis, and future research. *Technology in Society*, *74*, 102321. doi:10.1016/j.techsoc.2023.102321

Zaki, G. F., Wozniak, J. M., Ozik, J., Collier, N., Brettin, T., & Stevens, R. (2018, November). Portable and reusable deep learning infrastructure with containers to accelerate cancer studies. In *2018 IEEE/ACM 4th International Workshop on Extreme Scale Programming Models and Middleware (ESPM2)* (pp. 54-61). IEEE.

Zaydi, H., Zaydi, M., & Bakoury, Z. (2023). AI and IoT working for healthcare. In Computational Intelligence for Medical Internet of Things (IoT) Applications (pp. 3–32). Elsevier. doi:10.1016/B978-0-323-99421-7.00018-0

Zeng, X., Wang, F., Luo, Y., Kang, S. G., Tang, J., Lightstone, F. C., Fang, E. F., Cornell, W., Nussinov, R., & Cheng, F. (2022). Deep generative molecular design reshapes drug discovery. *Cell Reports Medicine*, *3*(12), 100794. doi:10.1016/j.xcrm.2022.100794 PMID:36306797

Zhang, J., Liu, S., Chen, M., Chu, H., Wang, M., Wang, Z., Yu, J., Ni, N., Yu, F., Chen, D., Yang, Y. I., Xue, B., Yang, L., Liu, Y., & Gao, Y. Q. (2023). Unsupervisedly Prompting AlphaFold2 for Accurate Few-Shot Protein Structure Prediction. *Journal of Chemical Theory and Computation*, *19*(22), 8460–8471. doi:10.1021/acs.jctc.3c00528 PMID:37947474

Zhang, J., Xie, Y., Wu, Q., & Xia, Y. (2019). Medical Image Classification Using Synergic Deep Learning. *Medical Image Analysis*, *54*, 10–19. doi:10.1016/j.media.2019.02.010 PMID:30818161

Zhang, Y., Diao, L., & Ma, L. (2020). Logistic regression models in predicting heart disease. *Journal of Physics: Conference Series.*

Zhao, J. (2020). Privacy-Preserving Machine Learning in Healthcare. *IEEE Transactions on Computational Social Systems*, *7*(5), 1331–1344.

Zhao, L. (2023). A Hybrid Deep Learning-Based Intelligent System for Sports Action Recognition via Visual Knowledge Discovery. *IEEE Access : Practical Innovations, Open Solutions*, *11*, 46541–46549. doi:10.1109/ACCESS.2023.3275012

Zhao, Y. C., Zhao, M., & Song, S. (2022). Online health information seeking among patients with chronic conditions: Integrating the health belief model and social support theory. *Journal of Medical Internet Research*, *24*(11), e42447. doi:10.2196/42447 PMID:36322124

Zhou, H., & Kan, C. (2021). Tensor-based ECG anomaly detection toward cardiac monitoring in the internet of health things. *Sensors (Basel)*, *21*(12), 4173. doi:10.3390/s21124173 PMID:34204575

Zhu, H., Cheng, C., Yin, H., Li, X., Zuo, P., Ding, J., Lin, F., Wang, J., Zhou, B., Li, Y., Hu, S., Xiong, Y., Wang, B., Wan, G., Yang, X., & Yuan, Y. (2020). Automatic multilabel electrocardiogram diagnosis of heart rhythm or conduction abnormalities with deep learning: A cohort study. *The Lancet. Digital Health*, *2*(7), e348–e357. doi:10.1016/S2589-7500(20)30107-2 PMID:33328094

Zhu, J., Chai, Z., Song, Z., Chen, Z., & Shi, Q. (2023). A Fuzzy-Boundary Enhanced Trident Network for Parcel Extraction in the Urban-Rural Area. *IEEE Journal of Selected Topics in Applied Earth Observations and Remote Sensing*, *16*, 2654–2667. https://doi.org/10.1109/JSTARS.2023.3247875

About the Contributors

Umesh Kumar Lilhore is a distinguished academician and researcher with extensive expertise in the field of Computer Science and Engineering (CSE). Holding a Post Doctorate in CSE along with a Master's and Doctoral degree in the same domain, Dr. Lilhore boasts over 20 years of enriching experience in both teaching and research. Currently serving as a Professor in the esteemed School of Computing and Research, Dr. Lilhore has made significant contributions to academia and the research community. His prolific research output includes the publication of over 100 scholarly articles in prestigious SCI and Scopus indexed journals, showcasing his profound insights and contributions to advancing the frontiers of knowledge in CSE. Dr. Lilhore's scholarly endeavors extend beyond traditional research publications. He has also demonstrated exceptional editorial skills, having edited more than 10 acclaimed books indexed in Scopus and Web of Science (WoS), published by renowned publishers such as Wiley, IGI Global, De Gruyter, IEEE, and Springer. Moreover, Dr. Lilhore's innovative spirit is evidenced by his extensive patent portfolio, comprising more than 50 patents across various domains within CSE. His inventive contributions have played a pivotal role in advancing technological innovation and addressing contemporary challenges in Machine Learning, Deep Learning, and Cloud Computing. Throughout his illustrious career, Dr. Lilhore has been a catalyst for academic excellence, nurturing the next generation of scholars and fostering a culture of innovation and inquiry. His multidimensional expertise, spanning research, teaching, editorial, and patenting domains, underscores his commitment to pushing the boundaries of knowledge and making transformative contributions to the field of Computer Science and Engineering.

Sarita Simaiya is a distinguished Professor at the School of Computing Science & Engineering (CSE) at Galgotias University, Greater Noida. Boasting over 17 years of teaching and 8 years of research experience, Dr. Sarita has held esteemed positions at various prestigious universities and colleges in India and abroad. With a Ph.D. and M.Tech, BE in CSE, Dr. Sarita completed postdoctoral research at the Institute of Advanced Computing, University of Louisiana at Lafayette. His extensive publication record includes articles in reputed, peer- reviewed national and international Scopus journals and conferences.

M. Poongodi received the B.Tech. degree in information technology (IT) from Anna University, Chennai, the M.E. degree in computer science (CSE) from St.Peters University, and the Ph.D. degree in information security from Anna University. She has teaching experience of more than five years. Her many cited publications in highly indexed journals talks about her vast knowledge and skill set in the area of blended areas network security, the IoT, machine learning, and deep learning. Her research interest is also extended in the areas of network analysis using social networking, mobile computing, Web services, 4G communication, cloud computing, and information security through anomaly detection. She is a renowned expert in networks field and a mass stunning speaker who has inspired a lot of students on network simulation through her hands on experience sessions. Many students have been done their B.E., M.E., M.Tech., and MCA projects under her guidance. She is with Hamad Bin Khalifa University and having expertise in many research areas.

Vishal Dutt (vishaldutt53@gmail.com), is pursuing a Ph.D. in Cryosphere with Remote Sensing from Punjabi University, Patiala, India and received MCA from Maharshi Dayanand Saraswati University, India. He is working as a technical trainer at Chandigarh University, Punjab, India, blending academia and industry expertise. He's actively involved in cutting-edge research in computer engineering, also excelling as a trainer in Research and Development since 2016. With over 8 years of teaching and research experience, he boasts 50+ publications in prestigious national and international journals, conferences, and book chapters, including SCI and Scopus-indexed journals. Vishal has contributed to editing numerous books and is actively engaged in three more publications with Wiley. Furthermore, he offers peer review services for esteemed publishers like Elsevier, Springer, and IEEE Access, focusing on research areas including Remote Sensing, Cryosphere, Data Science, Data Mining, Machine Learning, and Deep Learning.

* * *

C. V. Suresh Babu is a pioneer in content development. A true entrepreneur, he founded Anniyappa Publications, a company that is highly active in publishing books related to Computer Science and Management. Dr. C.V. Suresh Babu has also ventured into SB Institute, a center for knowledge transfer. He holds a Ph.D. in Engineering Education from the National Institute of Technical Teachers Training & Research in Chennai, along with seven master's degrees in various disciplines such as Engineering, Computer Applications, Management, Commerce, Economics, Psychology, Law, and Education. Additionally, he has UGC-NET/SET qualifications in the fields of Computer Science, Management, Commerce, and Education. Currently, Dr. C.V. Suresh Babu is a Professor in the Department of Information Technology at the School of Computing Science, Hindustan Institute of Technology and Science (Hindustan University) in Padur, Chennai, Tamil Nadu, India. For more information, you can visit his personal blog at .

Simhadri Chinna Gopi received his B.Tech degree in Computer Science and Engineering from JNTU Kakinada University, India in 2010. He completed his M.Tech, in Computer Science from the KL University, India in 2012. Currently, he is pursuing Doctor of Philosophy (Ph.D.) in the field of Computer Science and Engineering, VIT-AP University, Andhra Pradesh, India. His research interests include Digital Image Processing, Machine Learning and Deep Learning.

Amarendranath Choudhury is an Assistant Professor and Head of the Department of Zoology at Patharkandi College (affiliated under Assam (Central) University). Dr. Choudhury received his Ph.D. in Exercise Zoology (Neurochemistry) from Assam University and completed a Diploma course in 'Design Thinking for Innovation' from University of Virginia. He has been a Scientist in Bioassay Division at Dr. Reddy's Laboratories Limited from 2017 to 2020. Since 2013, he has published more than 40 peer-reviewed articles and obtained more than 500 citations. His current Google Scholar H-index is 12 (i10 index = 13). His research expertise includes Classical Zoology, Neurochemistry, Bioassay development and execution, Adherent and Suspension Animal Cell line culture, multiplex biomarker detection among other common biological measurement techniques. Dr. Choudhury is Associate Editor of The Neuroscience Chronicles Journal and actively serves as a Reviewer for more than 15 journals from reputed publishing houses. He is a Fellow Member of the International Parkinson and Movement Disorder Society, Indian Academy of Neuroscience, Indian National Science Academy, FORCE11: The Future of Research Communication, and International Natural Product Science Task Force. Dr. Choudhury was Globally ranked 3rd Position among the reviewers from the Multidisciplinary Research Section.

Sonia Deshmukh is working as an Assistant Professor in the Department of Computer Science and Information Technology at the KIET Group of Institutions, Delhi-NCR. She is doing her doctorate from the University of Delhi, Delhi, India. Her current research interests include quantum-inspired computing, multi-objective optimization, and process mining.

Piyanka H. has 8+years of experience in the Teaching in Computer Science and Engineering. She is currently working as Associate Professor in PES University Bangalore, Karnataka, India. Her area of interest are AI, ML,DL, IMAGE Processing, Cloud Computing, Smart City, Health Care Sectors, Energy Consumption, IoT and Data analytics. She has several publications in national and international conference and journals.

Prabhjyot kaur Haryal received her (B.Sc.) degree in Computer Science from RDVV University, India in 2006. She completed her (MCA) from RGPV University, India in 2009. Currently, she is pursuing Doctor of Philosophy (Ph.D.) in the field of Computer Applications from Lovely Professional University, Punjab, India. Her research interests include Digital Image Processing, Deep Learning and Computer Graphics.

Mangaiyarkkarasi J. is currently working as an Associate Professor of Physics in NMSS Vellaichamy Nadar College, Nagamalai, Madurai- 625 019, Tamil Nadu, India. She has 23 years of teaching experience. Her major research interest includes synthesis of ceramic materials, powder X-ray analysis and electron density studies. She has published 10 research papers in the refereed International journals and three book chapters. She has prepared study materials (UG& PG Physics) for Madurai Kamaraj University Distance Education Course.

Aih akr is pursuing her doctoral degree In Chemistry In the field of Biodiesel Production from waste material from Banasthali Vidyapith, Rajasthan. Ms. Kakkar completed her masters in Chemistry from Thapar Institute Of Engineering and Technology in the year 2020. She has done her project under Dr. Soumen Basu. Prior to that, she has completed her Bachelor's in Science from MCM DAV College, Chandigarh.

Rta Komalasari is a lecturer at YARSI University. Her current work is focused on Securing Healthcare Futures: Robust Federated Learning with Explainable Artificial Intelligence for Smart Healthcare Systems.

Hari Kishan Kondaveeti received his B.Tech degree in Information Technology from Acharya Nagarjuna University, India in 2009. He completed his M.Tech, in Computer Science and Engineering from the JNTUK University, India in 2012 and then joined the Department of CS & SE, AUCE

(A), Andhra University, India and got a Doctor of Philosophy (Ph.D.) in the field of Computer Science and Engineering. He worked as Research Associate in a research project funded by Naval Science and Technological Laboratory, India when he was at Andhra University. Currently, he is working as Associate Professor at the School of Computer Science and Engineering, VIT-AP University, Andhra Pradesh, India, and acting as a Coordinator of Engineering Clinics. He is an IBM Certified Data Science Professional and NASSCOM Associate Analyst certified faculty and handling multiple Data Analytics courses. His research interests include Digital Image Processing, Machine Learning, Data Analytics, Remote Sensing, and IoT. In recent years, he is focusing on collaborating actively with researchers in several other disciplines and trying to develop interdisciplinary projects.

Sudesh Kumar is working as Associate Professor with Department of Chemistry, Banasthali Vidyapith, Banasthali since 2018 before this he act as Assistant Professor in same department from 01.12.2010. Dr Kumar did Ph.D. in2008 from Maharshi Dayanand Saraswati University, Ajmer, India. Dr. Kumar completed post doctorate from Indian Oil Corporation Limited (Research & Development) Center, Faridabad, India. Prior to joining Banasthali Vidyapith, Banasthali he had been associated to MDSU Ajmer, IOCL, Faridabad and Laxmi Devi Institute of Engineering and Technology, Alwar (Rajasthan). He has more than 55 research papers in indexed journals, 20 book chapters and 04 books in credit. His major research area includes Corrosion Chemistry, Heterocyclic Chemistry, Polymer Degradation, and Advanced Oxidation Process for Removal of Laboratory Waste and Water Chemistry. He has also established Micro Chemistry lab for Bachelor Students at Department of Chemistry, Banasthali Vidyapith, Banasthali in 2018. He is also engaged in online education with National Council of Educational Research and Training (NCERT) and National Programme on Technology Enhanced Learning (NPTEL) for online education. Recently, filled 13 patents in the field of solar energy harnessing water purification system, Agriculture, Artificial Intelligence.

Vtavayi Valli Kumari is professor of computer science and systems engineering, Andhra University. She is an active consultant to several government/public sector/private organisations. She successfully completed six consultant projects for Naval Science and Technological Laboratories and two projects of DST, Govt of India. She has successfully managed the computerisation of Integrated Common Entrance Test (ICET) for MCA/ MBA in AP State, on behalf of Convener and APSCHE from 2009 to 2011 and Education Common Entrance Test (EdCET) from 2012 to 2014. She is a member of IEEE, ACM, CRSI and CSI. She is the founder Vice-Chair of IEEE Vizag Bay Subsection. She is also the Executive Member of Andhra Pradesh State Knowledge Mission and state nodal officer for Digital India Week, 2015.

Jve reo hse professional portfolio can be explored at , boasts an impressive career as a university professor and accomplished researcher, amassing over a decade of expertise spanning Nanomaterials, Marketing, and Business. His international reach extends far and wide, with roles as an International Consultant and Business Coach, impacting regions across Europe, including Spain, the UK, and France, as well as in Asia, with notable engagements in China, Thailand, and India.

Mnjula Rao, with over 22 years of experience in teaching Computer Science and Engineering, currently holds the position of Associate Professor at NMAMIT, NITTE (Deemed to be University) in Karkala, Udupi, Karnataka, India. Her areas of expertise include AI, ML, DL, Image Processing, Smart Transportation, Smart City, Health Care Sectors, Energy Consumption, IoT, and Data Analytics, with numerous publications in national and international conferences and journals.

Punam Rattan is an Associate Professor at Lovely Professional University, India, specializing in Computer Applications. She holds dual master's degrees in Computer Applications (MCA) and Business Administration (MBA), and a Ph.D. in Computer Application from IKG Punjab Technical University. With 20 years of experience, Dr. Rattan in a seasoned academician. She is a prolific author, having published three books and over 30 research papers in well-known conferences and journals like LEEE Xplore, SCOPUS, and SCl-indexed publications. Dr. Rattan's research focuses on Data Mining and Machine Learning, making significant. contributions to these fields. Furthermore, she actively mentors six scholars in Data Mining, Machine Learning, and Blockchain, with one scholar having already submitted her thesis under her guidance. Dr. Rattan has also demonstrated her organizational skills by hosting numerous conferences, workshops, conclaves, and seminars. With her expertise, scholarly accomplishments, and dedication to education, Dr. Punam Rattan continue to be an influential figure in Computer Applications and contribute significantly to academia and research.

K. Hemant Kumar Reddt is currently affiliated with VIT-AP University in Vijayawada, AP, Dr. Hemanth Kumar Reddy possesses over 16 years of experience post M.Tech, including 10+ years post-PhD and 11 years dedicated to research. He has an impressive publication record, contributing to 17 SCI papers, 8 SCOPUS papers, 5 book chapters, and 33 conference papers. Recognized for his excellence, he received the Best Researcher Award from Biju Patnaik University of Technology, Odisha, in 2020. Dr. Reddy serves as an Associate Editor for the Journal of Intelligent and Fuzzy Systems (JIFS) [SCIE] and regularly reviews submissions for IEEE IoT, IEEE System Journal, Springer, Elsevier, and IGI Global Journal.

Ygsh Kumar Sharma, presently working as a Professor in the Department of Computer Science and Engineering at Koneru Lakshmaiah Education Foundation (K L Deemed to be University), Vaddeswaram, Guntur District, AP. He has 18 years of teaching and 10 years of research experience. He completed his Ph.D. in Computer Science in 2014. In his research career, he published more than 173 Papers in National and International reputed journals; he published 08 patents & 11 Books in National & International Publications. Under his guidance, 14 research scholars were awarded Ph.D. Degree.

GgnTarl is currently working as Assistant Professor in CSE Department at KIET Group of Institutions, Ghaziabad. He has more than 13 years teaching experience. He done his B.Tech and M.Tech from Maharishi Dayanand University, Rohtak.

Index

E

F

G

H

I

M

P

R

S

T

V

Z